Germs and governance

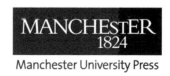

Manchester University Press

SOCIAL HISTORIES OF MEDICINE

Series editors: David Cantor, Elaine Leong and Keir Waddington

Social Histories of Medicine is concerned with all aspects of health, illness and medicine, from prehistory to the present, in every part of the world. The series covers the circumstances that promote health or illness, the ways in which people experience and explain such conditions, and what, practically, they do about them. Practitioners of all approaches to health and healing come within its scope, as do their ideas, beliefs, and practices, and the social, economic and cultural contexts in which they operate. Methodologically, the series welcomes relevant studies in social, economic, cultural, and intellectual history, as well as approaches derived from other disciplines in the arts, sciences, social sciences and humanities. The series is a collaboration between Manchester University Press and the Society for the Social History of Medicine.

Previously published

Migrant architects of the NHS *Julian M. Simpson*

Mediterranean quarantines, 1750–1914 *Edited by John Chircop and Francisco Javier Martínez*

Sickness, medical welfare and the English poor, 1750–1834 *Steven King*

Medical societies and scientific culture in nineteenth-century Belgium *Joris Vandendriessche*

Vaccinating Britain *Gareth Millward*

Madness on trial *James E. Moran*

Early Modern Ireland and the world of medicine *Edited by John Cunningham*

Feeling the strain *Jill Kirby*

Rhinoplasty and the nose in early modern British medicine and culture *Emily Cock*

Communicating the history of medicine *Edited by Solveig Jülich and Sven Widmalm*

Progress and pathology *Edited by Melissa Dickson, Emilie Taylor-Brown and Sally Shuttleworth*

Balancing the self *Edited by Mark Jackson and Martin D. Moore*

Accounting for health: Calculation, paperwork and medicine, 1500–2000 *Edited by Axel C. Hüntelmann and Oliver Falk*

Women's medicine *Caroline Rusterholz*

Germs and governance

The past, present and future of hospital infection, prevention and control

Edited by

Anne Marie Rafferty, Marguerite Dupree
and Fay Bound Alberti

MANCHESTER UNIVERSITY PRESS

Published by Manchester University Press
Altrincham Street, Manchester M1 7JA

www.manchesteruniversitypress.co.uk

British Library Cataloguing-in-Publication Data

A catalogue record for this book is available from the British Library

ISBN 978 1 5261 4078 4 hardback

First published 2021

Typeset by
Deanta Global Publishing Services

Contents

List of figures   *page* vii
List of tables   ix
Notes on contributors   x
Foreword – Professor Dame Sally Davies   xvi
Acknowledgements   xviii
List of abbreviations   xx

Introduction – Marguerite Dupree, Anne Marie Rafferty
and Fay Bound Alberti   1

I Policy and infection control

1 Hospital infections and the role of the community
   before MRSA, 1930–1960 – Flurin Condrau   27
2 Cleanliness costs: the evolving relationship between
   infection and length of stay in antibiotic-era
   hospitals – Sally Sheard   51

II Infection control: Nurses and medical students

3 Pus, pedagogy and practice: how 'dirt' shaped surgical
   nurse training and hierarchies of practice, 1900–1935
   – Pamela Wood   81
4 Septic subjects: infection and occupational illness in
   British hospitals, c. 1870–1970 – Claire L. Jones   104
5 Learning the art and science of infection prevention
   and control: a practical application – Susan Macqueen   128

III Practice and infection control: Focus on gloves

6 Wax paste and vaccination: alternatives to surgical
  gloves for infection control, 1880–1945 – Thomas Schlich 151
7 The evolving role of gloves in healthcare – Jennie Wilson 172

IV Practice and infection control: In the laboratory

8 Constructing the 'Sanitary Officer': the Pathologist's
  role in infection prevention and control at St
  Bartholomew's Hospital, London, 1892–1939 –
  Rosemary Cresswell   193
9 Infection control from the laboratory to the clinic:
  John H. Bowie and the Royal Infirmary of Edinburgh,
  c. 1945–1970 – Susan Gardiner   219

V Into the future

10 Infection prevention and control in the twenty-first
   century: the era of patient safety – Neil Wigglesworth   247
11 Infection control and antimicrobial resistance: the
   past, the present and the future – Alistair Leanord   257

Conclusion: using the past – Marguerite Dupree, Anne
Marie Rafferty and Fay Bound Alberti   270

Index   291

Figures

1.1 Phyllis Rountree in 1958. (Credit: State Library of
    New South Wales, MLMSS 6482)   *page* 37
1.2 British pathologist and bacteriologist Mary Barber.
    (Credit: Barretts Photo Press Ltd)   37
3.1 From H. C. Rutherford Darling, *Surgical Nursing
    and After-Treatment*. (J. & A. Churchill, 1947)   89
4.1 F. Nightingale and Sir H. Verney; Claydon House.
    (Credit: Wellcome Collection, CC BY)   109
4.2 Group portrait, Royal Infirmary Edinburgh, 1904.
    (Credit: Wellcome Collection, CC BY)   112
4.3 Nurses sterilising badges, King's College Hospital,
    c. 1960. (Credit: King's College London Archives,
    KH/NL/PH9/5)   116
5.1 Rose bushes in the sink used for decontamination
    of respiratory equipment on the cardiac ward at
    GOSH in 1980. (Credit: Susan Macqueen)   136
5.2 Cubicle for decontamination of ventilator tubing on
    the cardiac ward at GOSH in 1980. (Credit: Susan
    Macqueen)   137
6.1 W. S. Halsted operating in 1904. (Credit: Wellcome
    Collection, CC BY)   154
7.1 Clinical situations where gloves should or should
    not be worn. (Credit: World Health Organization
    Guidelines on Hand Hygiene in Health Care, 2009)   177
7.2 Drivers of glove use behaviour. (Credit: J. Wilson,
    A. Bak and H. P. Loveday, 'Applying human factors
    and ergonomics to the misuse of nonsterile clinical
    gloves in acute care', *American Journal of Infection
    Control*, 45 (2017). doi: 10.1016/j.ajic.2017.02.019)   179

7.3   A nurse carrying out observations on a patient.
       (Credit: Heart of England NHS FT, CC BY)				180
8.1   The 'Washington-Lyon Steam Disinfector' as
       depicted in W. Robertson and C. Porter, *Sanitary
       Law and Practice: A Handbook for Students*
       (1905). (Credit: Wellcome Collection, CC BY)				200
9.1   Bacteriological testing at the Royal Infirmary of
       Edinburgh, 1959–1970. (Adapted from Royal
       Infirmary of Edinburgh and Associated Hospitals
       annual reports, 1958–1970, Lothian Health
       Services Archive, LHB2/3/3–13)				226
11.1 MRSA in Scotland. (Source: Health Protection
       Scotland)				263
11.2 Relative frequency (%) of patients within each of
       the epidemiological categories (n=256). (Source:
       A. Banks *et al.*, 'Sentinel community Clostridium
       difficile infection (CDI) surveillance in Scotland,
       April 2013 to March 2014', *Anaerobe*, 37
       (2016), 49–53)				265
11.3 Types of HAI outbreak and incident 2016–2017				266

Tables

7.1 Evidence for role of hands in transmission of
    Staphylococcus aureus in a newborn nursery   *page* 173
7.2 Risk of cross contamination and appropriateness
    of glove use. Data from observation of clinical
    practice in two hospitals in England   177
7.3 Examples of touch sequences during observed
    episodes of care   178
7.4 Examples of attitudes towards the use of non-sterile
    clinical gloves   182
11.1 Distribution of HAI types in acute adult inpatients
    (including independent hospital inpatients) in 2005,
    2011 and 2016   261

Notes on contributors

Fay Bound Alberti is a writer and cultural historian, with specialisms in the histories of gender, medicine, emotion and the body. Her books include *Matters of the Heart: History, Medicine and Emotion* (Oxford: Oxford University Press, 2010); *This Mortal Coil: The Human Body in History and Culture* (Oxford: Oxford University Press, 2016) and *A Biography of Loneliness: The History of an Emotion* (Oxford: Oxford University Press, 2019). Fay is currently working on a book about the emotional and cultural histories of face transplants. She is a Future Leaders fellow at the Foundation for Science and Technology, Reader in History and UKRI Future Leaders Fellow at the University of York, where she is also Co-director of the Centre for Global Health Histories.

Flurin Condrau is Professor of the History of Medicine at the University of Zurich, Switzerland. Previously, he has held positions at the universities of Sheffield and Manchester. He has published widely on the history of infection, with particular focus on cholera, tuberculosis and, more recently, hospital infections. Among his publications are 'The Patient's view meets the clinical gaze', *Social History of Medicine*, 20, 2007, 525–540 and co-edited volumes *Tuberculosis Then and Now* (Montreal: McGill-Queen's University Press, 2014) and *Therapeutic Revolutions: Pharmaceuticals and Social Change in the Twentieth Century*, with Jeremy A. Greene and Elizabeth Siegel Watkins (Chicago; London: The University of Chicago Press, 2016).

Rosemary Cresswell's first book, *Bacteria in Britain, 1880–1939* (London: Pickering and Chatto, 2013), investigated the use of bacteriology in hospitals, workplaces and local communities, and her PhD on this topic was funded by the AHRC. Recently funded projects include 'Crossing Boundaries: The History of First Aid in Britain and France, 1909–1989', supported by the Arts and Humanities Research Council. In connection with this project, she is writing the history of the British Red Cross and was awarded a Bodleian Libraries Sassoon Visiting Fellowship in 2017 in order to research sections relating to war, health and humanitarianism. She has also published research relating to the history of colonial nursing. Rosemary has held postdoctoral research roles at the University of Oxford and at King's College London, and a temporary lectureship at Imperial College London, and between 2012 and 2020 was Senior Lecturer in Global History at the University of Hull. Rosemary recently joined the University of Warwick as a Research Fellow. She has formerly published as Rosemary Wall.

Marguerite Dupree has been a core staff member of the Centre for the History of Medicine at the University of Glasgow since 1986 and Professor of Social and Medical History. She is co-author with Anne Crowther of *Medical Lives in the Age of Surgical Revolution* (Cambridge: Cambridge University Press, 2007). She was co-organiser (with Brian Hurwitz) of a conference in 2012 to mark the centenary of Lister's death, and co-editor of a special issue, 'Learning from Lister', of *Notes and Records of the Royal Society*. Most recently, she has been co-holder, with Anne Marie Rafferty, of a Leverhulme Trust project grant for research into the history of infection control in British hospitals, *c.* 1870–1970. Among her other books and articles are publications on the history of hydropathic establishments, on medical practitioners and the business of life assurance, and on issues of service integration in the National Health Service (NHS), 1948–1974. She is also the author of books and articles on family history – *Family Structure in the Staffordshire Potteries 1840–1880* (Oxford: Oxford University Press, 1995) – and on the history of government-industry relations in Britain in the nineteenth and twentieth centuries (editor, *Lancashire and Whitehall: The Diary of Sir Raymond Streat, 1931–1957*, 2 vols (Manchester: Manchester University Press, 1987).

Susan Gardiner graduated PhD in the History of Medicine in November 2017. Based in the Centre for the History of Medicine at the University of Glasgow, Susan was a key member of the Leverhulme Trust-funded project entitled 'From microbes to matrons: infection control in British hospitals, *c.* 1870–1970', working alongside a project team comprising scholars from both the University of Glasgow and King's College London. Susan's research focused on infection control practice in Scottish hospitals in the early 'antibiotic era', *c.* 1928–1970. Using the Glasgow Royal Infirmary and the Royal Infirmary of Edinburgh as case studies, she undertook extensive archival research which she combined with oral histories. In addition to submitting her thesis within the three-year timeframe, Susan disseminated her research findings through journal publications. She also presented at six academic conferences held in world-leading institutions and in overseas locations during her studies.

Claire L. Jones is a lecturer in the History of Medicine at the University of Kent. Her research centres on the cultural, economic and social history of medicine and health in Britain post-1750, with particular emphases on the relationship between medicine and commerce, and ways in which this relationship affects professional social structures, consumption and material culture. She has published numerous articles on this topic, and her first monograph on the development of medical industry in Britain is *The Medical Trade Catalogue in Britain, 1870–1914* (London: Pickering and Chatto, 2013). Between 2014 and 2016, she was also Research Associate on the 'From microbes to matrons' Leverhulme-funded project, where her research focused on the ways in which systems of wound infection control affected professional structures, doctor-nurse relationships and hospital practices.

Alistair Leanord is a medical microbiologist at Glasgow Royal Infirmary and Director of the Scottish Microbiology Laboratories, Glasgow, who has a research interest in healthcare-associated infections and antimicrobial resistance using genome sequencing, informatics and interventional infection control. This work has led to the formation of the Scottish HAI Prevention Institute (SHAIPI). He has been recognised by the University of Glasgow where he is Honorary Professor of Microbiology. Previously, over the last five years, he was the HAI Medical Adviser to the Scottish government, advising and implementing Scotland's response to the UK antimicrobial resistance (AMR) strategy. Currently he is Chair of the UK Advisory Committee on Antimicrobial Prescribing, Resistance and Healthcare Associated Infection (APRHAI).

Susan Macqueen has been in infection prevention and control (IPC) since 1980 and, until her retirement in 2011, was Director of IPC at Great Ormond Street Hospital for Children NHS Trust, London.

She has worked at the UK Department of Health (1989) and been a member of the Expert Advisory Panel to the National Audit Office on the Management and Control of Hospital Acquired Infection in Acute Trusts in England (1998), the Expert Advisory Panel on the Department of Health Communicable Disease Strategy (1998), the Department of Health CJD Incidents Panel (2000–2003), the Advisory Group on the National Guidelines for the Prevention of Hospital Acquired Infection – EPIC Study (1998–2003) and the Department of Health Select Committee on Antimicrobial Resistance – SACAR (2001–2005). Susan was Chair of the Infection Control Nurses Association (ICNA, now Infection Prevention Society) from 1997 to 2000 and has been a national and international advocate for best practice in HCAI. Her sharing of work in programmes in Europe as well as Jordan, Oman, Russia and Japan has aimed at improving standards of practice in reducing HCAI. She was awarded an OBE in 1999 for her work in IPC. Publications include *The Great Ormond Street Hospital Manual of Children's Nursing Practices* with Elizabeth Anne Bruce and Faith Gibson (Chichester: Wiley Blackwell, 2012) and *The Children's Nurse: The True Story of a Great Ormond Street Nurse* (London: Orion, 2013). Susan continues to teach Management of Healthcare Acquired Infections on an MSc online module at Greenwich University, London.

Dame Anne Marie Rafferty is Professor of Nursing Policy, former Dean of the Florence Nightingale Faculty of Nursing and Midwifery, King's College London and President of the Royal College of Nursing. She is a historian and health workforce and policy researcher. She served on the Prime Minister's Commission on the Future of Nursing and Midwifery, 2009-10 and has been recipient of various awards: *Nursing Times* Leadership Award (2014); *Health Services Journal* Top 100 Clinical Leaders Award in 2015; 2017 nominated as one of 70 most influential nurses in the 70 years of the National Health Service. She co-led a Student Commission on the Future of the NHS supported by NHS England and was a member of the Parliamentary Review of Health and Social Care in Wales, 2018. She was elected Fellow of the Academy of Medical Sciences 2019 and Member of the National Academy of Medicine in the US in 2020. She was PI of the project 'From Microbes to Matrons' with Marguerite Dupree. Her publications span a textbook with Robert Dingwall and Charles Webster, her DPhil supervisor, *An Introduction to the Social History of Nursing* (London: Routledge, 1988); a monograph, *The Politics of Nursing Knowledge* (London: Routledge, 1996); co-authored *Nurses of all Nations* with Barbara

Brush, Joan Lynaugh, Meryn Stuart and Nancy Tomes (Philadelphia: Lippincott, 1999); and edited collections with Jane Robinson and Ruth Elkan on *Nursing, History and the Politics of Welfare* (London: Routledge, 1996), Hilary Marland, *Midwives, Society and Childbirth* (London: Routledge, 1997) and Sioban Nelson, *Notes on Nightingale* (Ithaca, NY: Cornell University Press, 2010).

Thomas Schlich, MD, is James McGill Professor in the History of Medicine, McGill University, Montreal, Canada, Department of Social Studies of Medicine. He has double qualification as physician and historian and has held previous research and research teaching positions in Cambridge, England, and in Stuttgart and Freiburg, Germany. Thomas' research interests include the history of modern medicine and science (eighteenth to twenty-first centuries), medicine and technology, surgery and body history. His previous books include *The Origins of Organ Transplantation: Surgery and Laboratory Science, 1880–1930* (Rochester, NY: University of Rochester Press, 2010); *Surgery, Science and Industry: A Revolution in Fracture Care, 1950s–1990s* (Houndmills and New York: Palgrave, 2002). Thomas is editor of *The Palgrave Handbook of the History of Surgery* (London: Palgrave Macmillan, 2018) and is currently working on a monograph on the history of modern surgery, 1800–1914.

Sally Sheard is the Andrew Geddes and John Rankin Professor of Modern History at the University of Liverpool, with a primary research interest in the interface between expert advisers and policymakers. She is currently leading a seven-year Wellcome Trust-funded project, 'The Governance of Health: Medical, Economic and Managerial Expertise in Britain since 1948'. Her latest book is *The Passionate Economist: How Brian Abel-Smith Shaped Global Health and Social Welfare* (Bristol: Policy Press, 2013). She has also written on the history of hospitals, the finance of British medicine and the development of the NHS. Sally has extensive experience of using history in public and policy engagement and has worked with local health authorities and government organisations. She has written for and presented television and radio programmes, including the 2018 BBC Radio 4 series *National Health Stories*.

Neil Wigglesworth qualified as a nurse in 1987, and following a clinical career primarily in critical care nursing, he moved into the field of IPC in 1995. Neil has worked in a number of nurse specialist, management, research and nurse consultant roles in the speciality as well as in Public Health/Health Protection and was appointed to the role of Deputy Director, IPC at Guy's and St Thomas' NHS Foundation Trust in March 2015 and Director in January 2019. Neil is the immediate past President of the Infection Prevention Society, current Chair of the International Federation of Infection Control and a former editor of the *Journal of Infection Prevention*. He has a particular interest in Quality Improvement approaches and in particular, Human Factors/Ergonomics (HFE).

Jennie Wilson has a first degree in microbiology, a master's in Public Health and a PhD in surveillance and is a registered nurse. She has thirty years' experience in IPC. She has worked as a senior IPC practitioner in NHS Trusts in London and was a key player in establishing the first national surveillance programmes on HCAI in England at the Health Protection Agency. She led the Surgical Site Infection Surveillance Service for ten years and developed HCAI surveillance and research initiatives in the United Kingdom and Europe. Jennie is currently Professor of Healthcare Epidemiology at the Richard Wells Research Centre at the University of West London. She is a lead author of the Epic guidelines on the preventing HCAI, and her research interests include prevention of HCAI, in particular urinary tract and respiratory tract infections, dehydration in the elderly, hand hygiene and the use of clinical gloves. She has published widely on many aspects of HCAI and is author of *Infection Control in Clinical Practice*, now in its third edition.

Pamela Wood is a retired nurse academic. Her career in New Zealand and Australia focused on teaching research to postgraduate students in a broad range of health professions and developing a research culture in schools of nursing and health. She is known internationally, particularly for her research in nursing history, and has published extensively on the history of nursing and health. Pamela's PhD in History from the University of Otago explored the meaning of 'dirt' in nineteenth-century colonial New Zealand and the way this shaped people's understanding of how a healthy, civilised settlement should be formed. Pamela's contributed chapter in *Germs and Governance* extends this exploration of the meaning of 'dirt' to the early twentieth-century world of the surgical nurse and efforts in infection control. Pamela is currently writing a cultural history explaining what it meant to be a New Zealand nurse at the time of empire, 1880–1950.

Foreword

Long before the global Coronavirus pandemic began in January 2020, it was clear that infection control continues to be one of the twenty-first century's most challenging health problems. Throughout my nine years as Chief Medical Officer (CMO) for England and the Chief Medical Advisor to the UK government I stressed the growing dangers of antimicrobial resistance (AMR), and I am proud to continue to serve as the United Kingdom's special envoy on AMR, working to build on global momentum on AMR.

This volume, in bringing together historians, healthcare professionals and policymakers, is prescient in its emphasis on the whole range of infection prevention and control (IPC) policies and procedures used to minimise the risk of spreading infections in hospitals and healthcare facilities, in addition to drug therapies. A historical perspective reveals the continuing importance of a broad spectrum of IPC practices, technologies and personnel – from handwashing to personal protective equipment to all levels of hospital staff. Because cures are limited, the need to devote adequate resources to all aspects of IPC emerges clearly from the following pages, just as much as the need to fund the search for new classes of antibiotics and vaccines.

Germs and Governance captures a crucial transition in understanding IPC policies in health history since the mid-nineteenth century, including first, the growing recognition of the role of microbes in creating infection and disease, and second, an emphasis on managing microbes, in which the governance arrangements of the hospital and healthcare providers play a prominent, yet little studied, role in mediating policy and practice. The volume offers the integration of historical and contemporary evidence, and a plurality of voices and experiences in hospital infection control, which give the book a greater range and scope than the existing literature. It looks beyond the antimicrobial drug revolution to focus on the other technologies and personnel of infection control. One key example is the history of nursing education and practice, which is a neglected aspect of research into infection control, but there are other examples including the roles of economics, standardisation, national governments and ideas of 'dirt' and 'blame'. Other topics include the long history of methicillin-resistant *Staphylococcus aureus* (MRSA) and its community origins; case studies of resistance to and rationales for the use of surgical gloves; the reciprocal roles of bacteriologists, pathologists and matrons in managing infection control; occupational health of hospital staff; high-level and micro politics of research into patient safety and case studies of early nursing practice of hygiene, neonatal intensive care and paediatrics in the 1980s; and the rise of disposables, central supply and sustainability.

The geographic focus here is on England and Scotland, but the contributors writing before the COVID-19 pandemic recognise that, as emphasised in my final annual report as CMO, infection prevention and control is a global issue. They make wider comparative references to other countries, including the United States, Europe, Canada, Australia and New Zealand.

There cannot be a more pressing moment to engage with this subject and look back in order to take forward the learning and lessons for the future.

Professor Dame Sally Davies
May 2020

Acknowledgements

This book arose from a two-day symposium, 'From microbes to matrons: the past, present and future of hospital infection control and prevention', held at the Royal College of Surgeons of England and King's College London. The symposium brought together thirty policymakers, health professionals and historians from the United Kingdom and abroad. The editors would like to thank all of the participants and all who presented papers; they are especially indebted to the enterprise and energy of Dr Claire L. Jones, who organised the symposium, and to Clare Hitchcox, who assisted her, and to the Wellcome Trust Small Grants Scheme and the Society for the Social History of Medicine for funding for the symposium. We are particularly grateful to the eleven contributors who developed their papers into the following chapters, to the anonymous referees who made this a better book and to David Cantor, the editor for the Social Histories of Medicine Series, for his encouragement and patience, steering the journey from symposium to book. The support of the team at Manchester University Press, including Thomas Dark and Lucy Burns, has been exemplary. Finally, we thank Professor Dame Sally Davies for her Foreword.

This symposium and book are part of a project, 'From microbes to matrons: infection control in British hospitals, 1870–1970', funded by a Leverhulme Trust Research Project Grant (RPG-2013–157) awarded to two of the editors, Professors Anne Marie Rafferty and Marguerite Dupree. They would like to record their thanks to King's College London and the University of Glasgow for jointly hosting the project and especially to the Leverhulme Trust for the award which made it possible to bring together the research team of Drs Claire L. Jones, Susan Gardiner and Iain Hutchison, subsequently joined by Drs Julie Hipperson, Agnes Arnold-Forster and Fay Bound Alberti. It has been a pleasure to work with each of the members of the team. We thank them for their hard work, dedication and good humour. We are also grateful to the members of the project's advisory board who both met formally with the project team and provided informal advice: Professors Roger Kneebone and Flurin Condrau, and Drs Rosemary Cresswell and Carol Pellowe.

In addition, much deserved thanks go to Professor Malcolm Nicolson for his co-supervision of Susan Gardiner's PhD thesis; the members of the Centre for the History of Medicine and Economic and Social History Subject Area for a congenial, supportive academic home, and the School of Social and Political Sciences for administrative support at Glasgow University; and the Florence Nightingale Faculty of Nursing, Midwifery and Palliative Care and administration at King's College London.

We would also like to thank archivists and librarians for their invaluable assistance, including Alistair Tough, the NHS Greater Glasgow and Clyde Archivist, for his expert guidance through the resources in his care; the staff of the Glasgow University Archives and Special Collections; the Lothian Health Services Archive; the Royal College of Physicians and Surgeons of Glasgow; the Bodleian Library, Oxford; the Science Museum, London; the London Metropolitan Archives; the Wellcome Library; the interview collections in the Royal College of Nursing and Kingston University; and Dr Geoff Browell, Head of Archives and Research Collections, and staff at King's College London, who not only facilitated use of the collections but also hosted our online exhibition.

Finally, Dr Fay Bound Alberti stepped into the role of co-editor with boundless enthusiasm, breadth of expertise, skill and dexterity in attention to detail. Our heartfelt thanks go to her for her patience, generosity and support for the project despite many calls on her time.

Anne Marie Rafferty and Marguerite Dupree
May 2020

List of abbreviations

AHA	American Hospital Association
AMR	antimicrobial resistance
APIC	Association for Practitioners in Infection Control
Barts	St Bartholomew's Hospital, London
BSI	bloodstream infection
CBA	cost-benefit analysis
CDC	Centers for Disease Control and Prevention
C. diff	*Clostridium difficile*
CHIP	Comprehensive Hospital Infection Project
COI	cost of illness
CPE	carbapenemase-producing Enterobacteriaceae
CPHL	Colindale Public Health Laboratories
CRE	carbapenem-resistant Enterobacteriaceae
CSSD	Central Sterile Supply Department
DH	Department of Health
DHSS	Department of Health and Social Security
DRG	diagnosis related group
E. coli	*Escherichia coli*
ENB	English National Board
ESDDT	Edinburgh Standard Disk Diffusion Technique
GI	gastrointestinal infection
GOSH	Great Ormond Street Hospital
GRI	Glasgow Royal Infirmary
HAI/HCAI	hospital-acquired infection/healthcare-associated infection
HEI	Healthcare Environment Inspectorate
HFE	human factors and ergonomics

HIC	Hospital Infection Committee
HII	high-impact intervention
HIPE	Hospital In-Patient Enquiry
HIV	human immunodeficiency virus
ICLN	infection control link nurse
ICN	infection control nurse
ICNA	Infection Control Nurses Association
ICT	infection control team
ICU	intensive care unit
IHI	Institute for Healthcare Improvement
IPC	infection prevention and control
IV	intravenous
KCH	King's College Hospital
KPC	*Klebsiella pneumoniae* carbapenemase
LSHTM	London School of Hygiene and Tropical Medicine
MRSA	methicillin-resistant *Staphylococcus aureus*
NAO	National Audit Office
NHS	National Health Service
NNIS	National Nosocomial Infection Study
NSCG	non-sterile clinical gloves
PHP	public health profiles
PPE	personal protective equipment
PPS	Point Prevalence Survey
QALYs	quality-adjusted life years
RIE	Royal Infirmary of Edinburgh
RSV	Respiratory Syncytial Virus
SARS	Severe Acute Respiratory Syndrome
SENIC	Study on the Efficacy of Nosocomial Infection Control
SP	Standard Precautions
SURPASS	Surgical Patient Safety System
TSC	Theatre Service Centre
UP	Universal Precautions
UTI	urinary tract infection
WHO	World Health Organization
WTP	willingness to pay

Introduction

*Marguerite Dupree, Anne Marie Rafferty
and Fay Bound Alberti*

Infection control and antimicrobial resistance: a global problem and its narrative

Infection prevention and control is one of the twenty-first century's most challenging problems, as indicated by global concerns about antimicrobial resistance (AMR) – a danger, according to many, comparable in size and complexity to climate change and warfare.[1]

The idea of a 'therapeutic revolution' – beginning with the development and increasing availability of 'miracle' drugs, that is sulpha drugs in the 1930s and antibiotics in the 1940s, to prevent and treat bacterial infection,[2] and ending in their declining efficacy and the failure to develop any new classes of antibiotics since the 1980s – is the subject of a large body of literature. Neither the recent emphasis on contemporaries' awareness of resistance to these drugs since their discovery, represented by Alexander Fleming's warning in his 1945 Nobel Prize acceptance speech,[3] nor recognition that it was a convoluted process, undermined the linear narrative 'from utopia to dystopia'.[4]

This narrative has become so ubiquitous that there is now a large number of studies about the rise of AMR aimed explicitly at a lay audience, demonstrating how high profile and highly emotive the issue has become.[5] This fear of 'superbugs' and politics of disgust harmonises with the 'affective turn' today.[6] The importance and power of the collective memory and the lived experience of patients, family and staff touched by the consequences of AMR have been moving to the fore, and are now the touchstone for scholarly accounts, news reports, television documentaries and the ability of hospitals and healthcare communities to develop new processes.[7] Taken together with the continuing interest from healthcare practitioners in understanding the origins of the present situation, this represents the emergence of a cultural perspective on infection prevention and control that stretches beyond the normal emphasis on the biomedical nature of infection. The main theme running through this literature and commentary is the desire to understand both how we have reached the current situation where resistance to these 'miracle drugs' is so dangerous, and where it will lead us in the future.

A similar narrative underlies the emergence of AMR as a global and national policy issue. Following the lead of the European Union (EU) internationally in addressing AMR with a monitoring and surveillance approach and an action plan in 2011, the World Health Organization (WHO) published its own action plan in 2015, and in 2016 a United Nations (UN) declaration to combat AMR was signed by 193 countries, confirming the importance of the problem and the rise of AMR as a global policy issue; the UN published a follow-up report in 2019.[8] At the national level, although Brexit now threatens the loss of EU safety controls, surveillance and innovations in this area,[9] the United Kingdom (UK) was an early follower of the EU. The UK developed a five-year plan for 2013–2018 to set a course of action to try to tackle multiple components of AMR; it commissioned an independent review on AMR under the chairmanship of Lord O'Neill, which published an influential final report in 2016; and in January 2019, the UK published a new five-year action plan for 2019–2024, together with a vision for 2040.[10] Reports indicate that 'superbugs' (species resistant to antimicrobial treatment) are responsible for approximately 700,000 deaths per year worldwide, and 5,000 deaths per year in the UK alone. Research suggests that deaths worldwide will rise to 10 million per year by 2050 if unchecked.[11] Of particular concern are the gram-negative *Escherichia coli* and carbapenemase-producing (CPE) bacteria and multidrug-resistant yeast, such as *Candida auris*, which are difficult to monitor and have few treatment options, together with the prospect of the rapid development of new resistant strains.[12] In addition to the huge cost in terms of human life, the World Bank predicts that the cost of drug-resistant infections will rise to $100 trillion and drive an extra 28 million people into poverty around the world by 2050.[13] There is recognition that drug development is a priority but alone will not solve the problem. AMR is seen not just as an issue of overuse or under-dosage, but as a threat that spreads through soil, water and the food chain to what we eat and drink. So, policymakers advocate a 'holistic' or 'One Health' approach to tackling AMR, which integrates human and animal health and environmental components of the problem.[14] From the current, prevailing perspective, infection prevention and control are part of a package of approaches which policymakers advocate for tackling AMR.

Hospital infection control and the 'patient safety agenda'

This volume provides an alternative vision of infection prevention and control. Rather than ranging across many sites, it focuses on the hospital to examine the prevention and control of infection. Medical dictionaries define 'hospital infection' (or 'nosocomial infection' or 'hospital-acquired infection' (HAI)) as an infection acquired in a hospital; both hospitalised patients and hospital staff can contract a hospital infection.[15] 'Hospital infection prevention and control' are the policies and procedures used to minimise the risk of spreading infections, especially in hospitals and healthcare facilities. AMR is too narrow a window; the shift of focus from AMR to HAI means a wider spectrum of infections are considered, including not only gram-positive bacteria, for example Streptococcal infections, such as erysipelas, cellulitis, scarlet fever and puerperal fever, and antibiotic-resistant *Staphylococcus aureus* and *Clostridium difficile* infections, but also gram-negative bacilli, such as *E. coli* and fungal infections – important in high-tech hospital medicine, especially transplants and other immunosuppressant therapies, and increasingly drug resistant.[16] In short, antibiotics and other drug therapies are only one aspect of hospital infection prevention and control.

In the UK, failures in infection control and prevention have been the focus of high-profile hospital scandals: a cause of excess mortality carrying high political stakes for governments.[17] Regulators see issues surrounding hospital hygiene standards and cleanliness as symptomatic of wider systems failures, and as a principal measure of healthcare quality. Thus, hospital infections serve as a key performance indicator, and infection prevention and control are an important part of a wider patient safety agenda within hospitals.[18]

Foreshadowed in the 1970s by the criticisms in Ivan Illich's influential polemic, *Medical Nemesis*, in which he argued that modern medicine was a major threat to world health, and that hospitals in particular caused more sickness than health,[19] 'patient safety' has attracted international medical attention since the late 1990s following the publication of the US Institute of Medicine's report, *To Err is Human*.[20] In 2000, the Chief Medical Officer for England, Liam Donaldson, following *To Err is Human*, Australian research and a UK pilot study, estimated that between 60,000 and 250,000 National Health Service (NHS) patients each year suffered serious disability or death as a result of healthcare interventions.[21] Although recent work suggests the estimates are too high,[22] Donaldson's report threw light on the potential scale of the problem of patient safety in the UK. In response, like the report *To Err is Human*, Donaldson advocated drawing on experience built up over many years in understanding the reasons for non-medical accidents, disasters and system failures in industries, such as aviation and nuclear power generation. These industries had implemented improvements based on systematic learning from accidents and incidents, such as guidelines and checklists – techniques which could be applied to healthcare.[23]

Among the serious failures in healthcare Donaldson cited in 2000 were HAIs, about 15 per cent of which might be avoidable, and he estimated that they cost the NHS nearly £1 billion every year.[24] During the next fifteen years, hospital infection prevention and control became not only an indicator of problems of patient safety, but also, as the final two chapters show, embodied the 'patient safety' agenda utilising understanding of the system-based causes of failure, learning from them and providing adequate resources. Hospital infection prevention and control practices, policies and personnel contributed to the dramatic fall in antibiotic-resistant, gram-positive, bacterial methicillin-resistant *S. aureus* (MRSA) and *C. diff* infections since 2000 – a fall which is unique to the UK, though accomplished by different methods in Scotland and England.[25]

Hospital infection control and history

Issues surrounding hospital infection and drug-resistant infection are not new problems. They have long histories. Even though challenges faced at different times are historically contingent, those histories arguably are relevant to both AMR policy and current patient safety concerns. For example, a historical perspective has been mobilised to understand the evolution of the AMR policy agenda and to inform policymaking in the 'AMR Historical Foresight' project. The research highlights lessons from the past, draws on the history of comparable large-scale, complex problems with public health consequences and engages with 'scenario planning' to inform potential policy responses.[26] Also, the recent report of the UK government's 'Review on Antimicrobial Resistance' argued that British hospitals must 'return to the attitudes of the pre-antibiotic era, when infection prevention was recognised as a priority, because cures were limited'.[27]

There are few sustained accounts of the history of infection control in the institutional setting of the hospital, and two that exist are from the perspective of practitioners.[28] The only book-length study of the history of hospital infection control is G. A. J. Ayliffe and M. English's *Hospital Infection: From Miasmas to MRSA*. The authors are medical practitioners, and the book provides a contextual historical overview of infection control before moving on to contemporary discussions. The identification and control of HAIs also sit on the periphery of histories of hospital life and development and of individual hospital histories, background noise to the healing purpose and activities of the site.[29]

This volume does not claim to present an entire history of hospital infection control. Instead, the hospital acts as a microcosm to allow authors to focus on the normally peripheral or tacit details of infection control and place them at the centre. As a whole, the volume places less emphasis on the well-known story of antimicrobial drugs, and more on the personnel, practices and alternative technologies associated with infection control. Also, where much historical research has focused upon the debates and controversies surrounding competing ideas about the causes of infection, what is less well understood are the practices of hospital infection control and prevention and their history, particularly how these practices changed and how they shaped the associated costs and workload of systems of operative and post-operative wound management, in the operating theatre, the ward and the hospital as a whole.

The past, present and future of hospital infection control

The volume arises from a symposium which brought together historians, practitioners and policymakers to consider the past, present and future of hospital infection control. The aims were to facilitate interdisciplinary discussion of hygiene and cleanliness and the role of drugs and other therapeutics in tackling HAIs, and to consider the current relevance of past infection control practices. The symposium explored questions including: how have hospital hygiene methods and practices of infection prevention and control and post-operative wound care evolved and changed since the mid-nineteenth century? How have practitioners and policymakers responded to challenges in the past? How have policies relating to infection prevention and control been implemented in practice and with what degree of success? How have these methods and practices varied according to hospital and geographic location? Who have been the key players in hospital infection prevention and control?

Thus, this interdisciplinary volume includes work from eleven leading historians, healthcare professionals and policymakers who consider the history, practice and future of infection control since the mid-nineteenth century. The authors bring a wide range of expertise, and their experience ranges from that of the established professional to the PhD student. The authors provide a bridge between existing practitioner-based histories and new research by medical history and humanities scholars into the critical processes that constructed sepsis and infection and their prevention and treatment since the mid-nineteenth century. The authors move beyond discussions of drug therapies; they offer a mixture of perspectives which open up the complexities of infection control, as they developed and emerged in the hospital setting.

The authors use a wide variety of methods, approaches and sources to provide a broader scope for insights than is available in current literature. The methods include historical case studies, policy debates, comparative international approaches and firsthand practitioner accounts and reflections. They draw on approaches from history, anthropology, sociology, economics, statistics, policy studies and engineering, among others. Sources include oral history, contemporary journal articles and textbooks, hospital archives and patient records, government reports and participant observation.

Although the authors appreciate that infection prevention and control has become a global issue, the geographic focus here is on England and Scotland, with some wider comparative references to the United States, Europe, Canada, Australia and New Zealand.

The title, *Germs and Governance*, captures a crucial transition in understanding infection and control policies in health history: first, with the growing recognition of the role of microbes in creating infection and disease from the mid-nineteenth century; and secondly, through an emphasis on managing microbes, in which the governance arrangements of the hospital and healthcare providers play a prominent, yet little studied, role in mediating policy and practice. The book offers a more comprehensive integration of historical and contemporary evidence, and a plurality of voices and experiences in hospital infection control, which give it a greater range and scope than the existing literature. It also looks beyond the antimicrobial drug revolution to focus on the other personnel and other technologies of infection control. One key example is the history of nursing education and practice, which is a neglected aspect of research into infection control, but there are other examples, including the roles of the bacteriologist, economics, standardisation and national governments and ideas of 'dirt' and 'blame'.

A chronology

Before examining the chapters and emerging themes in this volume, a brief chronological summary provides a framework for background. In particular, it brings out the importance of the early twentieth century, a period often overlooked. The history of infection prevention and control in British hospitals since the mid-nineteenth century can be broadly divided into five periods.

In the first period, from 1870 to 1900, Florence Nightingale and Joseph Lister were the most prominent advocates of systems for improving hospital sanitary standards on the one hand, and operative and post-operative antiseptic techniques on the other. Traditionally in the literature, these two approaches are pitted against each other, but they, and the emerging asepsis, can also be regarded as complementary – though not without controversies. Both elaborate wound dressing and cleaning rituals developed in this and the next period, informed by the new bacteriological science. At the same time, the burden of the work fell largely on women as ward servants or scrubbers, student nurses, staff nurses and matrons, so that working women and nursing became crucial to the success of hospital infection control.

In Britain, hospital provision featured different types of hospitals with different policies toward infectious disease. Most of the general and specialist voluntary hospitals attempted to exclude infectious disease patients from admission and infectious disease from operating theatres and wards. As Matthew Newsom Kerr discusses in detail in his book, *Contagion, Isolation, and Biopolitics in Victorian London*, from the 1870s local authorities began to establish separate permanent infectious disease hospitals to isolate patients, in an attempt to prevent the infectious disease becoming epidemic in the community, replacing the earlier policy of creating ad hoc temporary infectious disease hospitals after the start of an epidemic. Such permanent infectious disease hospitals came to be separated from the Poor Law so that admission did not entail becoming a pauper, and these hospitals rapidly attracted patients from a broad social spectrum. At the same time, separate Poor Law infirmaries developed along the lines of general hospitals. Asylum patients, too, commonly suffered from outbreaks of infectious disease.[30]

The second period, from 1900 to 1930, was a period of consolidation and included a range of practical developments: types of gloves, more complex handwashing, wound care routines, caps, overalls, boots, surgical masks, commercial dressings, new antiseptics and methods of sterilisation. In infectious disease hospitals, techniques of isolation within isolation developed, with patients separated by disease and stage of disease, and techniques of 'barrier' nursing emerged.

The third period, from the 1930s to 1957, was the heyday of antibiotics, beginning with the introduction of sulphonamides in the 1930s and penicillin in the Second World War and ending with the flu pandemic of 1957, which coincided with the spread of antibiotic-resistant *S. aureus* 80/81. At the same time, during the 1930s, techniques of phage typing developed to enable the identification of specific strains of bacteria causing disease and of carriers without symptoms. Furthermore, in Britain from 1948, the previously separately administered types of hospitals – voluntary hospitals, local authority hospitals (which included infectious disease and Poor Law hospitals from 1929) and asylums – came under the administration of the NHS.

The fourth period, from the 1957 flu pandemic to 1970, saw the beginning of widespread recognition of antibiotic resistance and a rediscovery of hospital infection and, accordingly, resulted in a renewed emphasis on hygienic practice, risk assessment and surveillance and, at the end of the period, the first infection control nurses. Gradual changes in governance from ward to hospital-wide infection control committees facilitated the development of central sterile supply and disposables.

The fifth period, from approximately 1970, saw the professionalisation of infection prevention and control in the UK, alongside widespread Staphylococcal infections in hospitals both in the UK and abroad, despite antibiotics. The appointment of full-time infection control nurses, to control cross infections in hospital patients, began in Torbay in 1959. Their development as specialists led to ad hoc and then annual conferences, with international visitors by the end of the 1960s; in 1970, they formed the Infection Control Nurses Association (ICNA). After expanding the membership to include any health professionals employed in the field of infection prevention and control, the ICNA became the Infection Prevention Society (IPS) in 2006.[31]

Not only infection control nurses, but also members of the medical community in the UK concerned with infection prevention and control, professionalised. Consultant microbiologists, clinical and research scientists and nurses set up the Hospital Infection Society (HIS), now Healthcare Infection Society, in 1979, 'to create and disseminate a body of scientific knowledge about the prevention and control of hospital and other healthcare associated infections' through activities such as publishing *The Journal of Hospital Infection*.[32]

Throughout the period since 1970, there has been continued emphasis on the hospital environment, influenced by research in the United States in the 1970s and 1980s, notably the Study on the Efficacy of Nosocomial Infection Control (SENIC) project, which offered evidence to show that a third of HAIs were preventable and demonstrated the importance of designing different surveillance and control programmes for each infection site (i.e. surgical site infections, urinary tract infections, blood stream infections, pneumonia), instead of relying simply on overall hospital infection rates.[33] Also, particularly influential in the United States and UK was the Keystone ICU project launched in 2003 to improve patient safety in intensive care units (ICUs).[34] The comprehensive, unit-based, evidence-based interventions reduced the rate of catheter-related bloodstream infection by 66 per cent over eighteen months and sustained the reduction in morbidity and cost of care. The more than 100 ICUs in the study began by designating at least one physician and one nurse as team leaders who were instructed in the safety concepts and the interventions and then disseminated the information among their colleagues. The intervention involved the use of five evidence-based procedures recommended by the Centers for Disease Control (CDC), including handwashing, using full-barrier precautions during the insertion of central venous catheters, cleaning the skin with chlorhexidine, avoiding the femoral site if possible and removing unnecessary catheters. Among other measures, a checklist was used to ensure adherence to infection-control practices; colleagues were stopped if the practices were not followed; the removal of catheters was discussed at daily rounds; and teams received feedback regarding the number and rates of catheter-related bloodstream infections at monthly and quarterly meetings. At the same time, as noted previously, the wider patient safety movement, beginning in the 1990s, and UK government interventions also highlighted the continuing importance of hygienic practice, risk assessment and surveillance in hospitals in the face of high-profile hospital scandals and the longer-term challenges of antibiotic resistance and failure to develop new classes of antibiotics.

Thematic approach

Although chronology is important as a background, the chapters in this volume are presented thematically in order to transcend the linear narratives of discovery, milestones and prominent figures found in other volumes on infection control and antimicrobial drugs. A thematic approach creates an innovative mixture of historical case studies and contemporary reflections from practitioners and policymakers, which allow the reader to make connections between past, present and future, and to understand how developments in the history of infection control are understood, absorbed and acted upon 'on the ground' as part of a continuing endeavour to pin down knowledge about what practitioners did, rather than just what they said.

Exploring the historical contexts in which technologies such as gloves, sensitivity testing and central sterile supply were developed, used and popularised – as well as the ways relationships between communities and hospitals, costs and lengths of stay, and doctors, nurses and bacteriologists have informed and shaped infection control practices – the collection emphasises the richly diverse ways in which ideas about germs, infection and safety take shape in the laboratory, clinic and hospital in different periods.

Policy and infection control are the focus of the two chapters in Part I. After discussing their nineteenth- and early twentieth-century contexts, Flurin Condrau maps the major debates around the problem of infection in British hospitals between 1930 and 1960. He places particular emphasis on the location of infection in hospitals and the community, the changes in the monitoring systems and the professional groups involved. He explores the extent to which the problems of infection stayed within the walls of the hospital, arguing that, given the importance of neonatal wards for the spread of infections, it is necessary to look outside the hospital to understand the complex mechanisms around infection and the challenges for infection control. The way we 'frame' a problem like AMR is important; a focus on the hospital blindsided analysts to the community as a source of infection, and therefore mobilising responses were slower to develop. The major flu pandemic in 1957, coupled with the emergence of resistant *S. aureus* 80/81, contributed further to this problem, at the same time that bacteriologists played a major role in monitoring infection, utilising the new technology of phage typing.

Sally Sheard highlights the importance of a comparative perspective and the economics of infection control. Her contribution explores the recognition, among policymakers in post-war Britain and the United States, of a relationship between length of stay in hospital and infection, as well as the costs and consequences for care. From the 1960s, the Department of Health (DH) – Department of Health and Social Security (DHSS) until 1988 – in the UK periodically addressed issues around the efficient management and discharge of hospital patients. These efforts paralleled shorter lengths of hospital stays for all types of patients, but especially surgical and obstetric cases, which reflected a combination of advances in clinical performance, concerns about increasing NHS costs and the introduction of general management, particularly following the 1983 Griffiths Report. Further contributory factors included the transition from 'Nightingale' wards to small bed units, which had implications for nursing as well as clinical management. Many of these policy developments were linked to the concept of 'value for money' in the NHS and the introduction of cost-effectiveness analyses. However, changes to patient management in hospitals also had risks, such as the rise of HAIs.

Infection control initially escaped the increased economic analysis witnessed in most areas of hospital activity, such as bed occupancy rates and length of stay. Studies such as the SENIC project, mentioned already, that began in the 1970s in the United States, paid little attention to these relationships. But by the 1990s, researchers in the UK were observing that 93 per cent of the total additional cost incurred by surgical patients with an HAI could be attributed to an extended length of stay.[35] The recognition of the relationship came earlier in the United States with the introduction in the 1980s of a system of insurance payments by diagnosis related group (DRG), each with expected lengths of stay for which a hospital would not be reimbursed for exceeding due to HAI.

Part II focuses on nurses and infection control in the operating theatre and ward, with comparative reference to surgeons, medical students and other healthcare workers. Nursing is given particular importance, as the role of nurses in infection control traditionally has been neglected.[36] Their intimate involvement with patients and their operation within larger hospital teams makes nurses a fundamental touchstone for understanding the development and success of infection control measures.

In her chapter, 'Pus, pedagogy and practice: how 'dirt' shaped surgical nurse training and hierarchies of practice, 1900–1935', Pamela Wood points out that surgical success depended not only on the surgeon's operative skill in the face of difficult challenges during surgery, but also on the prevention of sepsis. Pre- and post-operative care was mostly directed at preventing or managing infection and was the professional sphere of the nurse. Training skilled surgical nurses was therefore vital to both the patient's recovery and the surgeon's success.

Central to sepsis was the presence of 'pus' – a substance once applauded as 'laudable pus' associated with healing but, especially from the later nineteenth century, laden not only with fears of gangrene and death but also with responsibility, reputation and blame. Wood builds on previous work relating to the surgical nurse's role in relation to the surgeon, by using the anthropological notion of 'dirt' to explore how sepsis, particularly in its most dangerous form of 'pus', was considered avoidable and shaped surgical nurse training and practice.

Historical evidence from British, Canadian, Australian and New Zealand nursing journals, surgical nursing textbooks, examinations and examiners' reports and nurses' memoirs shows that the notion of 'dirt' shaped the surgical nursing curriculum and the performance of that curriculum in practice. 'Pus' shaped pedagogy. It created a hierarchy of practice that connected ideas about the nature and gradient of dirt with the nurse's ranking and responsibility (the larger the particles of 'dirt', the lower the status of the nurse) and with wound dressing practice (attending to the 'clean' wound, before the 'dirty'). It also determined a social order of surgical relations in which skilled nurses were seen as the surgeon's supporters and, regardless of the cause, the focus of blame for infected wounds.

Blame and responsibility also feature in Claire L. Jones' chapter, 'Septic subjects: infection and occupational illness in British hospitals, *c.* 1870–1970'. Jones points out that historians have long equated the introduction of hygienic practices and systems of infection control in nineteenth- and twentieth-century British hospitals with the need to tackle high rates of infection among patient populations. Yet, little is known of the effect of these practices and systems on the health of the hospital staff. Cross infection and iatrogenic sources of infection have been studied with respect to patients, but the degree of exposure to risk for different types of health workers has been relatively neglected.

Despite this neglect, hospital registers, government reports, medical journals and various related sources demonstrate that many doctors, nurses and other hospital workers regularly became ill throughout their careers, some fatally, as a direct result of working on wards with infected patients. William Ogle, Superintendent of Statistics in the General Register Office between 1880 and 1893, for example, reported that mortality rates from erysipelas in the 1880s among medical men was 'very largely in excess of the average', while nurses during the same period were frequently taken off ward work after developing 'septic finger', a well-known nursing malady.

Jones examines the effects of HAI (and practices surrounding its prevention and control) on hospital staff during the nineteenth and twentieth centuries. She pays particular attention to the experiences of medical students and nurses, who were generally the most frequently exposed to infective organisms. By framing the analysis in terms of occupational risk, she argues that the introduction and implementation of hospital infection control procedures were not solely for the benefit of the patient, but also for the staff who treated them. Monitoring the health of the workforce, and differential exposure to risk, was not only used to measure hospital efficiency, but also formed an important if neglected part of hospital-wide policy to tackle infection.

A hospital-wide approach to infection control and the gradual and uneven process of change emerge from Susan Macqueen's unique participant practitioner's perspective into nursing education and practice in infection prevention and control. In her chapter, 'Learning the art and science of infection prevention and control: a practical application', she draws on her training in the 1960s, her time as a hospital paediatric nurse dealing with infection outbreaks and the contested nature of the knowledge underpinning infection prevention and control practice in paediatric practice. Macqueen recounts and reflects on her experiences as an infection prevention and control nurse, working at local and national level, beginning in 1980 at Great Ormond Street Hospital for Children NHS Trust in London, becoming Director of Infection Prevention and Control from 2004 to 2011 and contributing to government committees shaping guidelines.

Part III explores the history of key technologies for infection prevention and control by focusing on glove use from the late nineteenth century to the present.

In his chapter, 'Wax paste and vaccination: alternatives to surgical gloves for infection control, 1880–1945', Thomas Schlich examines the uptake of surgical gloves in the late nineteenth century. He shows it was a protracted process and explains the relative disinterest of many surgeons in this particular technology by situating it in the context of alternative strategies of surgical infection control. Exploring such alternative innovations shows that technological change in surgery and infection control does not happen in a vacuum. Technical solutions to particular problems are often in competition with alternatives. Schlich describes these failed alternatives in relation to surgical gloves, asking how giving more room to alternative solutions provides a deeper understanding of the histories of surgery and infection control. The sources used in this chapter are mainly published papers in medical and scientific journals of the time, which reflect discussions among surgeons. By focusing on surgical gloves, antisepsis and asepsis, and neglected or forgotten alternative technologies, this chapter brings a new dimension to existing historiographies.

The increasing use of non-surgical, non-sterile gloves since the 1980s and their unintended consequences are Jennie Wilson's concerns in her chapter, 'The evolving role of gloves in healthcare'. The hands of healthcare workers are recognised as a key vehicle for the transmission of healthcare-associated infection (HCAI).[37] There is evidence that they acquire transient micro-organisms through touch and that these are readily transferred to other surfaces and to patients. Prior to the emergence of AIDS in the early 1980s, the availability of gloves in healthcare settings was limited and mostly focused on sterile gloves for invasive procedures, as Schlich describes in Chapter 6. The implementation of universal precautions in response to the need to protect healthcare workers from blood-borne viruses saw the gradual increase in the use of non-sterile clinical gloves across all care settings. The use of personal protective clothing for direct contact with blood and body fluids on the basis that these may be heavily contaminated with pathogenic organisms now forms part of standard infection control precautions policy. However, recent evidence is emerging about the frequent overuse and misuse of non-sterile clinical gloves, and the recognition that inappropriate use may expose patients to significant risks of infection. The perception that gloves protect both the healthcare worker and the patient may counteract triggers for hand hygiene, and thereby increase the risk of transmission of HCAI. In addition, changing attitudes of healthcare workers to patients, touching and risk to self, as well as organisational factors that promote the use of gloves to counteract inadequate hand hygiene, appear to be key factors driving unsafe glove use.

Practice and infection control from the perspective of the laboratory, notably the sanitary officer/pathologist and bacteriologist, from the 1890s to the 1970s is the focus of Part IV. Rosemary Cresswell's chapter examines the emergence of the role of the pathologist in preventing and controlling infection at one London hospital between 1892 and 1939. She emphasises the importance of low rates of infection to the reputation of the hospital, which, like all voluntary hospitals, was dependent for funds on voluntary contributors, and the importance of the emerging role of the sanitary officer/pathologist in identifying and controlling infection. She also explores the pathologist's contested division of labour with the matron.

In 1892, Frederick Andrewes, the Demonstrator in Practical Medicine at St Bartholomew's Hospital (Barts), London, was appointed as the Sanitary Officer. The new role included receiving reports from all doctors and nurses about cases of infectious disease at the hospital and notifying the Local Sanitary Authority, looking after the condition of sanitary appliances and inspecting the sanitary circumstances of the hospital. The successful candidate had to be qualified in medicine and have a diploma in Public Health. Andrewes continued to be the Sanitary Officer when he was appointed as the Pathologist to the Hospital in 1897, and maintained both roles until his retirement in 1928. Although Andrewes was appointed Sanitary Officer first and Pathologist to the Hospital five years later, his successors in the 1920s and 1930s inherited both roles simultaneously, the activities having become intertwined. Using archival sources, including journals and minutes from Barts,

Cresswell investigates the role of the sanitary officer in relation to the matron. She argues that the role of the pathologist as sanitary officer at Barts highlights pathologists' much earlier involvement in hospital management, patient care and infection control than has been presented within the key historiography of infection prevention and control, such as Ayliffe and English's *Hospital Infection: From Miasmas to MRSA* and Kathryn Hillier's seminal paper.[38]

Susan Gardiner continues the consideration of the hospital laboratory and its clinical infection control work in her chapter, 'Infection control from the laboratory to the clinic: John H. Bowie and the Royal Infirmary of Edinburgh, *c.* 1945–1970'.

The position of the bacteriologist in the twentieth-century hospital has recently attracted considerable attention from historians. The emerging picture is that rising rates of antibiotic-resistant infections and new methods for their control (e.g. phage typing and infection control committees) were catalysts to bacteriologists becoming authorities in the field of hospital infection control in the 1950s and 1960s. Gardiner builds on and modifies aspects of the literature by providing a broader understanding of the daily work of bacteriologists in the mid-twentieth-century hospital, and a deeper insight into their role in the control of infection. By using the Royal Infirmary of Edinburgh (RIE) as a case study, she also remedies the lack of scholarly work on the history of hospital infection and its control in twentieth-century Scotland.

Concentrating on the period *c.* 1945 to 1970, Gardiner focuses largely on the role of the RIE's Senior Bacteriologist, John H. Bowie, who provided much of the impetus for many new and improved infection control strategies. She examines infection control practice in the laboratory, exploring both how and why laboratory work changed and took on increasing importance at the hospital during this period. This she achieves by discussing improvements in antibiotic sensitivity testing and the rising demand for bacteriological testing for various other reasons. She then shifts her attention to the commanding role of the bacteriologist in the development of numerous new ward-based infection control procedures, from methods for soiled dressing disposal to sterile supply.

Gardiner uses a range of primary source materials, including medical literature, hospital annual reports, minutes of meetings of the RIE's infection control committee and newly created oral history interviews with clinicians and nurses who worked at the hospital. She argues that, in the mid-twentieth century, bacteriological expertise became increasingly important to the control of hospital infection, and that the work of bacteriologists notably changed and expanded. They performed several important duties and were crucial to the development of a range of new strategies for infection control in both laboratory and clinic. It is for these reasons that they merited being authorities on infection control.

In Part V, two prominent current infection prevention and control practitioners, one in England and Wales and the other in Scotland, recount and reflect on their experiences in the recent past and on national differences, and each suggests directions for infection prevention and control in the future.

Neil Wigglesworth focuses on England and Wales from the perspectives of his current post as Deputy Director, Infection Prevention and Control, Guy's and St Thomas' NHS Foundation Trust and as recent President of the Infection Prevention Society 2016–2018 in his chapter, 'Infection prevention and control in the twenty-first century: the era of patient safety'.

Wigglesworth points out that infection prevention and control (IPC) is a constant challenge in an ever-changing context. Practices have evolved as part of changing societal and healthcare culture, developments in medicine and other health professions and regulatory frameworks. He reflects on the impact of these influences in recent years, including where specific successes have been achieved, and describes the key infection prevention challenges now and in the near future. Specifically, Wigglesworth considers the rise and fall of MRSA and *C. diff*, as well as the current threat from multi-resistant gram-negative bacteria, including carbapenemase-producing Enterobacteriaceae (CPE). He also explores how infection prevention can embrace and engage with the wider patient safety agenda to continue developing. Given the economic and political conditions in England since 2009, and the global financial crisis, he suggests the likelihood of further major investment in IPC appears remote. In addition, he argues that the national focus on AMR has not resulted in a renewed focus on IPC, despite IPC featuring as a major component of the UK AMR Strategy. In this context, IPC needs to identify opportunities for further large-scale improvement. Recent work in areas such as safety culture, quality improvement, and human factors and ergo-nomics may present opportunities for collaboration to improve patient and public safety.

Alistair Leanord, Professor of Infection and Immunity at Glasgow University and HAI Medical Advisor to the Scottish Government, also draws on his experience over the past fifteen years in his chap-ter, 'Infection control and antimicrobial resistance: the past, the pre-sent and the future'. He highlights the process of policy change and implementation, and differences and similarities between England and Scotland.

From a senior participant observer perspective, he examines the emergence of recent policy around infection control in Scotland and the ways it differs from developments in England. With spe-cific reference to MRSA and *C. diff*, he considers the reasons why policy and implementation can lag behind knowledge about infec-tion control, as well as challenges associated with human factors. He begins with an account from Scotland in 2002, before estab-lishing infection control as a national priority, and he traces the development over the next fifteen years in which infection control became the subject of a rigorous and joined-up government policy, and rates of infection from MRSA and *C. diff* fell dramatically in Scotland and in England for different reasons. He also considers the ways in which 'migration' and 'localism' have become key words in policy development. He ends with some reflections on the future of infection control, based on experience, evidence and developing technologies.

Notes

1 Matt Hancock, UK Health and Social Care Secretary, quoted in 'Antimicrobial resistance: UK launches 5-year action plan and 20-year vision', www.gov.uk/government/news/antimicrobial-resistance-uk-launches-5-year-action-plan-and-20-year-vision (accessed 31 Jan 2019). 'Superbugs "are as dangerous as climate change"', *The Times*, 30 Apr 2019, 2.

2 J. E. Lesch, *The first miracle drugs: how the sulfa drugs transformed medicine* (New York: Oxford University Press, 2007); F. Condrau, 'Standardising infection control: antibiotics and hospital governance in Britain, 1948–1960', in C. Bonah, European Science Foundation (eds),

Harmonizing drugs: standards in 20th-century pharmaceutical history (Paris: Editions Glyphe, 2009), 327–339; J. A. Greene, F. Condrau and E. S. Watkins (eds), *Therapeutic revolutions* (Chicago and London: University of Chicago Press, 2016), 2.

3 R. Bud, *Penicillin: triumph and tragedy* (Oxford: Oxford University Press, 2009); F. Condrau and R. Kirk, 'Negotiating hospital infections: the debate between ecological balance and eradication strategies in British hospitals, 1947–1969', *Dynamis*, 31 (2011), 385–405.

4 S. H. Podolsky and A. K. Lie, 'Futures and their uses: antibiotics and therapeutic revolutions', in Greene, Condrau and Watkins (eds), *Therapeutic revolutions*, 19; S. H. Podolsky, *The antibiotic era: reform, resistance, and the pursuit of a rational therapeutics* (Baltimore: Johns Hopkins University Press, 2015); S. B. Levy, *The antibiotic paradox: how miracle drugs are destroying the miracle* (New York; London: Plenum Press, 1992); Bud, *Penicillin: triumph and tragedy*; D. Greenwood, *Antimicrobial drugs: chronicle of a twentieth century medical triumph* (Oxford: Oxford University Press, 2008); N. Gualde (trans. S. Rendall), *Resistance: the human struggle against infection* (Washington: Dana Press, 2006).

5 Levy, *The antibiotic paradox*; M. McKenna, *Superbug: the fatal menace of MRSA* (New York: Free Press, 2010).

6 See, for example, P. Clough and J. Halley (eds), *The affective turn: theorizing the social* (Durham, NC: Duke University Press, 2007); R. Porzig-Drummond, R. Stevenson, T. Case and M. Oaten, 'Can the emotion of disgust be harnessed to promote hand hygiene? Experimental and field-based tests', *Social Science & Medicine*, 68:6 (2009), 1006–1012; P. Harding, 'Pandemics, plagues and panic', *British Journalism Review*, 20 (2009), 27–33; M. Honigsbaum, *The pandemic century: one hundred years of panic, hysteria and hubris* (London: Hurst & Co, 2019) has also written on fear and panics in relation to flu.

7 Greene, Condrau and Watkins (eds), *Therapeutic revolution*, 2; see, for example, Angela Rippon, 'The truth about antibiotics', BBC ONE, accessed when broadcast 30 Jan 2019, www.bbc.co.uk/programmes/b0c1nl68.

8 Interagency Coordination Group on Antimicrobial Resistance, *No time to wait: securing the future from drug-resistant infections – report to the Secretary-General of the United Nations* (Apr 2019), www.who.int/antimicrobial-resistance/interagency-coordination-group/en/ (accessed 30 Apr 2019).

9 See, for example: 'No-deal Brexit could see UK locked out of EU infectious disease surveillance data, chief medical officer warns', *Pharmaceutical Journal* (13 Feb 2019), www.pharmaceutical-journal.com/20206154.article?firstPass=false (accessed 15 April 2019); House

of Lords, *Leaving the EU: Antimicrobial resistance* (Aug 2018), https:// lordslibrary.parliament.uk/research-briefings/lln-2018-0087/.

10 See 'Tackling drug-resistant infections globally: final report and recom- mendations – the review on antimicrobial resistance chaired by Jim O'Neill' (May 2016), https://amr-review.org/sites/default/files/160518_ Final%20paper_with%20cover.pdf; HM Government, 'Tackling antimi- crobial resistance 2019–2024: The UK's five-year national action plan' (24 Jan 2019), https://assets.publishing.service.gov.uk/government/uploads/ system/uploads/attachment_data/file/773130/uk-amr-5-year-national-acti on-plan.pdf; 'Contained and controlled: the UK's 20-year vision for anti- microbial resistance (AMR)' (24 Jan 2019), www.gov.uk/government/pub lications/uk-20-year-vision-for-antimicrobial-resistance (accessed 31 Jan 2019).

11 'Tackling antimicrobial resistance 2019–2024', 29. Caveats associated with these estimates should also be recognised: see, for example, M. E. A. de Kraker, A. J. Stewardson and S. Harbarth, 'Will 10 million people die a year due to antimicrobial resistance by 2050?', *PLOS Medicine*, 13 (2016), e1002184.

12 'Contained and controlled', 6; K. Forsberg, K. Woodworth, M. Walters *et al.*, '*Candida auris*: the recent emergence of a multidrug-resistant fun- gal pathogen', *Medical Mycology*, 57 (Jan 2019), 1–12. https://doi.org/ 10.1093/mmy/myy054 (accessed 15 Apr 2019).

13 'Contained and controlled', 3–4.

14 'Tackling antimicrobial resistance 2019–2024', 3, 7–8. The importance of antimicrobial resistance in animals is clear from Claas Kirchhelle, *Pyrrhic progress: the history of antibiotics in Anglo-American food production* (New Brunswick, NJ: Rutgers University Press, 2020).

15 *Oxford Concise Medical Dictionary*, 8th edition (Oxford: Oxford University Press, 2010), 505, cited in S. Gardiner, 'Answering Ackerknecht: infection control practice in Scottish hospitals in the early "antibiotic era", 1928–1970' (PhD thesis, University of Glasgow, 2017), 2. Healthcare- associated infection (HCAI) is a related term introduced in 2002 that includes HAI and some infections previously considered as community- acquired infections (CAI), such as bloodstream infections acquired in outpatient facilities and nursing homes. See N. D. Friedman, K. S. Kaye, J. E. Stout *et al.*, 'Health care-associated bloodstream infections in adults: a reason to change the accepted definition of community-acquired infec- tions', *Annals of Internal Medicine*, 137 (2002), 791–797; T. Cardoso, M. Almeida, N. D. Friedman *et al.*, 'Classification of healthcare-associated infection: a systematic review 10 years after the first proposal', *BMC Medicine*, 12 (6 Mar 2014), https://bmcmedicine.biomedcentral.com/ articles/10.1186/1741-7015-12-40 (accessed 1 Feb 2019).

16 In addition to Forsberg, Woodworth, Walters *et al.*, '*Candida auris*', see, for example, CDC, '*Candida auris*: a drug-resistant germ that spreads in healthcare facilities', www.cdc.gov/fungal/candida-auris/c-auris-drug-resistant.html (accessed 1 Feb 2019).

17 Healthcare Commission, *Investigation into outbreaks of* Clostridium difficile *at Maidstone and Tunbridge Wells NHS Trust* (London, 2007); The Mid Staffs NHS Foundation Trust Public Inquiry, *Independent inquiry into care provided by Mid Staffs NHS Foundation Trust January 2005–March 2009, chaired by Robert Francis QC* (2010), House of Commons 375–1, www.midstaffspublicinquiry.com.

18 Healthcare Commission, *Investigation into outbreaks of* Clostridium difficile *at Maidstone and Tunbridge Wells NHS Trust*; P. Griffiths, A. Renz, J. Hughes and A. M. Rafferty, 'Impact of organisation and management factors on infection control in hospitals: a scoping review', *Journal of Hospital Infection*, 73 (2009), 1–14; The Mid Staffs NHS Foundation Trust Public Inquiry, *Independent inquiry into care provided by Mid Staffs NHS Foundation Trust*.

19 I. Illich, *Medical nemesis: the expropriation of health* (London: Calder and Boyars, 1975). Illich introduced the term 'iatrogenesis' to describe what he viewed as the relentless increase in disease induced by doctors.

20 Institute of Medicine, *To err is human: building a safer health care system* (Washington: Institute of Medicine and National Academy Press, 1999).

21 Patient Safety movement – Department of Health, *An organisation with a memory: report of an expert group on learning from adverse events in the NHS, chaired by the Chief Medical Officer* (London: Department of Health, 2000), 11; Francis Report; follow-up (2013). Atul Gawande, 'Checklists'; M. E. Lark, K. Kirkpatrick, K. C. Chung, 'Patient safety movement: history and future directions', *Journal of Hand Surgery*, 43:2 (2018), 174–178.

22 H. Hogan, F. Healey and G. Neale, *et al.*, 'Preventable deaths due to problems in care in English acute hospitals: a retrospective case record review study', *British Medical Journal Quality & Safety*, 21 (2012), 737–745.

23 *An organisation with a memory*, Chapter 3. For a wider audience, the surgeon, Atul Gawande, described the application of this perspective in the case of surgery in his book, *The checklist manifesto: how to get things right* (New York: Metropolitan Books of Henry Holt, 2009; London: Picador, 2010), esp. 148–168, and for the BBC in his 'Reith Lectures 2014: the future of medicine, lecture 2: the century of the system'. Also in this tradition of 'an opportunity for learning' regarding patient safety are Robert Francis' *Independent inquiry into*

care provided by Mid Staffs NHS Foundation Trust, and the follow-up National Advisory Group on the Safety of Patients in England, D. Berwick (Chair), *A promise to learn – a commitment to act: improving the safety of patients in England* (2013). For recent discussions, see, for example, M. Dixon-Woods and P. J Pronovost, 'Patient safety and the problem of many hands', *British Medical Journal Quality & Safety*, 25:7 (2016), 485–488; and Lark *et al.*, 'Patient safety movement'.

24 *An organisation with a memory*, p. viii.
25 See Neil Wigglesworth and Alistair Leanord in this volume. See also M. H. Wilcox, 'The start of another infection prevention learning curve: reducing healthcare-associated Gram-negative bloodstream infections', *Journal of Hospital Infection*, 97:3 (2017), 205–206.
26 The 'AMR Historical Foresight' project, Dec 2017 to Feb 2020, University of Exeter http://sites.exeter.ac.uk/amrhistoricalforesight/about-the-study/ (accessed 3 Dec 2018).
27 'Tackling drug-resistant infections globally', 23.
28 G. A. J. Ayliffe and M. English, *Hospital infection: from miasmas to MRSA* (Cambridge: Cambridge University Press, 2003); and S. Selwyn, 'Hospital infection: the first 2500 years', *Journal of Hospital Infection*, 18, supplement A (1991), 5–64.
29 L. Abreu and S. Sheard (eds), *Hospital life: theory and practice from the medieval to the modern* (Oxford: Peter Lang, 2013); Laura Bowater, *The microbes fight back: antibiotic resistance* (Royal Society of Chemistry, 2017), 23.
30 M. Newsom Kerr, *Contagion, isolation, and biopolitics in Victorian London* (Basingstoke: Palgrave Macmillan, 2017). See also, G. M. Ayers, *England's first state hospitals and the Metropolitan Asylums Board 1867–1930* (London: Wellcome Institute for the History of Medicine, 1971); H. Tebbutt, 'On the bacteriology of asylum dysentery', *Journal of Hygiene*, 12 (1912), 218–226.
31 www.ips.uk.net/about/history/ (accessed 15 Feb 2019).
32 The HIS also provides grants and bursaries to support work in the field, and awards the Diploma in Hospital Infection Control (DipHIC) along with the London School of Hygiene and Tropical Medicine (LSHTM) and the Laboratory of HealthCare Associated Infection (LHCAI). www.his.org.uk/about/ and http://blog.wellcomelibrary.org/2009/07/hospital-infection-society/ (accessed 15 Feb 2019).
33 See R. W. Haley, D. Quade, H. E. Freeman, J. V. Bennett, 'The SENIC Project: Study on the Efficacy of Nosocomial Infection Control (SENIC Project) – summary of study design', *American Journal of Epidemiology*, 111 (1980), 472–485; J. M. Hughes, 'Study on the Efficacy of Nosocomial Infection Control (SENIC Project): results and implications for the

future', *Chemotherapy*, 34 (1988), 553–561; M. G. Daniel, 'A history of hospital infection control: the Study on the Efficacy of Nosocomial Infection Control [SENIC]', www.hopkinshistoryofmedicine.org/sites/default/files/SC%20Michael%20Daniel.pdf (accessed 15 Feb 2019).

34 P. Pronovost, D. Needham, S. Berenholtz *et al.*, 'An intervention to decrease catheter-related bloodstream infections in the ICU', *New England Journal of Medicine*, 355 (2006), 2725–2732, www.nejm.org/doi/full/10.1056/NEJMoa061115 (accessed 1 Feb 2019).

35 See, for example, R. Coello, H. Glenister, J. Fereres *et al.*, 'The cost of infection in surgical patients: a case-control study', *Journal of Hospital Infection*, 25 (1993), 239–250.

36 Exceptions include Christine Hallett, *Containing trauma: nursing work in the First World War* (Manchester: Manchester University Press, 2009); David Justnam, 'A study of nursing practices used in the management of infection in hospitals, 1929–48' (unpublished PhD thesis, University of Manchester, 2014); David Justnam, '"Those maggots – they did a wonderful job": the nurses' role in wound management in civilian hospitals during the Second World War', in J. Brooks and C. E. Hallett (eds), *One hundred years of wartime nursing practices, 1854–1953* (Manchester: Manchester University Press, 2015), 189–210.

37 Editors' Note: we have retained the authors' use of the term HCAI as appropriate for the period of their research.

38 Ayliffe and English, *Hospital infection*; K. Hillier, 'Babies and bacteria: phage typing, bacteriologists, and the birth of infection control', *Bulletin of the History of Medicine*, 80 (2006), 733–761.

Part I

Policy and infection control

1

Hospital infections and the role of the community before MRSA, 1930–1960

Flurin Condrau

Introduction

The historiography of hospital infections conceptualises most bacterial infections occurring in hospitals as inherently institutional. This chapter challenges this notion and argues that from very early on, microbiologists working inside and outside hospitals began to understand the link between the hospital and the community when explaining outbreaks of infections in hospitals. Looking at discussions in Britain and elsewhere in the era of the *Staphylococcus aureus* crisis after the Second World War, this chapter draws particular attention to key sites of hospital-community transfer, that is neonatal infection, as well as influenza. It argues that in both examples, the institutional nature of hospital infections remains unclear, and the community needs to be seen as a crucial site for infection control in hospitals.

This chapter builds on my previous work, which has explored the debates around antibiotic use in hospitals between *c.* 1930 and 1960, particularly controversies over the aim of eradication of Staphylococcal strains versus their ecological management.[1] This chapter elaborates my work further by showing the potential of looking beyond the hospital walls to begin to understand the complexities of infections due to Staphylococci and Streptococci. It uses two case studies of hospital-community interaction in different types of hospital settings: the question of newborns as the hospital birth increasingly became the norm; and the time-specific crisis of the Asian Flu outbreak in 1957, in relation to which many patients entered and subsequently left general hospitals. From our current perspective, the end point seems clear: the community has acquired a major role in explanations of the prevalence of Staphylococcal and Streptococcal infection.[2] Yet the historical literature has largely overlooked this.

Part of the reason for this neglect is that historians have tended to fail to mention the problem of infection – sourced from the community or the institution – within the emerging historiography of hospitals since the 1960s. It is not mentioned in Michel Foucault's *Birth of the Clinic*, which emphasised the clinical gaze to analyse the separation of medical thought from patient identity.[3] Nor is it evident in Erwin H. Ackerknecht's classic study, *Medicine at the Paris Hospital*, which examined the basis of Paris hospital medicine and argued the centrality of the lesion.[4] Nor is it considered in Nicholas Jewson's influential work, which argued that hospital medicine represented a distinct form of medicine.[5] These studies set the tone for a so-called new hospital history bereft of infections. Best exemplified by Brian Abel Smith's seminal study, first published in 1964, hospital histories have often failed to differentiate between types of hospitals, and hence the complicated place of infections within them.[6] Even relatively recent hospital histories tend to sideline infections, focusing instead on the development of the hospital system under the framework of the emerging medical sciences, the social structure of hospital patients, the finances and provision of hospitals and debates around the therapeutic effectiveness of hospital medicine.[7]

As well as the way hospital histories have been written, a further explanation of why historians have neglected the issue of hospital infection is the way the history of disease has been written. For historians, the term 'hospital infection' has only recently acquired the status of a disease. It appears that in the vast historiography of disease histories, single-disease narratives have dominated.[8] This is the case for most studies concerning the history of tuberculosis.[9] It holds for the historiography of cancer as well, which has been shaped by analyses of sub-types of cancer usually dealt with on a case-by-case basis.[10] And this trend culminated in two successful book series following specific disease 'biographies'.[11] Attempts to overcome this single-disease narrative have resulted in long trans-disease histories that do not, in my view, question the notion that diseases are distinct entities.[12] A productive way to overcome this limitation appears to be the focus on symptoms, as in a recent book on fever.[13] Co-infection, the interaction of diseases with each other, remains an innovative and promising approach.[14] The term hospital infections, however, refers to a wide number of medical problems that are linked together because these are infections caused by bacteria acquired in hospitals. The disease vector has given the name, which seems unusual. In many ways, the term hospital infection owes its power to two, at times contradictory, interpretations of what hospitals are. One is to regard hospitals as places of medical care, which by their very nature further health and well-being. Quite another is to regard hospitals, as Ivan Illich has done, as sites of a new, industrial medicine which expresses, rather than battles, the evils of modern society.[15] The former attitude comes in various guises, one linked more to Nightingale's often-cited request 'to do the sick no harm'. Illich's analysis of modern healthcare went further as he discussed iatrogenic diseases – diseases caused by, rather than cured by, medical treatment. As such, hospital infections can be regarded as primary examples of problems caused by modern healthcare. This, then, firmly frames the debate of hospital infections as problems of hospitals, where they are caused rather than merely acquired. The fundamental question of this chapter is to question whether this is an accurate reflection of debates around Staphylococcal and Streptococcal infection in the era of 1930–1960. The end point, as it were, seems clear: in a contemporary perspective, the community has acquired a huge role in explaining the prevalence of Staphylococcal and Streptococcal infection.[16] Interestingly, the historical literature has largely overlooked this issue. This certainly includes my own work. But, it is also true for Kathryn Hillier's groundbreaking contribution that sparked a lot of interest in the subject, mainly due to her focus on the importance of phage typing as a tool to identify specific strains of Staphylococci in hospitals around the world.[17] Hospital infections, in this view, are important triggers for new ways of knowing.[18] Christoph Gradmann's recent analysis has combined several interests such as antibiotic resistance and infection, but is held together by its focus on hospitals.[19] Again, the problem of hospital infections appears to be mainly a trigger for studying antibiotic resistance and its implications. In fact, it links well with several other publications, in which Gradmann explored the issues around resistance.[20] This work anticipates emerging historiography around antibiotics, such as Scott Podolsky's groundbreaking study.[21] My own work has explored the debates around antibiotic use in hospitals, where debates between eradication attempts and notions of ecological management of Staphylococcal strains in hospitals played out.[22] In many ways, this historiography reflects a tendency to see medicine and health issues most acutely realised in hospitals. While this is undoubtedly true, it generally leads historians to maintain high walls around most hospitals, privileging a hospital-centric perspective. Perhaps most convincingly, the history of psychiatry has developed ideas to diminish the separation between institution and community.[23] The purpose of this chapter, thus, is to show the potential of looking beyond the hospital to begin to understand the complexities of infection due to Staphylococci and Streptococci.

Background

Before focusing on the two case studies of hospital-community interaction from the period 1930 to 1960, it is helpful to look back to three aspects of infection control and hospital-community interaction since the mid-nineteenth century.

First, hospital infections were a concern of many advocates of the merits of hospitals. Florence Nightingale, for example, referred to the issue of contagious patients within hospitals when she made her oft-quoted statement in 1859 that hospitals 'should do the sick no harm'.[24] Comparing mortality within hospitals to the likely mortality outside hospitals, Nightingale concluded, was leading to a critical view of hospitals and their curative merit. But Nightingale went on to focus on hospital problems as problems of hygiene, and given the clinical interest of medicine in maintaining hospitals as sites of medical education and practice, the emphasis was not put on the likely impact that infection had on hospital organisation more generally.[25] Nightingale's concerns about the damage that infections might do to the status of hospitals thus stand in stark contrast to much of the hospital historiography since the 1960s.

Second, one of the ways in which concerns about hospital infection manifested themselves in the nineteenth century was in the segregation of fever patients. Patients thought to be suffering from fever or infectious disease tended to be excluded from voluntary hospitals, and in the early nineteenth century smallpox and fever hospitals were set up as temporary, emergency measures, often under the Poor Law, or as charity to the poor adjacent to an existing voluntary hospital as in Manchester or Glasgow, or separately as in the London Fever Hospital. They were replaced from the 1860s by permanent fever and smallpox hospitals, which started to emerge in Britain on a large scale.[26]

It is here that the general historiographical neglect of hospital infection begins to break down. The isolation in hospitals of patients suffering from contagious diseases, as distinct from the types of infectious diseases caused by lack of sanitation, has received considerable attention recently from historians, notably Matthew Newsom Kerr. He focuses on the emergence of the network of permanent infectious disease hospitals open to all and their role in public health throughout Britain, and especially in London, where they emerged under the auspices of the Metropolitan Asylums Board.[27] Beginning in the 1860s, by 1879, 296 out of 1,593 sanitary authorities in England and Wales provided a hospital for infectious diseases; by 1893 there were 400; and by the beginning of the First World War there were 755 fever hospitals and 363 smallpox hospitals. This 'great confinement' of infectious patients in the last decades of the nineteenth century did not coincide with a great rise of epidemics; in fact, typhus and smallpox epidemics were fading, though scarlet fever and typhoid remained prevalent but declining in virulence. The removal of people from homes which was associated with this growth of hospitals did not face resistance, while it would have fifty years previously. Newsom Kerr shows how this acceptance came about in London, and health authorities were able to get the public to accept and even expect treatment for infectious diseases in such institutions. The new institutions for the separate treatment of infectious diseases were dissociated from pauperism and a system of deterrence, deprivation and degradations. Most patients were admitted not as charity to themselves but in order to prevent them infecting others. Thus, for the good of public health, it was necessary to gain the cooperation of all classes and strip the hospitals of the overt signs of the Poor Law, paying close attention to ordinary comforts such as food, fittings and furniture. Hospital isolation had to act as a force of attraction to individuals, with health administrators facilitating and mobilising consent by employing tactics of persuasion and strategies of enticement.[28]

As a term to describe a public health strategy, 'isolation' in separate and special hospitals came to be fully accepted during the 1880s. These hospitals also came to be seen as a special place for the production of new aetiological knowledge with the main lesson that infectious diseases may be shut within wards and the public protected from their spread. The fever hospital was viewed as an effective means of improving public health, not simply ameliorating suffering. This separation itself made the infectious diseases more manageable.

The aim was not to annihilate infectious disease, but to prevent endemic infectious disease from becoming epidemic, and to enable its control before and not after it assumed epidemic proportions. At the same time, the fever hospital redefined the home as an unsuitable location for treating the most common infectious ailments.

As mentioned earlier, nosocomial infections, that is sickness originating as the result of hospital treatment, have always occurred in all hospitals.[29] Yet, in the 1890s, with fever hospitals increasingly directed at the general public and hospital physicians and nursing staff growing more sensitive to their own risk of illness, nosocomial infections came to be seen as an urgent issue that threatened the rationale of isolation. Between 1884 and 1904, at least 10 per cent of patients in London fever hospitals suffered from a disease other than the one certified on admission, although physicians in the London fever hospitals hesitated to consider this 'superadded infection' entirely a hospital creation. The response to the danger of 'superadded infection', such as convalescent scarlet fever patients who contracted diphtheria, was to redefine fever treatment, like many other medical and sanitary measures, as germ practice,[30] involving techniques of 'isolation within isolation' as a key organising principle, and the 'precise performance of asepsis'. The hospital was no longer considered merely a blockade but a mechanism of prevention in its own right, with its own internal territories and boundaries, both architectural and administrative, creating a deliberate geography of separation of acute and convalescent cases and smaller wards and paying careful attention to ward furnishings, creating impermeable surfaces, for example glass countertops, white enamelled iron, glazed tiles and highly polished wood floors, with walls and ceilings devoid of ledges or corners – all to eliminate any place where dust could collect and to make everything in the ward perfectly visible. In the later 1890s and 1900s, emphasis shifted from architectural isolation and the condition of places to the condition of bodies and aseptic hygienic behaviours, procedures and ritualised performance embodied in barrier nursing and bed isolation experiments, aiming to barricade each patient as a unique source of infection. Hospitals became a space possessing variable zones of concentration, infectivity and risk, and hospital hygiene became personal hygiene and vice versa for both patients and staff, especially nursing staff.

Yet, while the isolation hospitals quickly became, in the second half of the 1890s, important centres for testing and deploying new methods of treatment and diagnosis, and the introduction of antitoxin treatment led to a fall in diphtheria mortality by about half by 1900, bacteriological diagnosis failed to resolve problems of hospital infection and prolonged detention. It was difficult to distinguish between virulent and non-virulent bacilli, and scepticism remained about the extent to which laboratory screenings would have value in managing hospital infections related to diphtheria.

At the same time, the effectiveness of isolation in fever hospitals, particularly for scarlet fever, was the subject of controversy. A lack of consistent evidence and lack of understanding of the aetiology of scarlet fever[31] led to a longstanding debate over scarlet fever's period and mode of infectivity, which arose from the problem of 'return cases', that is cases of scarlet fever emerging in homes to which hospital patients had recently been discharged. Were they due to premature discharge, inadequate disinfection of homes or persistently high rates of infection in the community? The discussion ended up stressing that the value of the fever hospitals was not purely preventative. They offered the best treatment and chance for recovery in most cases, and they provided great convenience to affected families, as removal of the sick could be vital for assuring employment of a breadwinner, continuing a home business and school attendance of siblings. Arthur Newsholme, having served as Medical Officer of Health and later as the Chief Medical Officer of the Local Government Board, recognised this, and he argued that general sanitation and hospital sequestration worked to temper the scarlet fever germ and make the disease less fatal on average, despite continuing or increasing prevalence.

A similar debate in which Newsholme also participated took place at the same time over the hospital segregation of tuberculosis patients. Understanding the contagious nature of tuberculosis was a difficult undertaking, and defining the actual contagious cases remained a contested area of medical expertise, particularly in relation to the health risks of hospital staff in contact with such patients.[32] Hence, longer-term hospital care implied the challenge of cross infection, a problem clearly reflected in early twentieth-century medical writing. Newsholme also recognised the problem of cross infection in relation to the emerging sanatorium movement.[33] Taking Newsholme's arguments as a starting point, historians have argued for the merits of the sanatorium for isolation purposes.[34] However, short-term isolation in the sanatorium did not do much to influence the management of chronic tuberculosis, and most sanatoria were not even equipped to discern between infectious and non-infectious conditions.[35] Also, these institutions tried to select non-contagious cases, which they deemed more treatable by open air, rest or exercise. Often, patients with a clearly infectious condition were simply left to their own devices or were confined to Poor Law institutions.[36] There is robust evidence that tuberculosis wards in regular or chest hospitals remained half empty, for fear of inviting patients into hospitals risking cross infection in the wards.[37] So exclusion, rather than treatment, remained the stock answer in the case of some infectious diseases, while the response to many others was a strategy of 'isolation within isolation', by both physical means and aseptic ritual, with a goal of disease management reduction and acceptance of the probable failure of complete elimination.

A third feature of hospital infection is the recurrence of arguments about the possibility of the elimination of infection. Despite acceptance of the impossibility of complete elimination of cross infection in the early twentieth century, by the time of the establishment of the National Health Service (NHS) in Britain, its aim was to run hospitals as healthy institutions.[38] Developments in infection control were instrumental in this change. New ways of thinking influenced medical understanding of bacteria and infection on many levels.[39] One such trajectory was that sub-types of bacteria were linked to groups of diseases. For instance, Streptococci, presumed by Theodor Billroth and studied by Louis Pasteur, were seen to be responsible for conditions such as scarlet fever and puerperal fever.[40] Such understanding, together with the development of sulphonamides, facilitated the decline of maternal mortality rates in the 1930s.[41] One of the leading infection control specialists at the time, Leonard Colebrook, concluded in 1955 that puerperal fever caused by *Streptococcus pyogenes* was now almost unheard of.[42] Within twenty years, a serious infectious problem had almost disappeared.[43] It is interesting to note how many medical actors began to regard the period after 1945, probably until the mid-1970s, as a period akin to a 'Therapeutic Revolution'.[44] I have argued elsewhere how the expansion of hospital consultants and patients in hospital was made possible by an ever more intensifying use of the existing infrastructure, financed by cuts in non-medical staff.[45] Contemporary observers noted that overcrowding and procedural problems went hand in hand: 'Cross infections are as much due to overcrowding in busy wards as to the misuse of antibiotics and faulty technique on the part of the surgeon.'[46]

Hospital microbiologists, however, began to understand that hospitals were not just sites of occasional 'infection accidents'; they increasingly presented the hospital as a transmission vector for nosocomial infections. This association did not escape contemporary observers, who began to be interested in whether an infection-free hospital was even a realistic proposition. While German bacteriologists were largely following militaristic campaigns against bacteria, others began to see that complete eradication of bacterial strains was probably impossible. René Dubos, for instance, called the idea of disease eradication a mirage and suggested that 'nature will strike back'.[47] I have pursued these debates between eradication and equilibrium elsewhere. Here, suffice to say that such semantic contests were an expression of unresolved issues of managing disease processes, and the limitations of the success of control measures associated with either strategy.[48]

Newborns, hospitals and infection

For the purposes of this chapter, it is crucial to focus on exemplary cases of hospital-community interaction. To assess all departments of all hospitals in their relation to the community would be impossible, which is why I intend to focus on the hospital nursery. Maternity services were an important aspect of the early history of the NHS, and hospital births became the norm fairly soon after 1948.[49] The case for taking this particular angle is further strengthened by the historiography, which has emphasised the importance of the control of maternal mortality in the interwar period, and because Hillier's key contribution focused on the hospital nursery.[50] After the Second World War, thus, two distinct processes intersected in the hospital nursery: first, there were more births than ever before occurring in a hospital environment, which put a strain on hospitals, staff and general resources. Second, microbiologists examining the spread of hospital infections began to note that hospital nurseries were important sites for the spread of antibiotic-resistant strains.[51] Several authors have highlighted that this was not just an NHS question – for the hospital nursery was a key site fostering international collaboration among microbiologists, such as Phyllis Rountree, a research bacteriologist (1944–1961), later chief bacteriologist (1961–1971), on the staff of the Royal Prince Alfred Hospital in Sydney and Mary Barber, reader in bacteriology at St Thomas' Hospital Medical School (1948–1958), later reader (1958–1961) and professor of clinical bacteriology (1961–1965) at the British Postgraduate Medical School in London.[52] The hospital nursery not only became a key battleground for hospital bacteriologists trying to counter antibiotic-resistant microbial strains, but also facilitated important technical innovations, which in turn reshaped the way microbiologists conceptualised microbial disease strains.[53] The major innovation, according to Hillier, was phage typing as a means to differentiate between bacterial strains, a subject first written about by Wilson and Atkinson in a publication in the *Lancet* that triggered a new way of tracing bacteria.[54] It was important to know where the infecting strains came from to control hospital cross infection, whilst also propelling hospital bacteriologists and microbiologists into a leading role for infection control.[55] Hillier's task was to follow the phage typers in their search for specific strains; her job was not, however, to follow the babies. But the question was raised: what could be gained by following the health of babies through their pregnant mothers, and after birth?[56]

A *Lancet* editorial began to highlight the problem of infection in birthing wards in 1945, arguing that Staphylococcal infection was a 'common invader of the maternity unit'.[57] But *Staph* 80/81, the new strain discovered in the mid-1950s, represented a new crisis point for maternity units, as its increased pathogenic capacity

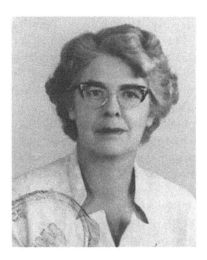

Figure 1.1   Phyllis Rountree in 1958.

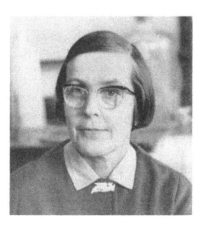

Figure 1.2   British pathologist and bacteriologist Mary Barber.

meant that older neonates represented the source of cross infection to newborns, and the assumption was generally upheld that there was a correlation between the length of stay in hospital and the prevalence of *Staph* 80/81 infection.[58] Indeed, the *Staph* 80/81 crisis highlighted the strain put on NHS infrastructure, with more and more births occurring in a hospital environment that had barely changed from the interwar years. Intensifying the use of maternity equipment, such as cots, made baby-to-baby transmission in the nursery ever more likely.[59] An initial examination of the likelihood of a transfer of *Staph* 80/81 from the hospital to the community was undertaken in 1955 by Phyllis Rountree. From an examination of blood donors in Sydney, Rountree concluded that the occurrence of *Staph* 80/81 in the community was negligible, and that it remained a hospital strain.[60] Further studies by Edinburgh bacteriologist John Gould revealed increasingly inconclusive evidence, and questions about the prevalence of *Staph* 80/81 outside hospitals were widespread.[61] How this transfer was supposed to happen remained unclear, as the technology of phage typing and the main advocates using it favoured the examination of pathways of micro agents within the walls of the hospital.[62]

The framing of *Staph* 80/81 as a hospital problem prevented the sustained analysis of its movement in the community. But this began to change in the second half of the 1950s, when an increasing number of studies began dealing with the question of whether *Staph* 80/81 had become a community problem, and if so, how. Blood donors, previously studied by Rountree, had begun to show an increased exposure to *Staph* 80/81.[63] *Lancet* editorials and articles serve as clear reminders of how abrupt this new understanding of the role of the community appeared in medical circles.[64] A further *Lancet* editorial, published in 1963, arrived at a wholly new conclusion: despite years of prominence in a hospital environment, Staphylococcal infections had firmly moved into the community.[65] In relation to hospital nurseries, California-based microbiologist Valerie Hurst commented early on: 'Although antibiotic resistant Staphylococci have been primarily a hospital problem, cumulative evidence indicates that resistant Staphylococci are no longer confined to hospitals and are increasing in the community at large … This problem has recently become serious because many hospital nurseries are now plagued with highly infectious *Staphylococcus*.

The phage type is variously reported as 80/81'.[66] The remark also reflects the increasingly international nature of the debate: while the issues arose locally, they were debated internationally by Rountree, Hurst and many others.

In 1960, the *Canadian Medical Association Journal* reported that, based on an extensive study in Australia, a third of all patients in general practice were carriers of *Staph* 80/81.[67] Between 1950 and 1960, then, the general consensus seems to have shifted: *S. aureus* changed its face from a hospital-related problem indicating governance issues within medicine, to a larger problem well beyond hospital infection control discussions.[68] The culprit, however, remained the hospital, and the main source of contamination was the nursery, with neonates appearing to carry infection out of the hospital and into the community.[69] The epidemiologic problem then became a question about which kinds of diseases were caused by *S. aureus* out in the community, where investigations revealed long infectious histories in babies without any clear root cause.[70] Interestingly, examinations of the epidemiology of *S. aureus* in the community emphasised the long-term nature of the problem, with one particular study tracing distinct phages over seven years within the same family.[71] A five-year follow-up study of a 1957 hospital nursery outbreak of *Staph* 80/81 revealed that after a considerable period of time, half of all families with a previous history of infection still showed Staphylococcal prevalence.[72] In other words, Staphylococcal infections turned out to have the same staying power and long-lasting issues in the community as they did in hospitals, showing equally persistent problems with infections. Yet, the hospital and the community differed in that hospital outbreaks continued to be analysed as acute outbreaks of infection with reference to hospital governance issues, while the infectious process in the community was increasingly understood as a chronic health problem without clear implications to healthcare organisation.[73] These nursery epidemics emphasised the importance of the hospital as a transmission vector for infection. One line of enquiry to develop this research would be to look at the role of the birthing family before entering the hospital. However, I will have to leave this to a more in-depth analysis of the changing role of hospital births after the Second World War, another theme worthy of a well-designed research project.

Crisis and infection during the 1957 influenza pandemic

Charles Rosenberg and other historians of medicine have pointed to infectious diseases as external shocks, which can be studied as tests for societies.[74] Similarly, one can argue that studying hospital infection at times of crisis might be useful to understand more broadly the history of infection. One such example of an external shock is the 1956–1957 influenza pandemic, also known as the 'Asian Flu Pandemic'. The virus type H2N2, known since the 'Russian Influenza Pandemic' of the late 1890s, appears to be a less virulent strain of the influenza virus.[75] And Asian Flu has certainly not received the historiographical or the media attention given to the 'Spanish Influenza' outbreak of 1918–1920.[76] One reason for this is that the Spanish Flu was one of the biggest mortality crises the world has seen, with more deaths likely caused by disease than occurring in the First World War. But, the key to understanding the role of an influenza pandemic for this discussion of hospital infections is, of course, not the viral infection itself, but its link to a secondary infection often affecting the respiratory tract, caused by *S. aureus*. Treatable by antibiotics, the secondary infection related to a flu pandemic had lost much of its potency after 1950, and contemporary observers immediately associated the relatively low mortality rate with the availability of antibiotic treatment.[77] But, a good proportion of all deaths in the United Kingdom as a result of Asian Flu were still caused by secondary infections, of which a substantial proportion must have been caused by *S. aureus*.[78] The Public Health Laboratory Service remained convinced that *S. aureus* was responsible for the vast majority of fatal cases of secondary infection during the Asian Flu Pandemic.[79] Clinical epidemiology revealed, in addition, that non-*Staph* related deaths occurred predominantly in older age groups, while Staphylococcal infections resulted in deaths in all age groups studied. There was a particular emphasis in children and young adults, who were unusual victims of the seasonal influenza.[80] In addition, the disease caused by *S. aureus* turned out to be more severe, leading to more deaths compared to non-*Staph* infections.[81]

The discovery of the penicillinase-producing *S. aureus* during the 1957 flu pandemic substantially undermined the confidence in antibiotics.[82] For influenza patients, having to go to the hospital implied an increased risk of acquiring a secondary infection which turned out to be hard to treat. The prevalence of *Staph* 80/81 in hospitals was, at the height of the *Staph* 80/81 crisis, so paramount that it seemed a very convincing explanation to suggest that the hospital was, yet again, the transmission vector for this deadly complication of influenza.[83] Numerous studies of influenza patients showed that on admission to hospital no *Staph* was present in the patient, but that the likelihood of an infection increased proportionally to their length of stay.[84] Hospital patients in Dundee showed Streptococci and *Haemophilus influenzae* in their sputum on admission, yet after a few days in hospital, Staphylococci in a resistant form were present in their samples.[85] However, soon enough the attention began to turn to the question as to whether or not patients with influenza were already carriers of Staphylococci. Within a relatively short time span, it was realised that *Staph* 80/81 was as much a community-acquired as it was a hospital-acquired infection. One microbiologist went so far as to suggest, 'The majority of *staphylococcal* infections are brought in rather than acquired in hospital, by patients admitted with influenza.'[86] Further studies, albeit based on small samples of patients associated with influenza, confirmed the causal role of community infection. This matched well with Hassle and Rountree's recognition that, in relation to septicaemia in Sydney, community-acquired *Staph* infection was more relevant to the epidemiology of *Staph* 80/81 than hospital-acquired infections: 'The chief factor responsible for the increase in Staphylococcal septicaemia in patients infected outside the hospital was the appearance of this new strain and its spread in the general community.'[87]

Conclusion

Medical microbiologists, clinical chemists and related professionals became routinely available in medical practice in hospitals around the time of the Second World War.[88] One way of explaining their growing significance lies in their specialist knowledge about bacteria in hospitals. Through the technique of phage typing of bacterial strains, microbiologists were able to prove they had the methods and the understanding to participate in the debate about infection control in hospitals in a meaningful way.[89] These microbiologists drove investigations into problems related to clinical practice; in particular, they studied the spread of bacteria, and the related concern of nosocomial infections connected to post-operative complications as well as infections related to clinical practice. Much of this research was built around antibiotic resistance, the mechanisms of which were only partly understood at the time.[90] In the clinical implementation of sulphonamides during the late 1930s, it had already become apparent that antibacterial medication could sometimes contribute to the emergence of resistant bacteria. But during later decades, this research reached a new level. Within the context of increased political attention on hospitals as the core of the NHS, microbiologists in Britain, as much as elsewhere, conceptualised their investigations within the confines of the hospital, an old battleground of hospital hygiene and reform.[91] Their work did not always align well with the interests of clinicians, as recent contributions, most notably by Scott Podolsky, have shown.[92] Here we see how the theme of this manuscript is closely related to wider issues dealt with in other contributions in this volume and the wider historiographic interest in hospital infections. 'Use the new drug while it lasts' – the crux of a 1952 *Lancet* editorial on the problem – has been cited by authors to suggest how interrelated problems of hospital care, the implementation of antibiotic therapy and the emergence of resistance were.

Everything changed with *Staph* 80/81. Through phage typing, it became possible to overcome the limitations of a local story; hospital infection became a global history. More importantly, *Staph* 80/81 turned out to be resistant against all forms of penicillin, triggering a huge crisis in infection control. At the time, nursing staff numbers in British hospitals had been cut, more surgeons appointed and more patients admitted. But, while the hospital infrastructure such as beds, floors and linen were initially blamed for transmission, it became apparent that nurses played a crucial role in hospital infection as they tended to patients and moved in and out of their wards. Trials of preventive application of antibiotic nasal creams were unpopular amongst staff, and even screening was met with fairly sharp resistance. Yet, nurses (and later also hospital visitors) played a role in breaking down the symbolic walls of the hospital. So, too, did babies, because they did not stay in hospitals but carried acquired bacteria out into the community. As long as babies were ill, isolation in hospital still provided a solution. However, umbilical cord and nasal carriage of *Staph* 80/81 began to be seen as a major link between the hospital and the community which shifted the ground for good. In other words, the story of infection in neonates is a story of the hospital boundary breaking down. Strains associated with the hospital environment began to proliferate within the community, decades before community-acquired methicillin-resistant *S. aureus* (MRSA) reopened the controversy.

But specific crisis points of hospitals, such as the 1957 influenza pandemic, probably contributed to an increasing audience for infection control and its specialists.[93] This argument was borne out during the Asian Influenza Pandemic of 1956–1957, which turned out to be a rather mild pandemic outbreak, with only around 20,000–30,000 people dying of Asian Flu in Britain. Staphylococcal infections in babies had already been studied in conjunction with the common cold. It appeared that a compromised immune system due to a viral infection increased the chances of a subsequent Staphylococcal infection. This idea was soon substantiated by follow-up research after the flu pandemic. A proportion of secondary infections were seen to be caused by *Staph* 80/81 and were therefore impossible to treat with antibiotics. It is difficult to ascertain with any degree of certainty the extent of this problem, but it is clear that research into the link between influenza and *Staph* 80/81 emphasised the hospital-community link in Staphylococcal infections. At first, microbiologists were left to ponder a new 'two-way traffic' system of infection: cases of *Staph* 80/81 were brought into and taken out of hospital at the same time. But later, they went further and acknowledged that the community was a major source of infection that affected the hospital. It appears that with the Asian Flu Pandemic, the conceptual framework for nosocomial infections had begun to change, as the role of the community had to be taken into account in order to understand the problem.

The evidence presented here gives historical depth to recent concerns about the role of the community in the spread of resistant microbacteria, and the ways the idea of hospital infection has blurred rather than helped our understanding of resistance travelling between hospitals and communities.[94] This argument, moreover, fits well within wider medical history, which locates the hospital at the intersection of medical, social and economic interests. If my reasoning has any merit, it points towards a more dynamic under-standing of the hospital-community relationship. A historical approach can successfully intertwine political, institutional and pro-fessional histories as it traces ideas about infection and institutions such as hospitals dealing with the problems and can draw together seemingly unrelated fields of inquiry to shed light on the complex problem of Staphylococcal infection. The historiography of infec-tion in the nineteenth century emphasised this complex framework for acute infections, such as those treated in fever hospitals, and the recent wave of studies in the history of antibiotics after 1945 arrives at similar conclusions.

Notes

I am hugely grateful to the editors of this volume and an anonymous referee for providing invaluable feedback. Any shortfalls of the text remain entirely my responsibility.

1 F. Condrau and R. G. W. Kirk, 'Negotiating hospital infections: The debate between ecological balance and eradication strategies in British hospitals, 1947–1969', *Dynamis*, 31 (2011), 385–405.

2 See, for example, Alistair Leanord's chapter, 'Infection control and antimicrobial resistance: the past, the present and the future', in this volume.

3 M. Foucault, *The birth of the clinic: An archaeology of medical percep-tion* (London: Tavistock, 1973, fr. 1963).

4 E. Ackerknecht, *Medicine at the Paris Hospital: 1794–1848* (Baltimore: Johns Hopkins Press, 1967).

5 N. Jewson, 'The disappearance of the sick man from medical cosmol-ogy, 1770–1870', *Sociology*, 10 (1976), S. 225–244; M. E. Fissel, 'The disappearance of the patient's narrative and the invention of hospital in medicine', in R. French and A. Wear (eds), *British medicine in an age of reform* (London: Routledge, 1991), 92–109.

6 B. Abel-Smith, *The hospitals 1800–1948: A study in social administra-tion in England and Wales* (London: Heinemann, 1964).

7 G. B. Risse, *Mending bodies, saving souls: A history of hospitals* (New York, Oxford: Oxford University Press, 1999) See also, for example, L. Granshaw and R. Porter (eds), *The hospital in history* (London: Routledge, 1989); S. Cherry, *Medical services and the hospitals in Britain 1860–1939* (Cambridge: Cambridge University Press, 1996); M. Gorsky, J. Mohan and M. Powell, 'British voluntary hospitals

1871–1938: the geography of provision and utilization', *Journal of Historical Geography*, 25 (1999), 463–82; K. Waddington, *Charity and the London hospitals 1850–1898* (Woodbridge: Boydell and Brewer, 2000); M. Gorsky, J. Mohan and M. Powell, 'The financial health of voluntary hospitals in interwar Britain', *Economic History Review*, 55 (2002), 533–557; L. Abreu and S. Sheard (eds), *Hospital life: Theory and practice from the medieval to the modern* (Oxford: Peter Lang, 2013); B. Doyle, *The politics of hospital provision in early twentieth-century Britain* (London: Pickering and Chatto, 2014).

8 A. Wilson, 'On the history of disease-concepts: The case of pleurisy', *History of Science*, 38 (2000), 271–319.

9 Just one example: C. McMillan, *Discovering tuberculosis: A global history 1900 to the present* (New Haven: Yale University Press, 2015).

10 C. Timmermann, *A history of lung cancer: The recalcitrant disease* (Basingstoke: Palgrave Macmillan, 2013); B. H. Lerner, *The breast cancer wars: Hope, fear, and the pursuit of a cure in twentieth-century America* (Oxford: Oxford University Press, 2003).

11 OUP's series launched in 2009: A. Scull, *Hysteria: The biography* (Oxford: Oxford University Press, 2009); JHU's series launched in 2007: R. M. Packard, *The making of a tropical disease: A short history of malaria* (Baltimore: Johns Hopkins University Press, 2007).

12 Two interesting cases are P. Baldwin, *Contagion and the state in Europe 1830–1930* (Cambridge: Cambridge University Press, 1999) and S. K. Cohn Jr., *Epidemics: Hate and compassion from the plague of Athens to AIDS* (Oxford: Oxford University Press, 2018).

13 C. Hamlin, *More than hot: A short history of fever* (Baltimore: Johns Hopkins University Press, 2015).

14 L. Engelmann and J. Kehr, 'Double trouble? Towards an epistemology of co-infection', *Medicine, Anthropology, Theory*, 2 (2015), 1–31.

15 I. Illich, *Medical nemesis: The expropriation of health* (London: M. Boyars, 1975).

16 L. G. Miller and S. L. Kaplan, '*Staphylococcus aureus*: A community pathogen', *Infectious Disease Clinics of North America*, 23 (2009), 35–52.

17 K. Hillier, 'Babies and bacteria: Phage typing, bacteriologists, and the birth of infection control', *Bulletin of the History of Medicine*, 80 (2006), 733–761.

18 J. V. Pickstone, *Ways of knowing: A new history of science, technology and medicine* (Manchester: Manchester University Press, 2000).

19 C. Gradmann, 'From lighthouse to hothouse: Hospital hygiene, antibiotics and the evolution of infectious disease, 1950–1990', *History and Philosophy of the Life Sciences*, 40:8 (2018), 1–25.

20 C. Gradmann, 'Re-inventing infectious disease: Antibiotic resistance and drug development at the Bayer Company 1945–1980', *Medical History*, 60 (2016), 155–80; C. Gradmann, 'Sensitive matters: The World Health Organisation and antibiotics resistance testing, 1945–1975', *Social History of Medicine*, 26 (2013), 555–574.
21 S. H. Podolsky, *The antibiotic era: Reform, resistance, and the pursuit of a rational therapeutics* (Baltimore: Johns Hopkins University Press, 2015).
22 Condrau and Kirk, 'Negotiating hospital infections', 385–405; F. Condrau, 'Standardising infection control: Antibiotics and hospital governance in Britain 1948–1960', in C. Bonah, A. Rasmussen and C. Masutti (eds), *Harmonizing 20th-century drugs: Standards in pharmaceutical history* (Paris: Glyphe, 2009), 327–339; F. Condrau, 'Krankenhausinfektionen und Antibiotikaresistenzen in englischen Krankenhäusern 1930–1960', *Therapeutische Umschau*, 72 (2015), 469–474.
23 P. Bartlett and D. Wright, *Outside the walls of the asylum: The history of care in the community 1730–2000* (London: Athlone, 1999).
24 F. Nightingale, 'Preface', *Notes on hospitals*, 3rd edition (London: Longman, Green, Longman, Roberts, and Green, 1863).
25 Condrau, 'Standardising infection control', 327–339.
26 M. Newsom Kerr, *Contagion, isolation, and biopolitics in Victorian London* (Basingstoke: Palgrave Macmillan, 2018).
27 Newsom Kerr, *Contagion, isolation, and biopolitics*. See also G. M. Ayers, *England's first state hospitals and the Metropolitan Asylums Board 1867–1930* (London: Wellcome Institute of the History of Medicine, 1971).
28 The discussion of the fever hospitals in this and the following four paragraphs is drawn from Newsom Kerr, *Contagion, isolation, and biopolitics*, Chapters 1, 5 and 7.
29 For another example from the nineteenth century, see H. Tebbutt, 'On the bacteriology of asylum dysentery', *Journal of Hygiene*, 12 (1912), 218–26; see also H. Pennington, 'Don't pick your nose', *London Review of Books*, 27 (2005), 29–31.
30 Historians have dealt with the emergence of germ theories on many levels; see M. Worboys, *Spreading germs: Disease theories and medical practice in Britain, 1865–1900* (Cambridge: Cambridge University Press, 2000).
31 While the cause was presumed to be a microbe, the exact role played by haemolytic *Streptococcus* remained unknown until the 1920s. see Newsom Kerr, *Contagion, isolation, and biopolitics*, Chapter 7.
32 K. A. Sepkowitz, 'Tuberculosis and the health care worker: A historical perspective', *Annales of Internal Medicine*, 120 (1994), 71–79.

33 A. Newsholme, 'The causes of the past decline of tuberculosis and the light thrown by history on preventive measures for the immediate future', in *Transactions of the International Congress on Tuberculosis in Washington 1908* (Philadelphia: W. F. Fell, 1908), 80–109.

34 L. G. Wilson, 'The historical decline of tuberculosis in Europe and America: Its causes and significance', *Journal of the History of Medicine*, 45 (1990), 366–396; L. G. Wilson, 'The rise and fall of tuberculosis in Minnesota: The role of infection', *Bulletin of the History of Medicine*, 66 (1992), 16–52.

35 L. Bryder, 'Correspondence', *Journal of the History of Medicine and Allied Sciences*, 46 (1991), 358–68; L. Bryder, '"Not always one and the same thing": The registration of tuberculosis deaths in Britain, 1900–1950', *Social History of Medicine*, 9 (1996), 253–266.

36 F. Condrau, 'The institutional career of tuberculosis patients in Britain and Germany', in J. Henderson, P. Horden and A. Pastore (eds), *The impact of hospitals in Europe, 300–2000* (Oxford: Peter Lang, 2007), 327–357.

37 A. A. Forder, 'A brief history of infection control – past and present', *South African Medical Journal*, 97 (2007), 1161–4; see also F. Condrau, *Lungenheilanstalt und Patientenschicksal. Sozialgeschichte der Tuberkulose in Deutschland und England während des späten 19. und frühen 20. Jahrhunderts* (Goettingen: Vandenhoeck & Ruprecht, 2000).

38 C. Webster, *The Health Services since the war, Volume 2: The National Health Service, 1958–1979* (London: Stationery Office, 1996), 16f.

39 S. Berger, *Bakterien in Krieg und Frieden. Eine Geschichte der medizinischen Bakteriologie in Deutschland, 1890–1933* (Göttingen: Wallstein, 2009).

40 J. Ferretti and W. Koehler, 'History of streptococcal research', in J. J. Ferretti, D. L. Stevens and V. A. Fischetti (eds), *Streptococcus pyogenes: Basic biology to clinical manifestations* (Oklahoma City: University of Oklahoma, 2016) (available online at www.ncbi.nlm.nih.gov/books/NBK333430/).

41 I. Loudon, 'Puerperal fever, the streptococcus, and the sulphonamides, 1911–1945', *British Medical Journal*, 295 (1987), 485–490.

42 L. Colebrook, 'Infection acquired in hospital', *Lancet*, 269 (1955), 885–891.

43 Risse, *Mending bodies – saving souls*.

44 J. A. Greene, F. Condrau and E. Watkins Siegel (eds), *Therapeutic revolutions: Pharmaceuticals and social change in the twentieth century* (Chicago: University of Chicago Press, 2016).

45 Condrau and Kirk, 'Negotiating hospital infections', 385–405.

46 J. C. Scott, 'Whose responsibility? Letters to the Editor', *Lancet*, 273 (1959), 578.

47 R. Dubos, *Mirage of health: Utopias, progress, and biological change* (London: Ruskin House, 1959).

48 Condrau and Kirk, 'Negotiating hospital infections', 385–405.

49 A. Davis, 'A revolution in maternity care? Women and the maternity services, Oxfordshire c. 1948–1974', *Social History of Medicine*, 24 (2011), 389–406; T. McIntosh, *A social history of maternity and childbirth: Key themes in maternity care* (London: Routledge, 2012).

50 Hillier, 'Babies and bacteria'; Louden, 'Puerperal fever'.

51 R. K. Shaffer, 'The challenge of antibiotic-resistant *Staphylococcus*: Lessons from hospital nurseries in the mid-20th century', *Yale Journal of Biology and Medicine*, 86 (2013), 261–270.

52 G. A. J. Ayliffe and M. P. English, *Hospital infection: From miasmas to MRSA* (Cambridge: Cambridge University Press, 2003), 154.

53 Hillier, 'Babies and bacteria'.

54 G. S. Wilson and D. Atkinson, 'Typing of staphylococci by the bacteriophage method', *Lancet*, 246 (1945), 647–649; 'Phage-typing', *Lancet*, 252 (1948), 263–264.

55 Hillier, 'Babies and bacteria', 737.

56 The following section benefits from the research of undergraduate students that I have supervised in Manchester; I am particularly grateful to Laura Calvert for her work on the transmission of *Staphyloccocus aureus* in the community.

57 'Editorial', *Lancet*, 246 (1945), 437.

58 See also Condrau, 'Krankenhausinfektionen'.

59 H. F. Eichenwald and H. R. Shinefield, 'The problem of staphylococcal infection in newborn infants', *Journal of Pediatrics*, 56 (1960), 665–674.

60 P. M. Rountree and B. M. Freeman, 'Infections caused by a particular phage type of *Staphylococcus aureus*', *Medical Journal of Australia*, 42 (1955), 157–161.

61 J. C. Gould and J. D. Cruikshank, 'Staphylococcal infection in general practice', *Lancet*, 273 (1957), 1157–1161.

62 L. Roodyn, 'Epidemiology of Staphylococcal infections', *Journal of Hygiene*, 58 (1960), 1.

63 V. Hurst and M. Grossmann, 'Antibiotic-resistant Staphylococci – familial infections caused by exposure of babies in hospital nurseries', *California Medicine*, 89 (1958), 107–110.

64 For example, 'Staphylococci in the family', *Lancet*, 275 (1960), 964–5; B. Donnison, W. A Gillespie, K. Simpson, R. C. Tozer, 'Spread of Staphylococci from hospital to community, *Lancet*, 275 (1960), 552.

65 'Staphylococcus Domesticus', *Lancet*, 282 (1963), 235.

66 V. Hurst, 'Staphyloccocus aureus in the infant upper respiratory tract, i: Observations on hospital born babies', *The Journal of Hygiene*, 55 (1957), 299–312, 299.

67 'Editorial: trouble in the nursery', *The Canadian Medical Association Journal*, 83 (1960), 1112–1113.

68 Eichenwald and Shinefield, 'The problem of Staphylococcal infection'.

69 Hurst and Grossman, 'Antibiotic-resistant Staphylococci', 107–110.

70 'Staphylococci in the family', 964–965.

71 Roodyn, 'Epidemiology'.

72 V. Hurst, M. Grossman, V. L. Sutter, J. Fennell, 'Five-year follow-up survey of an outbreak of Staphylococcal infection in a hospital nursery', *New England Journal of Medicine*, 270 (1964), 517–519.

73 A. J. Nahmias, M. H. Lepper, V. Hurst, S. Mudd, 'Epidemiology and treatment of chronic Staphylococcal infections in the household', *American Journal of Public Health*, 52 (1963), 1828–1843.

74 C. E. Rosenberg, 'Cholera in nineteenth-century Europe: A tool for social and economic analysis', *Comparative Studies in Society and History*, 8 (1966), 452–463.

75 M. Honigsbaum, *A history of the great influenza pandemics. death, panic and hysteria, 1830–1920* (London: I. B. Tauris, 2013).

76 See H. Phillips and D. Killingray, *The Spanish Influenza pandemic of 1918–1919* (London: Routledge, 2003).

77 N. C. Oswald, R. A. Shooter, M. P. Curwen, 'Pneumonia complicating influenza', *British Medical Journal*, 2 (1958), 1305–1311; E. J. L. Lowbury, 'Bacterial infection and hospital infection of patients with influenza', *Postgraduate Medical Journal*, 39 (1963), 582–586.

78 L. Robertson, J. P. Caley, J. Moore, 'Importance of *Staphylococcus aureus* in pneumonia in the 1957 epidemic of influenza A', *Lancet*, 2 (1958), 233–236; M. P. Jevons, 'Bacteria and influenza', *Lancet*, 270 (1957), 891; see also R. Bud, *Penicillin: Triumph and tragedy* (Oxford, New York: Oxford University Press, 2007), 119–120.

79 T.P.H.L. Service, 'Deaths from Asian influenza, 1957', *British Medical Journal*, 1 (1958), 915–919.

80 Lowbury, 'Bacterial infection', 582.

81 C. Giles and E. M. Shuttleworth, 'Post-mortem findings in 46 influenza deaths', *Lancet*, 270 (1957), 1224–1225.

82 D. B. Louria, H. L. Blumenfeld, J. T. Ellis *et al.*, 'Studies on influenza in the pandemic of 1957–58, II. Pulmonary complications in influenza', *Journal of Clinical Investigation*, 38 (1959), 213–265.

83 G. A. Gresham and M. H. Gleeson-White, 'Staphylococcal Bronchopneumonia in debilitated hospital patients', *Lancet*, 269 (1957), 651–653.

84 Robertson, *et al.*, 'Importance of *Staphylococcus aureus*', 233–236.
85 A Combined Study Group, 'Some aspects of the recent epidemic of influenza in Dundee', *British Medical Journal*, 1 (1958), 908.
86 Lowbury, 'Bacterial infection', 582.
87 J. E. Hassel and P. M. Rountree, 'Staphylococcal septicaemia', *Lancet*, 273 (1959), 213–217.
88 See other contributions in this volume.
89 Hillier, 'Babies and bacteria'.
90 Gradmann, 'Lighthouse to hothouse'.
91 Pennington, 'Don't pick'.
92 Podolsky, *The antibiotic era.*
93 R. Bud, 'From epidemic to scandal: the politicization of antibiotic resistance, 1957–1969', C. Timmermann and J. Anderson (eds), *Devices and designs: Medical technologies in historical perspective* (Basingstoke: Palgrave Macmillan, 2006), 195–211.
94 M. Z. David and R. S. Daum, 'Community-associated methicillin-resistant *Staphylococcus aureus*: Epidemiology and clinical consequences of an emerging epidemic', *Clinical Microbiology Reviews*, 23 (2010), S. 616–687.

2

Cleanliness costs: the evolving relationship between infection and length of stay in antibiotic-era hospitals

Sally Sheard

Hospital-acquired infection (HAI) – referred to as 'nosocomial' infection in US terminology – emerged as a specific policy concern in the mid-twentieth century, although it has a much longer recognition.[1] This chapter repositions the debate on the history of HAIs, which has to date been focused on scientific understanding of infection through the use of evolutionary paradigms, the development of new approaches such as clinical epidemiology and the enduring fascination with the discovery, use and abuse of antibiotics and associated rise of antimicrobial resistance (AMR).[2] Some of this historical research has marginalised or ignored (by choice or ignorance) the key issue that healthcare is a *commercial*, as well as a scientific-clinical, activity. These lacunae are particularly evident when historians discuss how responses to HAIs resulted in the formation of protocols and teams, which they invariably articulate as comprised of clinical/technical staff (surgeons, physicians, nurses, microbiologists and epidemiologists). There has been minimal recognition that hospital administrators and managers could (and did) play key roles in these developments because of the significant and increasing impact of HAIs on hospital costs, or of the role of economists at national policymaking levels.[3]

To present the history of hospital infection control, or wider AMR, as the result of scientific discovery, or episodic crisis, is naïve, but understandable, if one draws primarily on medical and/ or scientific primary literature.[4] This is literature often produced or co-produced by those whose reputations were built upon it – especially the microbiologists, clinicians and epidemiologists. It is found in elite medical journals such as the *British Medical Journal*,

Lancet, Journal of the American Medical Association and the *New England Journal of Medicine*, and in landmark monographs, such as Macfarlane Burnet's *Natural History of Infectious Diseases* and Wesley Spink's *Infectious Diseases: Prevention and Treatment in the Nineteenth and Twentieth Centuries*.[5] As hospital infection control emerged as a distinct discipline, it established its own culture and hierarchies – through new societies (national and international) and linked publications including the *Journal of Hospital Infection* and *Clinical Microbiology and Infection*. The emergence of managerial and economic literature on HAIs appears to have lagged behind its scientific and clinical counterparts. This was partly related to the relative priority of the issue for these disciplines, and also their publishing culture (less tied to producing peer-reviewed papers for an academic audience). I suggest that the history of this literature is critical. Publications (journal articles, textbooks, practical manuals) are integral to the explanation for the emergence and prioritisa-tion of economic components in HAI policies; they exemplify the problem of knowledge transfer between disciplines – in this case between non-clinical and clinical hospital employees. It also dem-onstrates that historians of science, medicine and health would ben-efit from actively seeking, and exploiting, a wider range of primary sources for their research on infections and infection control. It pro-vokes a reconsideration of our own (historian/social science) pub-lication choices (type of journal, monograph, policy briefing paper) to ensure efficient and effective knowledge transfer and mobilisa-tion, both within academia and, more importantly, into policymak-ing environments.

   This chapter demonstrates that increasing interest in the wider (and often hidden) costs of hospital care, beyond the immediate cost of treating the infected patient (usually the cost of the antibi-otics), played a key role in the introduction of hospital infection control policies. It shows that healthcare financing choices (fee-per-item; prospective v. retrospective payments) were critical in driving the shift in both state-funded and mixed-economy health-care systems from traditional 'blanket' infection surveillance and hygiene regimes to targeted interventions and management practices (individual and institutional) that drew on economic as well as clinical 'effectiveness' data. It establishes the parallel tra-jectories of intentional shortening of lengths of stay in hospitals (traditionally called convalescence) and the unintentional lengthening of stay due to HAIs. This was observed in all Western 'modern' hospitals, and the chapter uses examples from the United Kingdom and the United States to demonstrate the critical role of healthcare systems – their *modus operandi* and their governance culture – in determining the direction and pace of change in hospital infection control.

Hospital management for efficiency and effectiveness

Hospitals consolidated their dominance in the healthcare systems of high-income economies (and in public expectations) in the second half of the twentieth century. It was careful planning and media savviness that had Minister of Health Aneurin Bevan photographed alongside a bed-bound hospital patient on the first day of the British National Health Service (NHS) on 5 July 1948, rather than in a general practitioner's surgery. During the 1950s and 1960s, increasing numbers of patients were admitted to hospitals for tests, a greater proportion of births took place in hospital and there were more ambitious treatments, including renal dialysis and chemotherapy, that initially could only be delivered in a hospital environment. Yet, as the number of episodes of hospital care increased, the average length of hospital stay followed a different trajectory. After the basic science of physiological and psychological recovery had been established, patient management, especially for surgery, was increasingly viewed from an economic perspective. Medical, managerial and cultural expectations aligned so that recovery came to be seen as something to be achieved as quickly and efficiently as possible.

The history of hospital length of stay illuminates the fractured process of knowledge transfer both within and between national clinical cultures.[6] As early as 1886, the French surgeon Just Lucas-Championnière had expressed the belief that repair was more rapid and more complete when some early patient movement was permitted after surgery and that this also reduced the level of pain experienced.[7] By the end of the nineteenth century, early post-operative walking – early ambulation as it came to be known – was a common practice in European hospitals, with an extensive related scientific literature. However, a survey conducted in the 1920s suggested that most British, European and American doctors shared a 'traditional attitude of passive care' towards post-operative patients.[8]

In the interwar period, two main foci of research interest around convalescence/length of stay emerged: the role of nutrition and return to ambulation after surgery. This was reinforced by the quantity and severity of injuries sustained by troops during the Second World War, which triggered fresh investigations in how to repair human bodies as quickly and fully as possible. Hospitals were forced to critically examine their post-surgical regimes due to reduced bed capacity and staffing levels. British doctors and scientists were also beginning to challenge conventional post-surgical theory, but within a relatively conservative medical culture. In an editorial in 1945 entitled 'Keep moving please', the *Lancet* had urged a more permanent adoption of early movement, even if this was initially through exercises within bed.[9] A *British Medical Journal* editorial in 1948 generally supported early ambulation, but not early discharge: 'A surgeon would be in a difficult position if he allowed a patient to be discharged on the fourth day after appendectomy or the seventh day after cholecystectomy (as reported in some American Journals) and that patient subsequently developed a fatal embolism in the second week.'[10]

It is clear from the previous discussion that clinicians had been aware of length of stay as a management issue for some time, but almost invariably for the impact that it had on the patient, not the hospital. Robert Pinker used data collected by Henry Burdett for the British Hospitals Yearbooks to demonstrate that average lengths of stay shortened in both voluntary and public hospitals over the period 1921–1938, and speculates that for patients with infectious diseases this could have been due to the use of sulphonamides as well as improvements in clinical knowledge and practice.[11] The creation of the NHS in 1948, with its centrally funded system and hierarchical administration, facilitated the production of information to measure hospital activities. The initial massive overspend (£305 million) relative to Beveridge's estimate (£170 million), triggered a sustained interest in understanding how costs were apportioned, and could possibly be controlled.[12] The Hospital In-Patient Enquiry (HIPE) collected a sample of data which could now be used to investigate the efficiency and effectiveness of the service. But there was amazingly little information on what individual hospital procedures actually cost until a basic costing scheme was introduced in 1950. Even then, the data was not easy to interpret, and few analyses were returned from the Ministry of Health to the regional boards and their hospitals.

The 1956 Guillebaud enquiry into the cost of the NHS used a novel social accounting methodology, pioneered by the economist Brian Abel-Smith, working with the social administration guru Richard Titmuss. It opened up broader discussions on what constituted acceptable variability around NHS norms.[13] Yet even before the first significant economic analyses of the NHS, especially Martin Feldstein's 1963 study, 'Economic analysis – operational research and the National Health Service', the NHS at the regional level was responding to pressures on the service, through innovative schemes that brought together clinicians and administrators.[14] Controlled trials were being conducted in hospitals, with mixed motivations: to identify the most effective recovery process for the patient, but also the most efficient use of healthcare resources.

Parallel to concerns about variations in lengths of stay for specific procedures, such as hernia repair, appendectomy and hysterectomy, were also concerns about variability between clinicians and across NHS regions. Some of this was linked to factors such as bed supply, as the US economist Milton Roemer notably demonstrated with his theory that 'a built bed is a filled bed' (i.e. the more beds, the more use of them in insurance-funded healthcare systems).[15] There was also recognition that convalescence in hospital might reflect the relative availability of domestic care and patients' socioeconomic status. Yet there was an absurdly late recognition in the medical literature that reducing length of patient stays will actually increase the hospital's costs: as the patient through-put rate rises there will be more investigative procedures, meals, linen changes and so on. A study directed in Manchester in 1962 by the hospital administration expert Teddy Chester, and published by his researcher Beatrice Hunter, attempted to calculate the cost of each patient treated in a hospital (medical, nursing costs, food, laundry, share of the overheads, etc.).[16] Similar studies were being conducted in the US by Anne Scitovsky at the Stanford Research Center in California. Specific studies on the inpatient costs of heart disease were undertaken by the University of Louvain Medical School in France, Yale University and the World Health Organization. The common aim of these projects was to determine whether optimal use was being made of hospital resources. Efficiency was becoming quantifiable and separated from effectiveness.

As the NHS experienced significant financial crises and budget cuts in the 1970s, economists became more influential within its parent government organisation – the Department of Health and Social Security (DHSS) – especially those working from the newly established Economic Advisors Office.[17] In 1977, analysis of data from the HIPE calculated the average hospital stay at between seven and thirteen days. The average length of stay for general surgery in Britain was already on a downwards trajectory. It fell from 8.9 days in 1974 to 7.1 days in 1984; for appendectomies it fell from 14.9 to 11.9 days, and for inguinal hernias from 7.3 to 4.9 days.[18] The impact of new surgical techniques such as keyhole surgery in the 1980s facilitated shorter lengths of stay and more day surgery. Its widespread adoption also forced changes in hospital practices: patients now required tuition in changing dressings and domestic wound care.

In the US, where a significant percentage of the population have traditionally relied on private health insurance, there was an earlier and more proactive engagement with health economics. This reflected the marketised nature of the healthcare business, in which pricing mechanisms could be used overtly to control demand and supply. The creation of Medicare in 1966 introduced a limited public provision, but always within the broader philosophy of a mixed economy of healthcare. Even non-profit hospitals had to respond to wider fluctuations in demand.[19] Length of US hospital stays appear to have fallen faster than in the UK for most specialities. For example, the average hospital stay for hernias in 1985 was three days.[20]

Hospital-acquired infection and delayed recovery

The knowledge that HAIs delay patient recovery and have a cost is longstanding. Even Florence Nightingale recognised the causative relationship between HAIs and length of hospitalisation in the mid-nineteenth century.[21] Yet, this relationship, and more importantly, the potential to use it to improve hospital efficiency, emerged surprisingly late as a topic of interest and research in twentieth-century clinical literature.

HAIs in the mid-twentieth century were partly a reflection of the success of medicine. More patients were being processed through an often static number of hospital beds and subjected to more intrusive diagnostic and surgical interventions which increased the risk of infections – from staff (hidden carriers of *Staph* organisms); from equipment (especially urinary and cardiac catheters); from other patients (interactions in wards and use of shared facilities).[22] From the mid-1940s, antibiotics offered another way to treat infections (original and HAI), alongside sulphonamides and isolation practices. Hospitals adopted protocols in which patients were routinely given pre-operative antibiotics as deliberate efficiency strategies that reduced the need for some laboratory screening tests and helped to minimise length of stay post-operatively.[23] Rising levels of HAIs were also integral to the emergence of AMR, which Alexander Fleming and colleagues had predicted at the dawn of the antibiotic era in 1939.[24] In the 1950s, hospital clinicians and scientists such as Mary Barber and her team at the Hammersmith Hospital in London pioneered antibiotic combinations to halt the spread of multiple resistant Staphylococcal infections on their surgical wards.[25]

British acute hospitals responded to rising rates of HAIs with a variety of initiatives, including new surveillance regimes that moved beyond the traditional records of wound infections maintained by ward staff and surgeons.[26] The Staphylococcal outbreaks of the 1940s and the 1950s stimulated routine recording of infections to detect outbreaks. In 1959, the Torbay Hospital and the Royal Devon and Exeter hospital introduced proactive surveillance by creating a new role of infection control sister (ICS) or infection control nurse (ICN), who visited wards to detect infections and worked with laboratory staff to use phage typing of samples from wounds and noses to identify carriers.[27]

In 1957, Suzanne Clarke at the Virus Research Laboratory at Lodge Moor Hospital in Sheffield, England, published a paper on sepsis in wounds, with particular reference to *Staphylococcus aureus*, which explicitly analysed the relationship between infection and length of stay. She noted, 'The average length of stay in hospital of patients whose wounds were infected with *S. aureus* was found to be five days longer ... however, many patients stayed in hospital for more than the usual length of time for reasons not connected with Staphylococcal infection. These patients then, owing to their long stay in hospital, acquired *S. aureus* in their wounds.'[28] Clarke calculated that each patient with a Staphylococcal wound sepsis 'wasted' an average 8.1 bed-days.

An indication of the increasing concern about hospital infection control was the publication of the first British textbook in 1960, by Robert Williams, (Arthur) Robert Blowers, Lawrence Garrod and Reginald Shooter: *Hospital Infection: Causes and Prevention.*[29] A scrutiny of the index shows no interest in the costs of HAIs. The preface to the second edition published in 1966 noted the identification of new penicillinase-resistant penicillins, and increases in non-Staphylococcal infections. It contained a new chapter on hospital architecture and design that recognised that trying to exclude infections from the operating room would 'probably be more costly than can be justified by any possible effect in preventing wound sepsis'.[30]

On the other side of the Atlantic, in the US, there was a parallel emerging awareness of the wider ramifications of uncontrolled hospital infection. Although in 1965 only 16 per cent of hospitals had some kind of surveillance programme for nosocomial (the preferred US term) infections, there was increasing interest, including in the relationship between infection and length of stay.[31] Larger acute hospitals began to employ infection control staff, and some undertook long-term epidemiological studies, such as those by Maxwell Finland at the Boston City Hospital in the 1950s.[32] The Communicable Disease Center (later the Centers for Disease Control (CDC)) established infection prevalence pilot studies in the 1950s in six community hospitals. The Foothills Hospital Wound Study was initiated in 1967 – an ambitious ten-year prospective study that analysed 62,939 surgical wounds. It found that infection extended a patient's hospital stay by an average of 10.1 days. This was later costed at $4,000 per patient for hospitalisation, not including loss of earnings and so on.[33]

In 1968, the American Hospital Association (AHA) published the first edition of its handbook *Infection Control in the Hospital*. Costs barely featured – just one brief mention in the introduction: 'The financial cost to the patient and to the hospital as a result of nosocomial infection is considerable. If a conservative 2 per cent of 30 million persons admitted to American hospitals each year develop nosocomial infections, which extend their average stay by one day, at a per diem rate of $50, this represents an annual cost of £30 million.'[34] The US CDC, based in Atlanta, Georgia, had already published a first set of nosocomial definitions, which was used in the Comprehensive Hospital Infections Project (CHIP) from 1969 to 1972 and in the National Nosocomial Infections Study (NNIS) from 1970 to 1974. The first international conference on nosocomial infections was held at the CDC in 1970, with around 200 delegates. The proceedings were published as a monograph which was distributed widely to US and Canadian medical schools and other healthcare organisations.[35] Two years later, the Association for Practitioners in Infection Control (APIC) was founded in 1972, with a linked journal.[36] From the early 1970s, more US hospitals started to introduce infection control programs, but with little apparent concern for their costs, as most charges were passed on to patients or their insurers.

In 1975, reacting to increasing pressure from the AHA and the Joint Commission on Accreditation of Hospitals, the CDC began the Study on the Efficacy of Nosocomial Infection Control (SENIC), with Robert Haley of its Bacterial Diseases Division in the Bureau of Epidemiology as the project director. It studied 338 US hospitals selected at random. Cost-benefit analysis (CBA) was built into the SENIC project from the planning phase onwards. Haley and his team assumed an average nosocomial infection rate of 5 per cent in the annual 37 million patient admissions to all US hospitals (acute, long-stay, community), which would result in around 2 million infections annually. Working on an average 1975 cost per infection of $600, this equated to $1 billion per annum.[37] Haley found that nosocomial infections increased the average length of stay, and that the employment of an ICN/physician could achieve an average 32 per cent reduction in infection rates.[38] The SENIC project's CBA calculated the costs for those hospitals that had an organised hospital-wide infection control programme: an ICN cost $12,000 per annum; with other costs for infection control physician cover, clerical assistance and so on, the total costs for intensive surveillance of 250 beds would be approximately $20,000 per annum. If this was scaled up to cover all 898,000 US hospital beds in 1975, the cost would be around $72 million. Thus, only 6 per cent of infections would have to be prevented to offset the costs of having a hospital infection control programme. Haley and his team published the SENIC results widely, but it had little immediate impact on hospital practices.[39] Alongside the SENIC project, other studies were conducted on the relationship between specific nosocomial infections and length of stay. For example, Givens and Ward found that urinary tract infections (many linked to use of catheters post-surgery) extended stays by an average 2.4 days, which in 1980 cost $558 per patient.[40] Epidemiologists not only had to battle with getting accurate costings; developing appropriate methodologies to handle multiple linked risk factors was a huge challenge. Working in Boston in the 1970s, Jonathan Freeman and John McGowan showed that surgical patients experienced the highest risk of acquiring HAIs, and proposed for 'cost-effectiveness' that infection control activities should be matched to surgical risk and predicted length of stay. However, one of their biggest challenges was in getting clinicians to routinely and accurately record HAIs in the first place. They suspected that reluctance to do this was linked to fear of 'legal consequences'.[41]

The US publication of two key hospital infection handbooks marked a sea change in interest. John Bennett and Philip Brachman edited *Hospital Infections*, the first edition of which appeared in 1979.[42] Mary Castle and Elizabeth Ajemian published the first edition of their *Hospital Infection Control: Principles and Practice* in 1980.[43] Bennett and Brachman noted the relationship between nosocomial infections and extended length of stay, and how the increased charges were usually redistributed among different cost centres rather than fully charged direct to the patient or their insurance company.[44]

The second international conference on nosocomial infections was held at the CDC in Atlanta, Georgia, in 1980, this time with around 1,400 delegates. The emerging professional support infrastructure of the APIC coincided with the expansion of the scientific database on infection control that the second international conference had initiated and was facilitated by the increasing use of computers. A slew of publications followed, exploiting the ability to analyse specific types of infections. A study by Haley (with Pinner and Blumenstein) published in 1980 showed that nosocomial urinary tract infections occurred most frequently but incurred only 15 per cent of the overall costs of the nosocomial infections. However, surgical patients who developed a post-operative wound infection accounted for 48 per cent of the overall costs for nosocomial infections but accounted for only one-third of the total infections. The most expensive site per infection was the lower respiratory tract, with 13 per cent of the total infections accounting for 29 per cent of the total costs.[45] There were wide variations: combined data from the SENIC and NNIS studies purported to show 19,000 deaths annually in the US directly attributable to nosocomial infections, and as a contributing factor in a further 58,000 deaths.[46] But a study by Platt *et al.*, published in the *New England Journal of Medicine* in 1982, estimated 300,000 deaths in the US per annum from nosocomial urinary tract infections alone.[47]

Other studies, such as that by Craven *et al.* in 1982, demonstrated that it was a good investment to fund educational conferences and journal publications to inform infection control practitioners of new research on cost-effective changes in infection control practices. Their research showed that there was no increased incidence of infection if respiratory or intravenous therapy tubing was changed either at twenty-four- or forty-hour intervals.[48] But sometimes the most basic hygiene policies remained the most effective. Isolation was confirmed as an appropriate strategy in intensive care environments.[49] Studies by Steer and Mallison, and by Condie, demonstrated that proper handwashing was the single most important infection control practice and could reduce nosocomial infections by 50 per cent.[50] The rising concerns about indiscriminate use of antibiotics were also finding their way into HAI cost-benefit studies, with increasing transatlantic recognition of related literature. Katherine Chavigny and Janet Fischer's 1984 paper in the *Journal of Hospital Infection* on HAI risk factors highlighted Price and Sleigh's study in Glasgow in 1970 in which the elimination of all antibiotics from a neuro-surgical ward almost halved the rate of HAIs.[51]

The impact of healthcare financing policies on HAIs

A key driver in changing US policy on treatment and prevention of nosocomial infections came in October 1983, when patients covered by Medicare had their costs reimbursed to hospitals under a new prospective payment system. This used 383 diagnosis related groups (DRGs) to calculate a fixed reimbursement rate for each hospital-based procedure or 'product', for example, appendectomy or hysterectomy.[52] Any additional hospital stay because of nosocomial infection was no longer automatically reimbursed. A study in Massachusetts found that the introduction of DRGs reduced hospital stays by an average 20 per cent.[53] Patients in adjacent beds in an American hospital having the same surgical procedure could find that they had different lengths of stay purely because they had different health (insurance) plans, with those covered by Medicare being discharged earlier than those with private or employer-paid health insurance.[54]

The impact of this change was clear when the second edition of Castle and Ajemian's *Hospital Infection Control: Principles and Practice* was published in 1987.[55] They noted that the pressure of the DRG system had initially led to fears that hospital administrators might perversely scale back infection control work to reduce overheads. In response, some infection control groups seized the initiative and conducted their own CBAs to justify their work. One group noted that they 'calculated that 26 nosocomial infections cost their institution more than $43,000, of which only $1,696 was reimbursable under the DRG system of payment. This was so effective in this institution the [infection control] program was expanded rather than reduced. The hospital expects to more than recover the cost of the expanded program.'[56] Costs of nosocomial infections were increasingly difficult to 'hide' in hospital budgets. However, Castle and Ajemian also noted in their textbook that handwashing, long established as the most effective infection control measure, remained 'the least practiced infection control measure in most hospitals'.[57]

Five years earlier, in 1975, the first edition of a British hospital infection handbook had also placed a new emphasis on costs as a reason to improve infection control. Graham Ayliffe, Edward Lowbury, Alasdair Geddes and J. D. Williams' *Control of Hospital Infection* included information on prices and suppliers for infection control products.[58] The Preface justified this with a historical quote from Wilson Jameson, Chief Medical Officer for England and Wales between 1940 and 1950, that hospital infection was 'a steady drain on the hospital purse and efficiency' and that costs as well as effectiveness needed to be considered.[59]

Increasingly, hospital infection control experts collaborated at the international level in an attempt to influence policy development. In 1977, an international workshop was held at Baiersbronn, Germany, at which Robert Haley presented some early SENIC results.[60] An international symposium was held at Trinity College Cambridge in 1979, with funding from ICI Pharmaceuticals. It brought together infection control practitioners and surgeons from hospitals in Gothenburg, Sweden; Oslo, Norway; and London, alongside staff from the Division of Hospital Infection at the Central Public Health Laboratory at Colindale, London.[61] A key proponent of targeted surveillance was Franz Daschner, an epidemiologist at the University Hospital, Freiburg, Germany, who was an active collaborator with US and UK colleagues in testing methods for determining economic costs.[62] He highlighted through a series of publications in the 1980s that German hospitals had no interest in infection control because insurance companies paid the same amount of money for each day spent in hospital, irrespective of the patient's type or severity of illness. In fact, the longer the hospitalisation, the higher the profit for the hospital. German hospitals also spent considerable amounts of money on routine floor and surface disinfection, which had no evidence base. Daschner's trials, which included reducing the frequency of changing surgical dressings, moving from wet razor-shaving to electrical shavers to prepare surgical sites, and suprapubic bladder drainage instead of traditional urinary catheterisation, had significant impacts on HAI costs. He used his participation at international meetings to urge infection control practitioners in other countries, especially the US, to move from continuous surveillance to surveillance by objectives for economic reasons. He also urged, 'It is of utmost importance to regularly inform doctors about the costs of antibiotics in general, treatment costs for specific infections, and the antibiotic consumption of the department or ward.'[63]

Economics was becoming a more prominent mode of analysis employed at national level in the UK, which facilitated studies that investigated the two-way relationship between HAIs and length of stay.[64] A study undertaken for the DHSS in 1987 calculated that HAIs caused an average additional stay of four days per patient, with a total cost to the NHS (England and Wales) of around £120 million.[65] This was the chronic, 'hidden' cost of HAIs: 'visible' outbreaks of methicillin-resistant *S. aureus* infection (MRSA) could cost around £250,000 per hospital.[66]

By the time Ayliffe *et al.* wrote the preface to the third edition of their handbook in 1992, economics was a much more prominent theme, with frequent references to costs and benefits. It noted a concern that

> high costs of hospital care have had an increasing influence on hospital practices and infection control staff have had to justify their policies and provide evidence of improved quality of care by audit of infection control practices. The increasing involvement of hospital managers and outside agencies in control of infection has led to a tendency for a return of rituals which previously had been eliminated from most hospitals. These are often associated with increased costs without benefit to patients or staff. Examples are microbiological sampling of the environment, increased use of disinfectants in the environment and of expensive single-use products.[67]

By the early 1990s, there was an infection *prevalence* rate of around 10 per cent for British hospital patients, mainly of the urinary tract, surgical wounds, lower respiratory tract and skin. The *incidence* rate for infections presenting after hospital admission was slightly lower – Glenister *et al.* in 1992 calculated it at 7.2 per cent for 3,326 patients admitted for general surgical, medical, gynaecology and orthopaedics specialties in a UK district general hospital. Ayliffe *et al.* commented in their 1992 handbook edition that now 'the importance of hospital infection can be considered both in terms of the patients' illness, and of the prolonged occupancy of hospital beds …. The cost of a prolonged stay is a convenient measure of the cost of infection, although it represents a reduction in the number of beds available from the waiting list rather than an actual increased cost to the hospital.'[68] In a section of the handbook entitled 'Balances of risks of infection and cost-effectiveness of preventive measures', they noted,

> decisions on measures required in a particular situation must be made in terms of possible benefits to patients, benefits to the hospital community, and the cost of measures. Cost benefit is obviously not a term to be used lightly when considering infection in patients or staff, but it is unfortunately a necessity …. A good selective surveillance system is likely to be more cost-effective than routine environmental

monitoring, or routine screening of faeces of catering staff or noses of theatre staff; routine monitoring of air or surfaces in operating theatres or pharmacies is an example of a test method which is not related to the risk of infection.[69]

By scrutinising the multiple editions of these key hospital infection control handbooks, published both in the UK and US, it is possible to track the emergence of cost/economics as a significant policy driver. It was also attracting new interest from academic health economists. In 1989, E. Currie and Alan Maynard at the York Centre for Health Economics published a study, 'Economics of Hospital Acquired Infections'.[70] A case control study published by Coello *et al.* in 1993 estimated that 93 per cent of the total additional cost incurred by surgical patients with an HAI could be attributed to an extended length of stay (the rest of the cost being antibiotics, biology tests and radiological investigations).[71] Many of these costs continued to remain 'hidden' in the UK NHS as they were not routinely specifically allocated to individual patients.

Jennifer Roberts, a health economist at the London School of Hygiene and Tropical Medicine (LSHTM), had a long-standing interest in the economics of infections. In 1993, she began working with colleagues at LSHTM and from Colindale Public Health Laboratories (CPHL) to set up a collaborative study to assess the socioeconomic burden of HAI, with funding from the UK Department of Health (DH). Her colleague Rosalind Plowman was subsequently appointed as Project Coordinator/Lead, and the findings were submitted to the DH in August 1997, followed by an extended period of review and discussion before the report was accepted for publication in September 1999. It estimated there were 5,000 deaths a year due to HAIs in the UK, and attempted to calculate the number of years of life lost by these patients. As an indication of the 'political urgency' around HAIs, the DH had issued guidelines in 1995.[72] Plowman had also co-authored *Hospital Acquired Infection*, a publication from the Office of Health Economics in 1997.[73] The DH-funded socioeconomic burden of HAI study resulted in spin-off publications, including a 1999 report by Plowman *et al.* which was published by the Public Health Laboratory Service and sent to all UK hospitals. This contained the most detailed breakdown of HAI costs to date, showing that hospital overheads, capital charges and management costs accounted for 33 per cent of the additional costs; nursing care accounted for 42 per cent and medical care for 6 per cent; operations and consumables 6 per cent; paramedics and specialist nurses 4 per cent; antimicrobials 2 per cent; other drugs 3 per cent; microbiology tests 1 per cent; other tests and investigations 3 per cent. It highlighted the impact on length of stay: acquiring an infection could mean an extra eleven days in hospital.[74] The British government was also becoming more concerned about the parallel issue of AMR, and in 2000 it introduced a new UK Antimicrobial Resistance Strategy and Action Plan.

In 2000, Jennifer Roberts established the Collaborative Centre for Economics of Infectious Disease at LSHTM, an ambition she had held for some time, and which facilitated a leading role for the UK in hosting international meetings and leading collaborative research. In 2001, the UK National Audit Office (NAO) commissioned a study: *The Management and Control of Hospital Acquired Infections in Acute NHS Trusts in England* from Roberts and Plowman, who worked with Karen Taylor, an NAO audit manager who had developed 'value for money' studies since the mid-1980s.[75] They brought complementary expertise, which was reflected in their linked publication *The Challenge of Hospital Acquired Infection*.[76] The NAO study republished the estimates produced by the earlier DH-funded study of 300,000 HAIs and their cost to the NHS of around £1 billion. The NAO report hypothesised that if infections could be reduced by 15 per cent it would release NHS resources valued at £150 million a year (although this did not take into consideration the costs of achieving the reduction, or variations linked to factors such as sites of infection, specialty, etc.). The NAO report generated considerable public attention, and called for more information to be collected and analysed on the extent, costs and impact of HAIs. It found that many NHS hospitals were not adequately prioritising resources to tackle HAIs, and made twenty-nine recommendations. Partly in response, the UK government established the Nosocomial Infection National Surveillance Scheme and linked it to new Clinical Governance and Controls Assurance initiatives that the DH introduced in the early 2000s.

In the US, there was a similar increasing willingness to translate HAIs into economic terms, and to use this to bring pressure to bear at national policy level. From October 2008 the Centers for

Medicare and Medicaid Services (CMS) no longer reimbursed hospitals for conditions not present on admission. Infections were now also required to be noted on hospital scorecards alongside financial data.[77] Journals on hospital infection control more frequently published papers that combined clinical, epidemiological and economic methodologies. Patricia Stone and colleagues conducted systematic reviews of the US literature in 2002 (covering the period 1990 to 2000) and in 2005 (covering January 2001 to June 2004). They found fifty-five eligible articles for the first ten-year period, but seventy for the second two-and-a-half-year period. They found that publications estimating the cost attributable to an infection were almost seven times more likely to be judged of higher quality than studies of the cost of interventions. They recommended the development of more sophisticated mathematical models, training of infection control professionals in economic methods and, significantly, training for journal editors and reviewers in economic methodologies.[78]

Finding the right language

Yet it was not until 2006 that the first publication entirely devoted to the economics of infection was published. *The Economics of Infectious Disease* was edited by Jennifer Roberts.[79] The book had two linked objectives: to introduce economic analysis and its application to those who were involved in infectious disease and its control, and to introduce economists to infectious disease and the challenges that it raised. Roberts's book resonated with fears that infectious disease was becoming more difficult and costly to control. There were threats of new and resurgent old pathogens, growing resistance of organisms to prophylactic therapies and antibiotics, and the spectre of bioterrorism. All of these had significant economic impacts, and the relationship was reciprocal: the state of the economy, especially investment (or lack of) in healthcare, water, sanitation, education and transport, could also enable infections to flourish.[80]

Roberts presented infection control activities through the language of economics. She suggested it was helpful to see the practice as having the features of a 'public good' – a good that is provided or consumed in common. But, alongside the potential benefits of tools such as CBA, quality-adjusted life years (QALYs), willingness to pay (WTP) and cost of illness (COI) measures, Roberts placed a warning: 'economic evaluations are not sufficient. Economists wanting to contribute to efficient policy formation must contribute to the governance debate and indicate the effects of different forms of governance of infectious disease.'[81]

Rosalind Plowman's chapter in Roberts's edited book used a literature review for the period 1975 to 2003 to draw attention to the wide range of estimates of HAI costs that could be generated according to the type of analytical tool employed (e.g. cost of illness; cost effectiveness; cost utility; CBA).[82] Other confounding factors included hospital-specific treatment patterns, the changing point at which patients were deemed fit for discharge and the difficulties of calculating the costs of HAIs when the patients reentered their communities (social care, informal care, district nursing services, loss of earnings, etc.). Plowman highlighted the significant disagreements that existed within the health economics community on the most appropriate methods for calculating HAI costs (concurrent; comparative; comparative with matching cases). Her chapter, and that of Nicholas Graves and Diana Weinhold – 'Complexity and the Attribution of Cost to Hospital Acquired Infection' – highlighted and epitomized, respectively, the opportunities and challenges of developing an accessible language in health economics to convey useful findings to policymakers.[83]

Conclusion

This chapter has set out two significant trends in hospital-based healthcare: (1) progressively shorter lengths of stay, especially for surgical procedures, and (2) increasing attention to HAIs (nosocomial infections in US terminology). It has demonstrated that the two issues are more linked than hitherto understood. By constructing an 'economic' history of hospital infection control, that is to say, by analysing when infection control practitioners turned their attention to the costs and benefits of practising infection control, we can see that the emerging relationship between HAIs and extended (and therefore more expensive) lengths of stay was an increasingly important factor in the adoption, albeit slow and uneven, of infection control practices and, vice versa, in fuelling attempts to reduce length of stay.

The early infection control studies in the US in the 1960s predate the use of DRGs in Medicare but appear to have been largely ineffective in achieving policy change, precisely because most hospitals operated as independent commercial enterprises, and there was a wide degree of discretion in how much (and how) they chose to reclaim HA1-associated costs from patients and insurers. Daschner's studies in the German healthcare system, in which all costs were reimbursed by insurance schemes, found a similar disinterest in reducing HAIs for economic reasons. In the UK, where there has been no 'market' to drive healthcare costs since the creation of the NHS in 1948, policymakers appear to have responded relatively late to the emergence of the association between HAIs and length of stay as a route into reducing hospital costs and improving efficiency. Despite increasing numbers of studies, perhaps the language of health economics, and internal debates and doubt about what they were measuring, meant that there was an ambiguity about the evidence base. This did not help the nascent hospital infection control experts demonstrate the authority necessary to convince policymakers, or individual clinicians, to take action.

Literature searches, for example in the journal *Hospital Infection Control and Prevention*, demonstrate that these concerns about the relationship between infection, length of stay and costs have often been cyclical. The creation of national and international organisations, such as academic societies and research centres, appears to be critical in establishing and maintaining an analytical focus. This study has also highlighted the importance of building ongoing relationships between clinicians, experts (usually academics) and policymakers. Roberts and Plowman at LSHTM are a prime example of the benefits of maintaining an ongoing collaboration, and acting as a bridge between different government organisations: in their case the UK DH, its arms-length body the Public Health Laboratory Service and the NAO. There are also 'costs' of a different sort involved in such collaboration: results can be taken by one body and repurposed, sometimes losing in translation the accuracy or intent of the original research.[84] Yet, even in the early 2000s, the narratives of studies were still often focused on the 'novelty' of HAI findings.[85] The recent costs of HAIs, in the US alone, are staggering: between $28.4 billion and $33.8 billion per annum.[86] A single surgical site infection (SSI) was estimated to cost as much as $60,000 per patient.[87] With the relentless rise of AMR, the need for proactive economic analyses is more pressing than ever, yet economists still appear to be some way off securing a routine place in the average hospital infection control team.[88]

Notes

1 S. Selwyn, 'Hospital infection: The first 2500 years', *Journal of Hospital Infection*, 18, supplement A (1991), 5–64. Nosocomial means 'hospital-acquired'. It is derived from 'nosocomium', the Greek/Latin term for hospital.

2 R. Bud, *Penicillin: Triumph and tragedy* (Oxford: Oxford University Press, 2007); S. Podolsky, 'Antibiotics and the social history of the controlled clinical trial', *Journal of the History of Medicine and Allied Sciences*, 65 (2010), 327–367; S. Podolsky, *The antibiotic era: Reform, resistance and the pursuit of rational therapeutics* (Baltimore: Johns Hopkins University Press, 2015); S. Podolsky, R. Bud, C. Gradmann *et al.*, 'History teaches us that confronting antibiotic resistance requires stronger global collective action', *Journal of Law, Medicine and Ethics*, 43:3_Supp (2015), 27–32.

3 Calculating the costs of infections and their impact on the economy is not a recent innovation. The technique of CBA was evident, if not named as such, in William Petty's seventeenth-century suggestion to move labourers away from plague-infected parts of London to Hampstead so they could continue working. Likewise, Edwin Chadwick's justification of sanitary improvements in the 1840s was based on calculations of the cost of ill-health and associated poverty. William Farr's work as the registrar general took the rationale a stage further and in 1885 put values on lives: from £5 at birth to £246 at age thirty, followed by a decline to £138 at fifty-five and £1 at seventy. See W. Petty, *Political arithmetick, or, A discourse concerning the extent and value of lands, people and buildings* (London: printed for R. Clavel and Hen. Mortlock, 1691); E. Chadwick, *General report on the sanitary condition of the labouring population* (London: HMSO, 1842). See also C. Hamlin, *Public health and social justice in the age of Chadwick* (Cambridge: Cambridge University Press, 1998); R. Fein, 'On measuring economic benefits of health programs', in Nuffield Provincial Hospitals Trust, *Medical*

history and medical care: A symposium of perspectives (Oxford: Oxford University Press, 1971), 181–217; J. Roberts (ed.), *The economics of infectious disease* (Oxford: Oxford University Press, 2006), Introduction.

4 F. Condrau and R. G. W. Kirk, 'Negotiating hospital infections: The debate between ecological balance and eradication strategies in British hospitals, 1947–1969', *Dynamis*, 31 (2011), 385–405; C. Gradmann, 'From lighthouse to hothouse: hospital hygiene, antibiotics and the evolution of infectious disease, 1950–1990', *History and Philosophy of the Life Sciences*, 40:8 (2018), 1–25.

5 F. M. Burnet, *The natural history of infectious disease* (Cambridge: Cambridge University Press, 1953); W. Spink, *Infectious diseases: Prevention and treatment in the nineteenth and twentieth centuries* (London: W. M. Dawson, 1978).

6 S. Sheard, 'Getting better faster: Convalescence and length of stay in British and US hospitals', in L. Abreu and S. Sheard (eds), *Hospital life: Theory and practice from the medieval to the modern* (Oxford: Peter Lang, 2013), 299–330.

7 J. Lucas-Championnière, *Bulletin et mémoires de la société de chir.*, 12 (1886), 560; *British Medical Journal*, 2 (1908), 981.

8 John Bryant, *Convalescence: Historical and practical* (New York: Sturgis Fund of the Burke Foundation, 1927), 1. I have not found literature to suggest that 'early ambulation' was attempted for non-surgical patients.

9 Anon, 'Keep moving please', *Lancet*, 1 (1945), 118.

10 Anon, 'Early rising after operation', *British Medical Journal*, 2 (1948), 1026–1027.

11 R. Pinker, *English Hospital Statistics 1861–1938* (London: Heinemann, 1966), 117.

12 T. Cutler, 'Dangerous yardstick? Early cost estimates and the politics of financial management of the National Health Service', *Medical History*, 47:2 (2003), 217–238; S. Sheard, 'A creature of its time: the critical history of the creation of the British NHS', *Michael Quarterly*, 8 (2011), 428–441.

13 R. M. Titmuss and B. Abel-Smith, *The cost of the national health service in England and Wales* (Cambridge: Cambridge University Press, 1956); S. Sheard, *The passionate economist: How Brian Abel-Smith shaped global health and social welfare* (Bristol: Policy Press, 2013), 84–89.

14 M. Feldstein, *Economic analysis, operational research and the National Health Service* (Oxford Economic Papers, 1963); M. Feldstein, *Economic analysis for health service efficiency: Econometric studies of the British NHS* (Amsterdam: North Holland Publishing Company, 1967).

15 M. Shain and M. Roemer, 'Hospital costs relate to the supply of beds', *Modern Hospital*, 92 (1959), 71–73.

16 B. Hunter, *The administration of hospital wards* (Manchester: Manchester University Press Studies in Social Administration, 1962).

17 E. Mackillop and S. Sheard, 'The politics of health policy knowledge transfer: The evolution of the role of British health economics academic units', *Evidence and Policy: A Journal of Research, Debate and Practice*, 15:4 (2018), 489–507.

18 Sheard, 'Getting better faster', 326.

19 D. Fox, 'Policy commercialising non-profits in health: the history of a paradox from the 19th century to the ACA', *Milbank Quarterly*, 93:1 (2015), 179–210.

20 Sheard, 'Getting better faster', 326.

21 F. Nightingale, *Notes on nursing* (London: Harrison, 1859).

22 L. Colebrook, 'Infection acquired in hospital', *Lancet*, 266 (1955), 885–891; E. J. L. Lowbury, 'Cross-infection of wounds with antibiotic-resistant organisms', *British Medical Journal*, 1:4920 (1955), 985–990.

23 R. I. Wise, E. A. Ossman and D. R. Littlefield, 'Personal reflections on nosocomial Staphylococcal infections and the development of hospital surveillance', *Reviews of Infectious Diseases*, 11 (1989), 1005–1019; Bud, *Penicillin: Triumph and tragedy*, 99–100.

24 I. H. Maclean, K. B. Rogers and A. Fleming, 'M. & B.693 and Pneumococci', *Lancet* 233: 6028 (1939), 562–568; W. M. M. Kirby, M. D. Douglas, M. D. Corpron and D. C. Tanner, 'Urinary tract infections caused by antibiotic-resistant coliform bacteria', *Journal of the American Medical Association*, 162 (1956), 1–4.

25 M. Barber, A. A. C. Dutton, M. A. Beard *et al.*, 'Reversal of antibiotic resistance in hospital Staphylococcal infection', *British Medical Journal*, 5165 (1960), 11–17.

26 J. W. D. Goodall, 'Cross-infection in hospital wards – its incidence and prevention', *Lancet*, 1 (1952), 807–812.

27 A. M. N. Gardner, M. Stamp, J. A. Bowgen and B. Moore, 'The infection control sister: A new member of the infection control team in general hospitals', *Lancet*, 2 (1962), 710–711. This was pioneered by the medical microbiologist Brendan Moore.

28 S. K. R. Clarke, 'Sepsis in wounds, with particular reference to *Staphylococcus aureus*', *British Journal of Surgery*, 44 (1957), 592–96. This was in line with earlier studies. See E. L. Eliason and C. McLaughlin, 'Post-operative wound complications', *Annals of Surgery*, 100 (1934), 1159–1176; Goodall, 'Cross-infection in hospital wards – its incidence and prevention', 807–12.

29 R. E. O. Williams, R. Blowers, L. P. Garrod and R. A. Shooter, *Hospital infection: Causes and prevention* (London: Lloyd-Luke Medical Books, 1st edition 1960; 2nd edition 1966). Robert Williams was Professor of Bacteriology and Consultant Bacteriologist at St Mary's Hospital Medical School, London, and a world expert on Staphylococcal infections. He was later Director of the UK Public Health Laboratory Service. (Arthur) Robert Blowers was Director of the Public Health Laboratory at Middlesbrough. Lawrence Garrod was Professor of Bacteriology and Bacteriologist at St Bartholomew's Hospital, London. Reginald Shooter was Bacteriologist at St Bartholomew's Hospital and Reader in Bacteriology in the University of London.

30 Williams, Blowers, Garrod and Shooter, *Hospital infection* (2nd edition 1966), 192.

31 M. Castle and E. Ajemian (eds), *The US/Canadian handbook hospital infection control* (New York: John Wiley, 2nd edition 1987), 309.

32 M. Finland and W. F. Jones Jr, 'Staphylococcal infections currently encountered in a large municipal hospital: Some problems in evaluating antimicrobial therapy in such infections', *Annals of the New York Academy of Sciences*, 65 (1956), 191–205, G. A. J. Ayliffe and M. P. English, *Hospital infection: From miasmas to MRSA* (Cambridge: Cambridge University Press, 2003), 186–199.

33 P. J. E. Cruse and R. Foord, 'The epidemiology of wound infection: A 10-year prospective study of 69,939 wounds', *Surgical Clinics of North America*, 60 (1980), 1. The costing figure is given in J. V. Bennett and P. S. Brachman (eds), *Hospital infections* (Boston: Little, Brown and Co., 1986 edition), 424.

34 American Hospital Association, *Infection control in the hospital* (Chicago: AMA, 1968). Referencing R. J. Weinzettel, 'Infection-control program reduced hospital stay, costs', *Hospital Topics*, 46:2 (Feb 1968), 53–56.

35 J. S. Garner, J. V. Bennett, W. E. Scheckler, *et al.*, 'Surveillance of nosocomial infections', in *Proceedings of the International Conference on Nosocomial Infections*, Atlanta, Centre for Disease Control, 1970 (Chicago: American Hospital Association, 1971); T. C. Eickhoff, 'Historical perspective: the landmark conference in 1970', *American Journal of Medicine*, 91, supplement 3B (1991), 3B–3S.

36 The *APIC Journal* was renamed the *American Journal for Infection Control* in 1980, edited by Mary Castle and Joseph Klimek.

37 R. W. Haley, 'Preliminary cost-benefit analysis of hospital infection control programs (the SENIC Project)', in F. Daschner and D. Adam (eds), *Proven and unproven methods in hospital infection control: Proceedings of an international workshop at Baiersbronn, Germany,*

24–25 September 1977 (New York: Gustave Fischer Verlag, 1978), 93–96.
38 R. W. Haley, D. R. Schaberg, S. D. Von Allmen and J. E. McGowan Jr., 'Estimating the extra charges and prolongation of hospitalisation due to nosocomial infections: A comparison of methods', *Journal of Infectious Diseases*, 141 (1980), 248; R. W. Haley, D. R. Schaberg, K. B. Crossley *et al.*, 'Extra charges and prolongation of stay attributable to nosocomial infections: A prospective interhospital comparison', *The American Journal of Medicine*, 70 (1981), 51–58; R. W. Haley, D. H. Culver, J. W. White *et al.*, 'The efficacy of infection surveillance and control programs in preventing nosocomial infections in US hospitals', *American Journal of Epidemiology*, 121 (1985), 182.
39 B. H. Raven, H. E. Freeman and R. W. Haley, 'Social science perspectives in hospital infection control', in A. W. Johnson, O. Grusky and B. H. Raven (eds), *Contemporary health services: Social science perspectives* (Boston: Auburn Publishing House, 1981), 137–176.
40 C. D. Givens and R. P. Wenzel, 'Cather-associated urinary tract infections in surgical patients; A controlled study on the excess morbidity and costs', *Journal of Urology*, 124 (1980), 646. See also M. S. Green, E. Rubenstein and P. Amit, 'Estimating the effects of nosocomial infections on the length of hospitalisation', *Journal of Infectious Diseases*, 145 (1982), 667.
41 J. Freeman and J. E. McGowan, 'Risk factors for nosocomial infections', *The Journal of Infectious Diseases*, 138 (1978), 811–819.
42 J. V. Bennett and P. S. Brachman (eds), *Hospital infections* (Boston: Little, Brown and Co., 1979).
43 M. Castle and E. Ajemian (eds), *Hospital infection control: Principles and practice* (New York: John Wiley, 1980).
44 Bennett and Brachman, *Hospital infections* (2nd edition 1986), 369.
45 R. W. Pinner, R. W. Haley and B. A. Blumenstein, 'High cost nosocomial infections', *Infection Control*, 3 (1982), 143.
46 Bennett and Brachman, *Hospital infections* (2nd edition 1986), 371.
47 R. Platt, B. F. Polk, B. S. Murdock *et al.*, 'Mortality associated with nosocomial urinary tract infection', *New England Journal of Medicine*, 307 (1982), 637.
48 D. E. Craven *et al.*, 'Contamination of mechanical ventilators with tubing changes every 24 or 48 hours', *New England Journal of Medicine*, 306 (1982), 1505.
49 G. A. Preston, E. L. Larson and W. E. Stamm, 'The effect of private isolation rooms on patient practices, colonisation and infection in an intensive care unit', *American Journal of Medicine*, 30 (1981), 614.

50 A. C. Steere and G. F. Mallison, 'Handwashing practices for the prevention of nosocomial infections', *Annals of Internal Medicine*, 83 (1975), 683; R. K. Albert and F. Condie, 'Handwashing patterns in medical intensive care units', *New England Journal of Medicine*, 304 (1981), 1465.

51 K. H. Chavigny and J. Fischer, 'Competing risk factors associated with nosocomial infection in two university hospitals', *Journal of Hospital Infection*, 5, supplement A (1984), 57–62; D. J. D. Price and J. D. Sleigh, 'The control of infection due to Klebsiella aerogenes in a neurosurgical unit', *Lancet*, 1 (1970), 1212–1215.

52 This had been trialled from 1980. A second DRG classification with 467 groups was introduced in 1984. See J. R. G. Butler and J. D. Thompson, 'The DRG Hospital Payment Scheme: some economic outputs', *Economic Analysis and Policy*, 14 (1984), 166–181.

53 A. M. Epstein, J. Bogen, P. Dreyer and K. E. Thorpe, 'Trends in length of stay and rates of readmission in Massachusetts: implications for monitoring quality of care', *Inquiry*, 28 (1991), 19–28.

54 R. S. Stern, P. I. Juhn, P. J. Gertle and A. M. Epstein, 'A comparison of length of stay and costs for health maintenance organization and fee-for-service patients', *Archives of Internal Medicine*, 149 (1989), 1185–1188.

55 M. Castle and E. Ajemian (eds), *Hospital infection control: Principles and practice* (New York: John Wiley, 2nd edition 1987).

56 B. E. Beyt and S. Troxler, 'Prospective payment and infection control', *Infection Control*, 6:4 (1985), 161. Quoted in Castle and Ajemian, *Hospital infection control*, 303–304.

57 Castle and Ajemian, *Hospital infection control* (2nd edition 1987), 306.

58 G. A. J. Ayliffe, E. J. L. Lowbury, A. M. Geddes and J. D. Williams, *Control of hospital infection* (London: Chapman and Hall, 1st edition 1975; 2nd edition 1981; 3rd edition 1992). Graham Ayliffe and Edward Lowbury had been Professors of Medical Microbiology at the University of Birmingham and Directors of the Hospital Infection Research Laboratory at Birmingham's Dudley Road Hospital. Lowbury was one of the first to identify antimicrobial cross infection, published as Lowbury, 'Cross-infection of wounds with antibiotic-resistant organisms', 985–990. Their colleague Alasdair Geddes was Professor of Infection at the University of Birmingham and Consultant Advisor in Infectious Diseases to the DH. The fourth editor-author, J. D. Williams, was Professor of Medical Microbiology at the Royal London Hospital Medical College and Consultant Microbiologist at the Royal London

Policy and infection control

Hospital. Nine further contributors were all based in Birmingham. Other members of their working party, listed in the acknowledgements, included several ICNs.

59 Ayliffe *et al.*, *Control of hospital infection* (1992 edition), xvii.
60 Haley, in Daschner and Adam (eds), *Proven and unproven methods*, 93–96.
61 S. W. B. Newsom and A. D. S. Caldwell, *Problems in the control of hospital infection* (London: Royal Society of Medicine and New York: Grune and Stratton, 1980).
62 F. D. Daschner, 'The cost of hospital-acquired infection', *Journal of Hospital Infection*, 5, supplement A (1984), 27–33.
63 F. D. Daschner, 'Cost-effectiveness in hospital infection control – lessons for the 1990s', *Journal of Hospital Infection*, 13 (1989), 325–336.
64 See, for example, R. A. Garibaldi, M. R. Britt, M. L. Coleman *et al.*, 'Risk factors for post-operative pneumonia', *American Journal of Medicine*, 70 (1981), 677–680; Haley, Schaberg *et al.*, 'Extra charges and prolongation of stay attributable to nosocomial infections', 51–58; M. J. Arbo, M. J. Fine, B. H. Hanusa *et al.*, 'Fever of nosocomial origin: Aetiology, risk factors and outcomes', *American Journal of Medicine*, 95 (1993), 505–512; A. Glynn, V. Ward, J. Wilson, L. Taylor *et al.*, *Hospital acquired infection: Surveillance, policies and practice* (London: Public Health Laboratory Service, 1997).
65 DHSS, *Hospital Infection Control: General Management Arrangements* (London: HMSO, 1988). Ayliffe *et al.*, in 1992, thought the actual average extra length of stay was more likely to be eight days.
66 North Thames Microbiology Subcommittee MRSA Working Party, 1987.
67 Ayliffe *et al.*, *Control of hospital infection* (1992 edition), xv.
68 *Ibid.*, 3.
69 *Ibid.*, 26–27.
70 E. Currie and A. Maynard, *Economics of hospital acquired infections. Discussion Paper 56* (York: Centre for Health Economics, 1989).
71 R. Coello, H. Glenister, J. Fereres *et al.*, 'The cost of infection in surgical patients: A case control study', *Journal of Hospital Infection*, 25 (1993), 239–250.
72 Department of Health and Public Health Laboratory Service, *Hospital infection control: Guidance on the control of infections in hospital*. Prepared by the Hospital Infection Working Group of the DH and Public Health Laboratory Service (London: DH, 1995). See also R. W. Haley, 'Cost-benefit analyses of infection control activities', in P. Brachman and J. Bennet (eds), *Hospital infections* (Philadelphia: Pippincott-Raven, 1998), 249–267.

73 R. M. Plowman, N. Graves, M. A. S. Griffin *et al.*, *Hospital acquired infection* (London: Office of Health Economics, 1997).
74 R. M. Plowman, N. Graves, M. Griffin *et al.*, *The socio-economic burden of hospital-acquired infection* (London: Public Health Laboratory Service, 1999). See also R. M. Plowman, N. Graves, M. Griffin *et al.*, 'The rate and cost of hospital-acquired infections occurring in patients admitted to selected specialities of a district general hospital in England and the national burden imposed', *Journal of Hospital Infection*, 47 (2001), 198–209.
75 National Audit Office, *The management and control of hospital acquired infections in acute NHS Trusts in England* (London: TSO, 2000).
76 K. Taylor, R. Plowman and J. A. Roberts, *The challenge of hospital acquired infection* (London: National Audit Office, 2001).
77 D. Reed and S. A. Kennedy, 'Infection control and prevention: A review of hospital-acquired infections and the economic implications', *The Ochsner Journal*, 9 (2009), 27–31.
78 P. W. Stone, E. Larson and L. N. Kawar, 'A systematic audit of economic evidence linking nosocomial infections and infection control interventions: 1990–2000', *American Journal of Infection Control*, 30 (2002), 145–152; P. W. Stone, D. Braccia and E. Larson, 'Systematic review of economic analyses of health care-associated infections', *American Journal of Infection Control*, 33 (2005), 501–509; E. N. Perencevich, P. W. Stone, S. B. Wright *et al.*, 'Raising standards while watching the bottom line: making a business case for infection control', *Infection Control and Hospital Epidemiology*, 28 (2007), 1121–1133.
79 Roberts (ed.), *The economics of infectious disease*.
80 *Ibid.*, 6–12.
81 *Ibid.*, 12.
82 R. Plowman, 'The economic evaluation of HAI', in Roberts (ed.), *The economics of infectious disease*, 129–157.
83 Nicholas Graves and Diana Weinhold, 'Complexity and the attribution of cost to hospital acquired infection', in Roberts (ed.), *The economics of infectious disease*, 103–116.
84 Author discussion with Rosalind Plowman, December 2018.
85 R. P. Shannon, B. Patel, D. Cummins *et al.*, 'Economics of central line-associated bloodstream infections', *American Journal of Medical Quality*, 21, supplement (2006); 7S–16S.
86 R. D. Scott, *The direct medical costs of healthcare-associated infections in US Hospitals and the benefits of prevention* (Atlanta: Centers for Disease Control and Prevention, 2009).

87 D. J. Anderson, K. S. Kaye, L. F. Chen *et al.*, 'Clinical and financial out-comes due to methicillin-resistant *Staphylococcus aureus* surgical site infection: A multi-center matched outcomes study', *Public Library of Science ONE*, 4 (2009). Duke University Medical Center study.

88 R. D. Smith and J. Coast, 'The economic burden of antimicrobial resist-ance: Why it is more serious than current studies suggest', Technical Report, London School of Hygiene and Tropical Medicine, 2012.

Part II

Infection control:
Nurses and medical students

3

Pus, pedagogy and practice: how 'dirt' shaped surgical nurse training and hierarchies of practice, 1900–1935

Pamela Wood

In the 1900–1935 period, surgical success depended not only on the surgeon's operative skill in the face of difficult challenges during surgery, but also on the prevention of sepsis. Pre- and post-operative care was mainly directed at preventing or managing infection, and was the relatively new professional sphere of the nurse. Training nurses to be skilled in surgical nursing was therefore vital to both the patient's recovery and the surgeon's success.

Central to sepsis was the presence of pus; a substance laden with fears of gangrene and death, and morally laden judgements of responsibility, reputation and blame. Substances carrying this kind of symbolic power are often those that in some way cross category boundaries. Pus epitomised a transgression of the wound from the category of healing tissue, to one of decaying flesh. The substance and power of pus can be understood through the anthropological notion of 'dirt'. This chapter uses the idea of 'dirt' to explore how sepsis, particularly in its most dangerous form of pus, shaped surgical nurse training and practice in the 1900–1935 period.

Nurse training, professionalisation and the emergence of germ theories

Two contextual factors are important to consider. First, nursing was consolidating its position at this time in the healthcare system of many countries. By 1900, nursing's importance was recognised in Britain, particularly through the influence of Florence Nightingale and the creation of the School of Nursing at St Thomas' Hospital in London in 1860. Nurses who trained there, such as Rebecca Strong and Isla Stewart, were appointed as matrons of other hospitals, where they established schools of nursing, increasing the number and quality of trained nurses. Others who trained elsewhere were similarly influential, such as Eva Lückes, who became Matron of the London Hospital in 1880.[1] This spread of well-qualified and influential nurses ensured that nurse training, and disciplined nursing practice, became embedded and valued in most major hospitals. Hospital leaders in different countries wrote to Nightingale, requesting a group of trained nurses for their own hospitals, and cohorts were sent when possible. Even at the farthest edges of the British Empire, senior medical staff were demanding from their trustees, as part of hospital reforms in the 1880s and 1890s, female nurses trained in the Nightingale system. Hospitals recruited them individually from Britain and elsewhere, and appointed them as matrons. Nursing schools were quickly established. One example is Isabella Fraser, who trained at the Edinburgh Royal Infirmary and was recruited from her position as Acting Lady Superintendent of Melbourne Hospital in Australia to become Matron of Dunedin Hospital in New Zealand in 1893. In both positions, she established a system of nurse training.

Throughout the period, alongside this spread of nurse training, nursing also transitioned, in part, from a vocation to a profession. At different times in different places, the early indicators of professionalisation were evident by the state registration and regulation of nurses; controlled and formalised training; and nursing organisations, conferences and journals. The first countries to establish state registration of nurses were South Africa in 1891 and New Zealand in 1901. From 1902, New Zealand was first to have a formalised national nursing curriculum in all its training hospitals, leading to state examinations for registration. In many countries, nursing organisations met to discuss nursing issues at conferences and were connecting with sister organisations in other countries through the founding of the International Council of Nurses in 1899. Nursing journals were established, for example in Britain, Ireland, Canada, South Africa, Australia, New Zealand and the United States, publishing material on professional and practice issues. A strong connection between editors ensured an international exchange of volumes, with several articles reprinted. During this time, then, nursing was an emerging profession with an international network and was defining its sphere of knowledge and practice.

The second contextual element relates to changing scientific and medical knowledge. By 1900, approaches to combatting sepsis were already shifting in emphasis from antisepsis to asepsis. In the mid-nineteenth century, surgeons had seen pus in a wound as 'laudable pus', laudable as it indicated healing.[2] From the 1860s, Lister had argued that wounds inevitably became contaminated in surgery through contact with air. The ever-present germs in the atmosphere of the operating theatre could only be combatted through 'antisepsis', particularly a continuous spray of carbolic acid and the use of antiseptics in wound care. Although initially ignored, belittled and sometimes ridiculed in England, his ideas and practice became widely followed in many countries. Surgeons now had a chance to prevent infection. In the later nineteenth century, a different approach was advocated. Lawson Tait believed that the presence of microbes was not inevitable, and that sepsis could be prevented by ensuring a clean environment. His argument of 'asepsis' demanded rigorous scrubbing of wards, furniture and operating theatres, and the sterilisation of equipment and materials through heat (boiling and steaming) rather than antiseptics. Hospital reforms in the late nineteenth century ensured a scouring of all crevices where microbes could lurk. By the beginning of the twentieth century, although the use of the carbolic spray had dwindled, surgeons tended to combine elements of the antiseptic and aseptic approaches. As one surgeon explained, 'we cannot boil the surgeon, cook the nurses, steam the patient. Thus, antiseptics are not quite indispensable, but their use is narrowed down to a small limit.'[3]

In the early twentieth century, sepsis remained a major focus of surgical practice and pre- and post-operative care, operationalised in procedures that were well-established and routine. Surgeons now had a means of combatting the microbe and had the skilled support of trained nurses who chose surgical nursing as the focus of their practice. Their combined attention meant that wounds could heal without infection. Conversely, the appearance of pus increasingly carried with it a sense of failure and shame. Surgeons who were worried that their professional reputations could be marred sought to shift the blame to the surgical nurse. They focused on both the trainee nurse, learning surgical nursing as part of a general nurse training, and the trained nurse selecting surgical nursing work. The power of sepsis as a driver for surgical nurse training and practice, and for determining professional relations between surgeons and nurses, can be explored through the anthropological notion of 'dirt'.

'Dirt' as an anthropological idea

The pus of septic wounds is a form of dirt, as it is understood in cultural anthropology. Mary Douglas explained that all cultures create categories to understand their world, and anything that does not fit into a category or crosses category boundaries is 'matter out of place' and is labelled as 'dirt'.[4] For example, fruit belongs to the category of food, but when it rots it transgresses category boundaries and becomes matter out of place, or dirt. A septic wound is no longer in the category of healthy or healing tissue – it has become rotting flesh or dirt, and is epitomised by pus. Julia Kristeva noted that a substance identified as dirty or disgusting is often unpleasant, slimy, sticky, difficult to remove and associated with decomposition and decay.[5] Pus and tenacious slough fit these characteristics. A key identifier, however, which is not included in these definitions, is that to be considered dirt the substance must first be *perceived* as problematic.[6] For Douglas, any matter out of place was identified as dirty and problematic. However, this indiscriminate classification is too broad. Matter out of place might be considered either a valuable resource or a source of contamination. Animal dung can be a useful garden manure, or a filthy and unwelcome contaminant inside a house. It is therefore only when it becomes problematic that it is identified as 'dirt'. Surgeons initially applied a similar differentiation to pus. Until the later nineteenth century, healing by 'second intention' following infection and suppuration (the formation of pus) was accepted as the likely course for any wound. Surgeons defined pus as 'laudable pus' if it was free-draining. In contrast, pus enclosed in an abscess or wound could seep into the blood stream and cause blood poisoning. Only this form of pus was considered problematic. Once antiseptic or aseptic measures were in common practice, however, pus in a wound was a distinct problem for surgeons and nurses, as well as the patient.

As Douglas explained, anything that challenges or transgresses category boundaries is considered powerful and dangerous.[7] In this 1900–1935 period, it is not surprising that sepsis was an important topic addressed in surgical nurse training, especially as surgeons had only recently acquired the means to combat it effectively, but its significance went further. Dirt in the form of a suppurating wound was symbolically powerful (and continues to be emotionally impactful, as Jennie Wilson explores in her contribution to this volume).[8] As a Guy's Hospital ward sister, M. N. Oxford, said in 1900 in her textbook *A Handbook of Nursing*, before the cause of infection was understood, 'the suppuration of wounds was the rule rather than the exception', but now 'it is certain that if a wound suppurates, someone is to blame'.[9] Nurses recognised the shame of the presence of pus. As one nurse, Gladys Tatham, declared in an article in the *British Journal of Nursing* in 1914, a suppurating wound was a 'disgrace'.[10] Pus also shaped pedagogy – a pedagogy that incorporated more than a curriculum of nursing knowledge and skills. It also embedded values, and shaped or reinforced hierarchies of practice, including a social order of surgical relations.

Curriculum design and delivery

Five elements need to be addressed when considering a curriculum: intention, delivery, content, assessment and the 'hidden curriculum', that is those lessons that are learnt but not openly intended, including the social transmission of norms, values and beliefs. The literature supporting training in surgical nursing in the early twentieth century shows that the curricular intention was to prepare knowledgeable, skilful and reliable nurses, who understood sepsis, could identify its signs and knew their role in its prevention and treatment. This training prepared nurses for responsibility before, during and after an operation, whether in hospital or a patient's home.[11] Well-trained nurses were seen as assets to surgeons in their challenging roles.

The nursing curriculum was delivered primarily on the ward. In most hospitals, new probationers, pupil nurses or nurse trainees, as they were variously called, started in a ward on their first day of training. They learnt their roles from senior nurses and ward sisters. Doctors gave occasional lectures, which nurses attended often in their own time, even if on night duty. Matrons and sisters from specialist wards followed up these lectures with their own. Lectures, however, did not always offer optimal teaching. New Zealand nurse Bridget Ristori, training at the small, rural Masterton Hospital in the 1920s, recorded that theoretical teaching was 'extremely poor', with few lectures given.[12] They had surgical nursing lectures from the hospital superintendent, who was 'a brilliant man but one of the world's worst lecturers'. She 'slept through most of his lectures' but 'kept awake in one by reading the romantic novel *The Sheik* under cover of a desk'.[13] Even by the 1930s, the curriculum for British nurses, set by the General Nursing Council, included a minimum of only ten lectures on surgical nursing, with nurses required to attend just eight.[14]

Improvements in the delivery of nurse training were gradually introduced. By the 1930s, many hospitals had a Preliminary Training School where nurses gained basic knowledge and skills before entering the wards. These were run by sister-tutors whose sole function was nurse training. To support the curriculum, moreover, matrons, other senior nurses and doctors wrote nursing textbooks, and edited and wrote for professional nursing journals.[15] They could therefore shape understandings of sepsis, nursing practice and surgeons' and surgical nurses' professional relations. Some textbooks were aligned with the specific curricula of agencies responsible for nursing qualifications. S. J. Woodall's British textbook *Outline of Surgical Nursing* was prepared 'strictly in accordance with the syllabus of the General Nursing Council'.[16] And the successive editions of *Surgical Nursing and After-Treatment* by the Sydney Hospital surgeon H. C. Rutherford Darling met the requirements of the Australasian Trained Nurses' Association, which covered all Australian states except Victoria.[17]

The supremacy of sepsis was evident in all surgical nursing textbooks, which were consistent in the importance they assigned to two things: an explanation of sepsis, and its underlying scientific bacteriological basis. A survey of several editions in 1900–1935 of sixteen British and Australian textbooks that were also used in other countries shows that sepsis was often addressed in the first chapters. London Hospital surgeon Russell Howard's textbook, for example, kept infection and pus, and its prevention, as the topic of the first chapter throughout multiple editions.[18] Similarly, Rutherford Darling's textbook itemised and addressed bacteriology, infection, inflammation, suppuration (pus formation) and sepsis in the first and third chapters in each edition.[19] The first three chapters of another textbook, by London surgeons Hamilton Bailey and R. J. McNeill Love, presented disinfection, sterilisation, bacteriology, specific infections, inflammation and wounds.[20] The history of antisepsis and transition to asepsis was often explained with pride.[21] Although the history of infection control is more accurately one of shifting, concurrent and conflicting beliefs rather than a continuous progression, surgeons were delighted to trace this history as a narrative of scientific and medical advancement. The superintendent of the Kingston General Hospital in Ontario, Canada, captured this trend with his comment in 1909 that 'surgery has passed from the night of infection and empiricism to the dawn of antisepsis and certainty; from antisepsis, with its limited field of operation, to the glorious noon-day of asepsis, with its broad operative field'.[22]

Textbooks also explained the classification of different forms of sepsis, from localised wound infection (from inflammation through to pus formation), to the systemic forms of sapraemia (localised bacteria, with circulation of toxins), pyaemia (circulation of infected clots, causing fresh abscesses) and septicaemia (circulation of bacteria).[23] The most virulent form of dirt – pus – was specifically described. Howard, for example, explained that pyogenic (pus-forming) microbes killed white cells and liquefied tissue 'in a manner similar to the digestion of food in the stomach', so the inflamed area filled with a liquid containing dead and dying cells. 'This liquid is pus, and suppuration is said to have occurred.'[24] Some surgeons gave visual pointers to recognising it. Wilfred Hadley at the London Hospital noted, 'Pus is a greenish-yellow fluid, composed of dead tissue cells killed by the poisonous effect of the micro-organisms.'[25] Laurence Humphrey at Addenbrooke's Hospital in Cambridge believed, even well into the twentieth century, that nurses should know earlier modes of treating wound infection as these were still in practice. These earlier modes expected and welcomed suppuration as a sign of healing by 'second intention'. He therefore differentiated the 'character of pus' by explaining that 'healthy or *laudable* pus is of yellowish colour and of a sweet, faint odour', whereas the 'discharge from an unhealthy wound or abscess is greenish-yellow or green, or dark brown or red, from decomposing blood, and the smell is unpleasant, offensive, or even putrid' (emphasis in original).[26] Information about sepsis and the nurse's role in addressing it were also detailed in nursing journal articles, available for both the nurse in training and for the continuing education of those already in practice.[27]

To bolster understanding of the new, scientific basis for preventing sepsis, separate textbooks on bacteriology were also written, reviewed and recommended. A review for one by a British doctor, G. Norman Meachen, for example, even appeared in New Zealand's nursing journal, *Kai Tiaki*.[28] Similarly, the rationale for practice was stressed. Marjorie Chambers, training at Christchurch Hospital in New Zealand in the 1920s, commented that 'the reasons for all our techniques were carefully explained'.[29] This was also evident in textbooks. A. N. McGregor, Assistant Surgeon at the Glasgow Royal Infirmary, had even noted in 1905 that 'intelligent appreciation' of the reasons for aseptic measures was needed, otherwise implementing those measures would be 'meaningless' and apt to be 'perfunctorily performed'.[30] The message continued throughout the 1920s and 1930s. As Charles Childe, Senior Surgeon at the Royal Portsmouth Hospital, noted in the preface to his third edition in 1920, a 'sound knowledge of the causes and means of introduction of infection' was needed as a 'foundation'.[31]

Surgical nurses' knowledge of sepsis and its prevention and treatment was stringently assessed. In final surgical nursing examinations for state registration in New Zealand or entry to the register of the largest professional nursing association in Australia, the Australasian Trained Nurses' Association, the prevention of sepsis was the most frequently occurring topic.[32] Candidates answered questions on wound healing, preventing infection, aseptic techniques, antiseptics and disinfectants and managing septic wounds. They usually showed good knowledge, but at times examiners worried that nurses were too zealous. One examiner remarked that some nurses prepared a patient for abdominal surgery so thoroughly that it was 'merely a question of which gave out first, the skin or the bowel'.[33]

Examiners' reports show that the surgeons setting final examination papers were aware of the need to set discriminating questions in order to identify well-prepared nurses. Their comments also show their concern to have not just knowledgeable, well-trained nurses but 'first-class' nurses who could draw on their practice experience in answering questions.[34] They chose topics that could be a 'good searching test of quality'.[35]

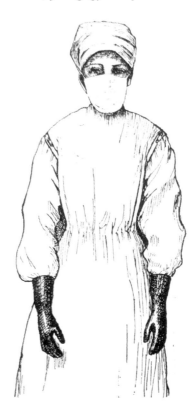

Figure 3.1 From H. C. Rutherford Darling, *Surgical Nursing and After-Treatment* (J. & A. Churchill, 1947).

Gladys Tatham's comment that a suppurating wound was a 'disgrace'[36] shows that certain moral values were embedded in the curriculum and reinforced in practice. Nurses were to learn, embody and demonstrate values such as conscientiousness, diligence, honesty, reliability and meticulousness. The connection between these values, the prevention of sepsis and the notion of 'dirt' can be seen not only in the requirement for scrupulous wound care but in the emphasis placed, for example, on the nurse's personal cleanliness. The nurse was to display these values in her bodily care and presentation – dirt in any form was not to be tolerated. In 1900, Sister M. N. Oxford considered any new probationer at Guy's Hospital needed to show habits of neatness and cleanliness to be considered 'good material for training'.[37] In 1920, M. A. Gullan, Sister Tutor at St Thomas' Hospital, warned that 'fastidious cleanliness' must be the nurse's 'undeviating purpose'. She should be 'so imbued with the spirit of cleanliness that she will keep herself and her clothing clean even while doing the dirtiest work'.[38] The nurse's bodily cleanliness, emphasised into the 1930s, had to address any dirty matter exuding from her body that was likely to give offence. Body odours and discharges were portrayed in the same terms as the 'unpleasant, offensive, even putrid' odour of pus.[39] Nurses must correct 'any cause of offensive odour, such as decayed teeth, discharging ears, and perspiring feet',[40] 'offensive nasal discharge', 'bromidrosis' (excessive, foetid sweating) or 'any other unhealthy taint'.[41] Offensive discharges seeped across bodily boundaries, becoming matter out of place. They met Kristeva's description of unpleasant, slimy and sticky matter and therefore elicited a disgust that tainted the nurse,[42] who had not displayed the moral value associated with cleanliness. She should 'practise cleanliness as a matter of honour. Every vestige of dirt, whether visible or not, must be removed.'[43] A nurse's disgusting odour, grubby person or unkempt presentation were physical signs of a disregard for the moral values essential in surgical nursing to prevent sepsis. Dirt – whether visible or not – brought moral disgust and alarm. The curriculum therefore emphasised cleanliness. The performance of the curriculum in practice also showed that the idea of 'dirt', focusing on sepsis, created hierarchies of practice, including an order of social relations.

Hierarchies of practice

The first hierarchy of practice connected three elements: the nature and gradient of dirt; surgical nurse ranking and responsibility; and wound dressing practice. As material identified as dirt became smaller in size and more specific, especially down to the microbial level, the seniority of nurses responsible for it conversely increased. Broadly defined, dirt that was visible in the ward environment and on the patient's body was therefore the responsibility of the junior nurse, whereas septic matter inside wounds – pus – harbouring the invisible microbe, was the senior nurse's responsibility. In the prevention of sepsis, junior nurses learnt 'medical asepsis' or general cleanliness and were therefore responsible for a clean ward and patient. Damp-dusting furniture, sweeping floors with damp tea leaves and ensuring clean, crisply made beds were their realm. A speaker at a nursing conference saw teaching potential in these tasks. A junior nurse would take much more interest in this, she said, if she realised that the cleanliness of her lampshades was as important as a senior nurse's correct aseptic treatment of a wound.[44] Junior nurses' responsibilities also extended to the patient's pre-operative bodily hygiene and the administration of what one nurse described as the 'ritual of the bowel-cleansing soap-and-water enema'.[45] For skin cleanliness, the junior nurse could remove 'gross dirt and grease' by giving the patient 'a hot bath and plenty of soap', but the operation site needed very careful preparation.[46] That was the province of the senior nurse.

Alison Bashford argued that while asepsis was revolutionary for most male surgeons who had now to think of themselves as 'potential polluters', it was not for female nurses 'who had thought of their work and themselves within a language of absolute purity for a generation and more'. Asepsis 'allowed for, rather than obliterated, nurses' sanitarian practices' that continued from the nineteenth century.[47] This was evident for the junior nurse's role, particularly with its emphasis on ward cleanliness. Humphrey reflected these sanitarian principles in advising nurses that the 'main predisposing causes to pyaemia are overcrowding, dirt, bad ventilation, and insecure drainage, some of which may be guarded against by the nurse'.[48] In contrast to Bashford's view, however, for the senior nurse asepsis meant a distinct shift in emphasis, focus and practice. Sanitarian practices were no longer sufficient. Senior nurses learnt 'surgical asepsis', combatting the microbe itself.[49] They learnt responsibility for operating theatre cleanliness, the sterilisation of surgical instruments and materials,[50] the strengths and uses of antiseptics (including new forms developed during the First World War)[51] and thorough preparation of the patient's operation site. Scrupulous preparation meant shaving, washing, drying, swabbing with disinfectant, painting with antiseptic and covering the site with a sterile dressing and binder.[52] Finally, for duty in the operating theatre, she scrubbed, soaked and wrapped herself. Having ensured her general bodily cleanliness, she followed finely detailed instructions for surgically cleaning her hands, nails and arms with soap, water, brush and disinfectant. By the 1930s, drawings or photographs illustrated how she should then garb herself with gown, head covering, mask, gloves and sometimes galoshes, until only her eyes were visible.[53] Just as her seniority made her responsible for the smallest-size element in the gradient of dirt – the microbe – so it directed her to the crevices of the patient,[54] and herself.[55]

Post-operatively, the senior nurse maintained vigilant watchfulness for signs of the microbe's suppurative success – wound sepsis.[56] In this, the nurse's role was frequently expressed in the military metaphor of a sentry, 'guarding ... patients from the attacks of organisms' and keeping 'a sharp lookout' for signs of complications like sepsis.[57] Military metaphors also encompassed changes in the wound. Sepsis was caused by 'invasion of the wound by microorganisms'.[58] Microbes were the enemy. As E. Stanmore Bishop, a surgeon at Ancoats Hospital in Manchester, noted in 1909, 'carelessness or thoughtlessness' could 'render aid to the enemy' and make 'the efforts of all the rest ineffective and useless'.[59] This message was reinforced throughout the time period. Even by the late 1930s, the invasion metaphor with its dangerous, destructive goal was also used, for example, by E. Divens, Sister-Tutor at the Dundee Royal Infirmary.[60] As she told a tutorial group at the British College of Nurses in 1931, 'the invasion of the micro-organisms may extend to the fixed tissue, and, by causing their destruction, enlarge the area of the wound'.[61] The 'slightest lapse into carelessness' was therefore 'fraught with danger'.[62]

The third dimension in this hierarchy of practice constructed by 'dirt' and reflecting the understanding of cross-contamination was the sequence and manner of attending to wound dressings. The nurse should always be 'working from "clean to dirty"'.[63] 'Clean dressings' – uninfected wounds – were done first. 'Dirty dressings' were septic wounds with what one nurse described as 'foul smelling discharge [that] nearly made me vomit'.[64] This was a physical embodiment of the revulsion and disgust engendered by septic matter,[65] particularly the 'offensive, or even putrid' stench of pus.[66] Dirty dressings were done last to 'prevent contamination of clean wounds'. If there was more than one dirty dressing, one nurse was designated as the 'clean nurse' and another the 'dirty nurse'.[67]

Surgical relations

A further hierarchy of practice was a social order of surgical relations based on septic blame.[68] This social order positioned and repositioned the surgical nurse in relation to the surgeon. It reflects the most striking aspect of the journal literature supporting surgical nurses' learning, in that their role was almost always presented as an adjunct to the surgeon, rather than in relation to the patient. Some historians have argued that this primary work relationship with the surgeon was that of an obedient, subservient handmaiden.[69] However, this one-dimensional view is not borne out by the literature referred to in this chapter, and a more complex professional relationship is evident.[70] Even surgeons pointed to views that had changed since the late nineteenth century: Russell Howard at the London Hospital explained in the preface to his 1908 surgical nursing textbook that 'modern nursing has passed beyond the stage of passive obedience'. Active strides in surgery, he said, demanded greater knowledge on the part of the nurse. While the direction of treatment remained in the surgeon's hands, he left the details in the hands of the nurse.[71] By the 1930s, the nurse's role was also being expressed as that of a team member, with success dependent on the combined efforts of all concerned.[72]

This recognition of the key role of skilled nurses marked a change in surgical attitudes; thirty years earlier, nurses had been mainly depicted – and valued – as supporters of the surgeon's heroic efforts.[73] There were, however, earlier exceptions: in 1894, the British surgeon Bedford Fenwick acknowledged that surgical success had come to be as dependent on the nurse's carefulness and cleanliness as on the surgeon's skill.[74] There is no way of knowing if Fenwick's statement was related to the fact that he was married to one of the most powerful nurses in Britain, and was writing in the nursing journal that she edited.[75] A more traditional and gendered statement of roles was given in the opening statement of Bishop's 1909 textbook. He started with the somewhat condescending compliment that of all 'pleasant relationships' he doubted if there was 'one more delightful' than that of a surgeon and 'the nurse he implicitly trusts, whose ever ready smile and cheerful face greet him on every occasion' and who gave him 'quiet, willing, enthusiastic help'. Perhaps mindful of his readership among surgical nurses, Bishop went on to acknowledge the debt he owed to the 'splendid nurses' for 'a great part of any success' he had achieved and hoped he could pass on to their successors some of the things they had taught him.[76]

Surgeons expected nurses to support their efforts through diligence, conscientious attention to detail and vigilance in watching for sepsis.[77] They were to have mental acumen and sound moral character.[78] Cleanliness in their person and in all their work was essential and should be automatic – 'matters of habit and not of thought'.[79] Their 'most desirable qualities' were 'thorough intelligence, tact, powers of observation, sympathy, and practical ability'. They should show 'strict obedience to instructions' and be 'absolutely loyal' to the surgeon.[80]

Despite their conscientious vigilance, wounds could still become infected. At least one surgeon simply acknowledged that a mistake could occur, stating that it was most important to find out why in order to prevent it happening again. In his 1921 textbook, Alexander Miles at the Edinburgh Royal Infirmary was clear that if sepsis occurred it was 'certain that someone has blundered': 'we all fail at times,' he added, and when this happened it was 'a great thing to know why we fail, and where we have made mistakes, so that we may avoid them in the future'.[81] Most, however, did lay blame, and most frequently laid it squarely on the nurse, regardless of what might have actually occurred during the operation to cause the infection. Septic wounds meant septic relations.

There was a gradient of suppurating blame. At its least condemnatory, sepsis identified nurses' practice as merely careless. A nurse's careless ways, however, directly undermined the surgeon's skill. As McGregor explained, division of labour was necessary in surgical work, and a nurse might 'think that her particular share is small, and of little importance'. She should remember, however, that 'as a chain has only the strength of its weakest link, so her carelessness or neglect may nullify the most stringent precautions adopted'.[82] As the gradient of blame increased in vehemence, the nurse was depicted as slipshod and lacking in moral fibre. At the most vituperative end of the gradient, the worst offending nurses were labelled as slovenly.

In each edition of his textbook, Childe blamed sepsis on nurses' 'slackness'. He first praised the surgical nurse as 'the partaker in the triumphs of every modern operation and literally the surgeon's "right-hand woman"', someone who contributed to the surgeon's success 'in no small degree, except possibly in regard to the skill of his anaesthetist'.[83] He seemed frustrated, however, that 'when a failure occurs … it is seldom that we are able to place our finger on the exact source of infection, and to state positively that such or such an error in the technique was the cause of it'. This was the 'unsatisfactory part of the business'. Nevertheless, it was clear from his gendered statements where he laid the blame. 'If we could bring the defaulter to book, we should possess a powerful weapon against "slackness" and should be in a position to expose the delinquent and convince her of her error. As, however, the reverse is the case … unless a woman has a conscience, she is unfit to undertake surgical work.' Without a conscience, suspicion could fall unjustly on others, 'who have faithfully done their duty'.[84] Perhaps he was concerned about the effect on his own surgical reputation. All aspects of nurses' practice were scrutinised. C. B. Keetley, a senior surgeon at the West London Hospital in 1908, for example, noted fourteen faults in the way nurses dealt with surgical instruments. By this time, the shift from reliance on chemical measures in sterilisation to the inclusion of heat (boiling and steaming) was in place. Clearly disenchanted with nurses' practice and knowledge, he admonished them, as though unskilled housewives, that 'you could not kill microbes, any more than you could cook puddings, by popping them into boiling water for a few seconds'.[85]

A slovenly approach in caring for the surgical patient came not only from a nurse's lack of diligence or moral fibre, but also from an over-reliance on antiseptics. Although (or perhaps because) nurses were expected to be thoroughly familiar with antiseptics, they sometimes disregarded other aspects of preventing sepsis. As H. L. Maitland, Honorary Surgeon at Sydney Hospital, bellowed in 1904, over-reliance on antiseptics was 'but a salve to an elastic conscience', a 'delusion', a 'snare' and was 'fraught with danger', not least to her own reputation as a surgical nurse.[86]

Nurses also contributed to this hierarchy of blame. New Zealand nurse Marjorie Chambers commented that working with other nurses on the ward 'taught us the most. One learns so easily from watching and helping other people, but sometimes we learned bad habits, short cuts in nursing techniques when we were all short of time and not being careful enough.'[87] In the 1930s, it was still routine for nurses to do even septic dressings by holding swabs in their fingers. Perhaps it was carelessness, or an over-reliance on antiseptics, that meant that one of the commonest reasons for nurses reporting sick was having a septic finger.[88] Even in 1889, an American nurse had cautioned that one little sin of omission or commission was 'sufficient to overthrow the most able surgeon's efforts'.[89] In 1908, a Canadian nurse warned that if nurses were careless, slovenly or foolhardy enough to handle pus, infected fingers would result.[90] Another, in Australia in 1921, warned nurses that wearing rubber gloves, when they had them, sometimes made them careless about handwashing, reducing it to a few seconds.[91] The view of the careless, slovenly nurse and her effect on the surgeon's success was apparent even at the end of this time period. As one noted in 1937, nurses should remember that the surgeon's 'skilled work' could be 'rendered of no avail' by some careless or unconscientious action on the part of a nurse.[92]

In general, the literature by both doctors and nurses placed the blame for sepsis on the surgical nurse. Nurses, however, sometimes blamed surgeons. One observed that 'once a man gets into a cap, gloves and gown he thinks he sterilizes everything he touches'.[93] Gladys Tatham, who thought suppuration was a disgrace, spread the blame more evenly. Suppuration showed faulty aseptic technique, she noted, by either the nurse or surgeon.[94]

Pus, pedagogy and practice

As this chapter has shown, pus shaped pedagogy and practice in the early twentieth century. In the context of changing scientific and medical knowledge, and at a time when nursing was defining its sphere of practice, the idea of 'dirt' expressed in understandings of sepsis moulded three things. First, it established the direction of a surgical nursing curriculum. Secondly, it created a hierarchy of practice that connected a gradient of dirt, surgical nurse experience and training, and wound dressing practice. And thirdly, it determined a social order of surgical relations, co-constructed by surgeons and nurses, in which the nurse was positioned through her scrupulous practice as the surgeon's supporter, or through her slovenly ways as undermining his heroic efforts. Nevertheless, surgeons' contribution of lectures, articles, textbooks and examinations shows their positive engagement in a pedagogy that would produce skilful, knowledgeable nurses, able to identify and take effective action against dirt in its most purulent form.

The combined histories of pus, pedagogy and practice offer points for consideration in the present. History lets us take the long view. It teaches an understanding of the context in which medical practices take shape and creates an awareness that knowledge continues to change. Our current evidence-based practices of sepsis control could be viewed with surprise, amusement, shock or bafflement by those looking back in twenty or thirty years' time. And as Thomas Schlich's contribution to this volume shows, there is nothing inevitable about the development and take-up of medical interventions. In engaging with history, we encounter, as the historian John Tosh reminds us, points of familiarity and difference.[95] Although the contexts of time and place are always different, a historical perspective allows us to distinguish between issues that are enduring and those that are transient. They offer a new perspective.

To this end, there were specific issues encountered in preventing and managing wound infection in the past that are worth considering today. As H. L. Maitland warned in 1904, the over-reliance on antiseptics was a dangerous delusion. Similarly, the Australian nurse's caution in 1921 that wearing rubber gloves could make nurses careless about handwashing is a message with relevance today. Over-reliance on antibiotics has created the current circumstance of antimicrobial resistance. In the same way, over-reliance on any method, such as using antiseptics or gloves, obscures other measures that should or could be taken to prevent or control infection.

In relation to education, the curriculum and pedagogical approach in the early twentieth century embedded values of diligence, vigilance and scrupulousness in nursing practice. These values are just as meaningful today and should be made explicit through nursing curricula. It is not sufficient merely to list them in a curriculum document; every nursing student should be able to explain and demonstrate how they translate them into action. This could be included in reflective practice processes and made explicit in their practice exemplars.

Perhaps most importantly, the history of infection control shows us that a culture of blame is not productive. Septic wounds caused septic relations. Despite the significant urge to blame that was evident in surgeons' and sometimes nurses' writing, at least one surgeon took a different stance. Alexander Miles reminded others nearly a century ago that everyone fails at times. When someone blunders, as he said, the crucial outcome is to learn from the error in order to avoid it in the future. What is needed today is this culture of curiosity – an urge to discover the reason for any infection so that practice can be improved. When coupled with commitment from every health professional to take responsibility for preventing infection, we can develop a culture of exquisite care.

Notes

1 For further information, see S. McGann, *The battle of the nurses: A study of eight women who influenced the development of professional nursing, 1880–1930* (London: Scutari Press, 1992).

2 C. Lawrence and R. Dixey, 'Practising on principle: Joseph Lister and the germ theories of disease', in C. Lawrence (ed.), *Medical theory, surgical practice: Studies in the history of surgery. Symposium* (London: Routledge, 1992), Chapter 6.

3 M. Herz, 'Asepsis', *Kai Tiaki*, 1 (1908), 85–86, 85.

4 M. Douglas, *Purity and danger: an analysis of concepts of pollution and taboo* (London: Routledge & Kegan Paul, 1966); M. Douglas, *Implicit meanings: Essays in anthropology* (London: Routledge & Kegan Paul, 1975). For recent examples of scholars' use of Douglas's definition, see H. Callaghan, 'Birth dirt', in M. Kirkham (ed.), *Exploring the dirty side of women's health* (London: Routledge, 2007), 9–29; P. J. Wood and M. Foureur, 'A clean front passage: dirt, douches and disinfectants at St Helens Hospital, Wellington, New Zealand, 1907–1922', in Kirkham (ed.), *Exploring the dirty side of women's health*, 30–43; S. van der Geest, 'Hygiene and sanitation: Medical, social and psychological concerns', *Canadian Medical Association Journal*, 187 (2015), 1313–1314; S. Newell, 'Researching the cultural politics of dirt in urban Africa', in S. Puri and D. A. Castillo (eds), *Theorizing fieldwork in the humanities* (New York: Palgrave Macmillan US, 2016), 193–211.

5 J. Kristeva, *Powers of horror: An essay on abjection* (New York: Columbia University Press, 1982).

6 P. J. Wood, *Dirt: Filth and decay in a new world arcadia* (Auckland: Auckland University Press, 2005).

7 Douglas, *Purity and danger*.

8 See Chapter 7.
9 M. N. Oxford, *A handbook of nursing* (London: Methuen & Co, 1900), 145.
10 G. Tatham, 'Sepsis – what it is, and how to avoid it', *British Journal of Nursing*, 53 (1914), 219–221, quotation on 219.
11 See for example J. McNaughton Christie, 'Second lecture delivered before Wellington Branch, N.Z.T.N.A.', *Kai Tiaki*, 7 (1914), 7–18.
12 B. Ristori, *Patients in my care* (London: Eleck, 1967), 38.
13 *Ibid.*, 38.
14 A. M. Jackson and K. F. Armstrong, *Teaching in schools of nursing* (London: Faber & Faber, 1934), 134.
15 *The British Journal of Nursing, Canadian Nurse, Australasian Nurses' Journal* (from Australia) and *Kai Tiaki* (from New Zealand) were the main historical nursing journals systematically surveyed in this research.
16 S. J. Woodall, *Outline of surgical nursing, adapted to the requirements of the general nursing council* (London: Law & Local Government Publications, 1925), n.p.
17 H. C. Rutherford Darling, *Surgical nursing and after-treatment: A handbook for nurses and others* (London: J. & A. Churchill, 1923, 1928, 1932, 1935, 1938). Victoria had its own organisation, the Victorian Trained Nurses Association, which administered examinations for that state.
18 R. Howard, *Surgical nursing and the principles of surgery for nurses* (London: Edward Arnold, 1908, 1920, 1926).
19 Rutherford Darling, *Surgical nursing* (1923, 1928, 1932, 1935, 1938).
20 H. Bailey and R. J. McNeill Love, *Surgery for nurses* (London: H. K. Lewis, 1938).
21 See, for example, E. Stanmore Bishop, *Lectures on surgical nursing* (Bristol: John Wright & Sons, 1909), 1–13; W. J. Hadley, *Nursing: General, medical and surgical* (London: J. & A. Churchill, 1902), 233–235; Howard, *Surgical nursing*, xix–xx. For nursing journal articles on the history of antisepsis and asepsis, see, for example, Herz, 'Asepsis'; 'The history of antiseptics, and the lessons to be learnt', *British Journal of Nursing*, 65:1732 (1921), 352–353; 'The evolution of surgical technique during the last half century', *British Journal of Nursing*, 43:1109 (1909), 23–24.
22 'The evolution of surgical technique during the last half century', 24.
23 See, for example, E. W. Hey Groves and J. M. Fortescue-Brickdale, *Textbook for nurses: Anatomy, physiology, surgery and medicine* (London: Hodder & Stoughton, 1915), 141.
24 Howard, *Surgical nursing*, 20.
25 Hadley, *Nursing*, 251.

26 L. Humphrey, *A manual of nursing: Medical and surgical* (London: Charles Griffin & Co, 1917), 162–163.

27 As some examples, see E. C. Ferguson, 'The operating room – equipment, care, supplies', *Canadian Nurse*, 18 (1922), 673–677; E. Stanmore Bishop, 'Lectures to nurses on antiseptics in surgery. Lecture III (continued)', *Nursing Record*, 3:74 (1889), 131; 'The importance of asepsis', *Australasian Nurses' Journal*, 12 (1914), 366–8, reprinted from the *Nursing Mirror*; Andrew Moorhead, 'Preparation of a patient for an abdominal operation and the after treatment of abdominal surgery', *Canadian Nurse*, 21 (1925), 354–5; 'Ante-operative and post-operative care', *Canadian Nurse*, 25 (1929), 191–3. Please note that it was common practice for no author to be identified in nursing journals from this period.

28 'New books for study and leisure hours', *Kai Tiaki*, 17 (1924), 60.

29 M. Chambers, *My life in nursing* (Tauranga: Moana Press, 1988), 15.

30 A. N. McGregor, *A system of surgical nursing* (Glasgow: David Bryce, 1905), 14.

31 C. P. Childe, *Surgical nursing and technique: A book for nurses, dressers, house surgeons, etc.* (London: Bailliere, Tindall & Cox, 1920), vii.

32 Pamela J. Wood, 'The enduring issue of assessing nursing knowledge: Surgical nursing final examinations in Australia and New Zealand, 1905–1930', *Contemporary Nurse*, 32:1–2 (2009), 109–122.

33 'State examinations', *Kai Tiaki*, 5:3 (1912), 12–18; 15.

34 'State examinations', *Kai Tiaki*, 21 (1928), 190–191.

35 'State examinations in medical, surgical, midwifery and maternity nursing held in December 1929', *Kai Tiaki*, 23:1 (1930), 65–88; 78.

36 Tatham, 'Sepsis', 219.

37 Oxford, *A handbook of nursing*, 4.

38 M. A. Gullan, *Theory and practice of nursing* (London: H. K. Lewis & Co, 1920), 5.

39 Humphrey, *A manual of nursing*, 163.

40 W. T. Gordon Pugh, *Practical nursing, including hygiene and dietetics* (Edinburgh: William Blackwood, 1937), 5.

41 A. M. Ashdown, *A complete system of nursing* (London: J. M. Dent & Sons, 1939), 3.

42 Kristeva, *Powers of horror*.

43 Ashdown, *A complete system of nursing*, 3.

44 F. Gill, 'Ward teaching', *Kai Tiaki*, 22 (1929), 181–185; 184.

45 I. Gill, *The lamp still burns: Nursing in Victoria 1936–1981 – an autobiographical account* (Bendigo: Bendigo College of Advanced Education, 1989), 92.

46 E. Divens, 'Healing and treatment of wounds', *British Journal of Nursing*, 79 (1931), 94–95 and 124–125; 124.

47 A. Bashford, *Purity and pollution: Gender, embodiment and Victorian medicine* (London: Palgrave MacMillan, 1998), 128.

48 Humphrey, *A manual of nursing*, 164.

49 Chambers, *My life in nursing*, 21.

50 Ferguson, 'The operating room'. See also Bishop, 'Lectures to nurses on antiseptics in surgery', 131; 'The importance of asepsis'. For examination questions on this topic, see 'State examination of nurses', *Kai Tiaki*, 4:3 (1911), 121–124; 'Examination questions and answers', *Australasian Nurses' Journal*, 4 (1906) 114–115; 'Answers to examination papers', *Australasian Nurses' Journal*, 7 (1909), 368–70; 'Answers to examination papers', *Australasian Nurses' Journal*, 9 (1911), 239–41; 'Answers to examination papers', *Australasian Nurses' Journal*, 10 (1912), 22–24; 'Answers to examination papers', *Australasian Nurses' Journal*, 12 (1914), 24–32. 'Answers to examination papers', *Australasian Nurses' Journal*, 12 (1914), 315–318; 'Answers to examination papers', *Australasian Nurses' Journal*, 13 (1915), 397–402.

51 See, for example, A. Miles, *Surgical ward work and nursing: A handbook for nurses and others* (London: Scientific Press, 1921), 10–19; Woodall, *Outline of surgical nursing*, 43–73; Rutherford Darling, *Surgical nursing* (1923, 1928, 1932, 1938), 142–146, 150–154, 162–167, and 162–166, respectively.

52 Moorhead, 'Preparation of a patient'; 'Ante-operative and post-operative care'; 'State examination of nurses', *Kai Tiaki*, 7 (1914), 151–155; 'State examination of nurses', *Kai Tiaki*, 13 (1920), 163–167; 'Examination questions and answers'; 'Answers to examination papers', *Australasian Nurses' Journal*, 10 (1912), 22–24; 'Examination for membership, 1916', *Australasian Nurses' Journal*, 15 (1917), 104–108; 'Australasian Trained Nurses' Association, examination for membership, best paper (unaltered)', *Australasian Nurses' Journal*, 18 (1920), 6–9.

53 See, for example, Childe, *Surgical nursing*, frontispiece; Rutherford Darling, *Surgical nursing* (1932), 140.

54 Divens, 'Healing and treatment of wounds', 124.

55 Bishop, *Lectures on surgical nursing*, 21.

56 For information about antiseptics, for example, see Howard, *Surgical nursing* (1908, 1920), 45–50 and 48–49, respectively.

57 See, for example, Divens, 'Healing and treatment of wounds'; C. MacLaurin, 'The nursing of abdominal operations', *Australasian Nurses' Journal*, 7 (1909), 385–90, reprinted from the *Nursing Mirror*; Tatham, 'Sepsis'. For military terms, see E. Bedford Fenwick, 'Elementary anatomy, as applied to nursing', *British Journal of Nursing*, 12 (1894), 291–292; MacLaurin, 'The nursing of abdominal operations'; 'The after care of operation cases: The general treatment of post-operative cases',

Australasian Nurses' Journal, 17 (1919), 381–6, reprinted from the
South African Nursing Record; Moorhead, 'Preparation of a patient';
H. J. Paterson, 'Lecture. The preparation for and after-treatment of
abdominal operations', *British Journal of Nursing*, 85 (1937), 68–69.

58 Hadley, *Nursing*, 250.

59 Bishop, *Lectures on surgical nursing*, 13.

60 Divens, 'Healing and treatment of wounds', 94–95.

61 *Ibid.*, 95.

62 *Ibid.*, 124.

63 Gullan, *Theory and practice of nursing*, 5.

64 Gill, *The lamp still burns*, 92.

65 See, for example, H. A. Chapman and A. K. Anderson, 'Things rank and
gross in nature: A review and synthesis of moral disgust', *Psychological
Bulletin*, 139 (2013), 300–327; V. A. Curtis, 'Dirt, disgust and disease:
A natural history of hygiene', *Journal of Epidemiology & Community
Health*, 61 (2007), 660–664.

66 Humphrey, *A manual of nursing*, 163.

67 Gill, *The lamp still burns*, 92.

68 P. J. Wood, 'Supporting or sabotaging the surgeon's efforts: portrayals
of the surgical nurse's role in preventing wound sepsis, 1895–1935',
Journal of Clinical Nursing, 18 (2009), 2739–2746.

69 T. M. Group and J. Roberts, *Nursing, physician control, and the medical monopoly: Historical perspectives on gendered inequality in roles,
rights, and range of practice* (Bloomington: Indiana University Press,
2001); J. A. Ashley, *Hospitals, paternalism, and the role of the nurse*
(New York: Teachers College Press, 1976); B. Melosh, *'The physician's
hand': Work culture and conflict in American nursing* (Philadelphia:
Temple University Press, 1982). For an overview and critique of such
historical interpretations, see, for example, Julie Fairman, 'Not all
nurses are good, not all doctors are bad …', essay review, *Bulletin of
the History of Medicine*, 78 (2004), 451–460.

70 Wood, 'The enduring issue of assessing nursing knowledge'.

71 Howard, *Surgical Nursing* (1908), vii.

72 Paterson, 'Lecture'.

73 'The importance of asepsis'; 'Professional review. Surgical nursing and
technique', *British Journal of Nursing*, 58:1505 (1917), 88–89; 88.

74 Fenwick, 'Elementary anatomy'.

75 This was Ethel Fenwick, Matron of St Bartholomew's Hospital 1881–
1887, founder of the British Nurses Association, founding president of
the International Council of Nurses and editor of the *Nursing Record*,
later the *British Journal of Nursing*.

76 Bishop, *Lectures on surgical nursing*, page facing verso.

77 M. E. Francis, 'Asepsis for the nurse', *Trained Nurse*, 2 (1889), 153 and 160.
78 E. Bolton, 'Teaching surgical nursing', *Canadian Nurse*, 29 (1933), 591–592.
79 H. L. Maitland, 'Lecture on asepsis (continued)', *Australasian Nurses' Journal*, 2 (1905), 120–122; 122.
80 Childe, *Surgical nursing*, 2–3.
81 Miles, *Surgical ward work and nursing*, 191 and 31.
82 McGregor, *A system of surgical nursing*, 17.
83 Childe, *Surgical nursing*, 1–2. See also his later editions. See also 'The surgical nurse', *Australasian Nurses' Journal*, 21 (1923), 264.
84 'The surgical nurse', 264.
85 C. B. Keetley, 'The care of surgical instruments', *Australasian Nurses' Journal*, 6 (1908), 304–307.
86 H. L. Maitland, 'Lecture on asepsis', *Australasian Nurses' Journal*, 2 (1904), 87–92, quotation on p. 91. See also E. Roberton, 'The origin of antiseptic methods', *Kai Tiaki*, 3 (1910), 23–27.
87 Chambers, *My life in nursing*, 21.
88 See, for example, G. Yeo, *Nursing at Bart's: A history of nursing service and nurse education at St Bartholomew's Hospital, London* (Stroud: Alan Sutton Publishing, 1995), 74.
89 Francis, 'Asepsis for the nurse', 153.
90 C. Aikens, 'The care of the hands', *Australasian Nurses' Journal*, 6 (1908), 237–239.
91 'Surgical training of nurses', *Australasian Nurses Journal*, 19 (1921), 126–127.
92 'Operating room procedures for nurses', *British Journal of Nursing*, 85 (1937), 80.
93 Amy A. Armour, 'What a pupil nurse should know when she leaves the operating room', *Trained Nurse and Hospital Review*, 6 (1914), 339–342.
94 Tatham, 'Sepsis', 219.
95 John Tosh, *The pursuit of history: Aims, methods and new directions in the study of modern history* (London: Routledge, 2013).

4

Septic subjects: infection and occupational illness in British hospitals, *c.* 1870–1970

Claire L. Jones

In 1936, Robert Handfield-Jones, Surgeon to the Outpatients Department at St Mary's Hospital London, opened his lecture on infections of the fingers and hand by asking his post-graduate audience to

> picture yourselves lying in bed with an infected hand and forearm. Three days ago, you had a simple infection in the distal segment of the finger, of which you thought little, and to-day, feeling desperately ill, you face the horror of a spreading lymphangitis up your forearm and arm, and you dare not think of the possibilities which may lie ahead.[1]

The dramatic opening of Handfield-Jones's lecture not only aimed to raise awareness among medical students of how dangerous infected fingers and hands could be for their patients, but was also a direct message about what they could expect if they themselves became infected and chose to ignore it. Handfield-Jones's message was all the more powerful given the fact that the hospital had lost one its 'most brilliant surgeons' that year as the result of a slight prick of a finger. 'It should need no such tragedy' continued Handfield-Jones, 'to bring home to us the importance of these infections.'[2]

Handfield-Jones's aim in his lecture then, and in its subsequent publication in the *Lancet*, was to encourage doctors to take seriously the well-known but largely ignored medical malady, septic finger. 'Septic finger' or 'poison finger', common terms used by nurses and doctors for a bacterial infection of the distal pulp, typically resulted from an open wound or cut on the hand or finger, and in the most serious cases, septicaemia could follow. Handfield-Jones's lecture reflected a wider and long-running concern within medicine and nursing that working with patients within the confines of a hospital could be a serious occupational risk. Indeed, two of the most famous medical figures to die from contracting an infection at work were Curt Schimmelbusch (1860–1895), German inventor of the Schimmelbusch anaesthetic mask, who died at the age of thirty-five due to a septic infection caught in the operating room, and Charles B. Lockwood (1856–1914), British pioneer of asepsis, who died from an infection he contracted in an operation on a patient with peritonitis.[3] Hand injuries were common among industrial workers, but surgeons and nurses, Handfield-Jones argued, faced their 'own peculiar dangers in the surgery, the operating theatre and the post-mortem room', as well as on the ward. Indeed, by the late nineteenth century, septic afflictions were relatively common; hospitals and surgeons like Handfield-Jones took steps to limit their effects on their medical workforce, including offering guidance stating that individuals should cease work on noticing a wound, should cleanse it and, by the 1930s, take a course of Prontosil injections. Surgery would be the treatment of last resort.

This chapter examines how doctors and nurses experienced septic finger, wound sepsis and related diseases (such as erysipelas) within the British hospital between 1870 and 1970. Its focus on sepsis, as opposed to other types of infection, is significant. Hospital staff were, of course, at risk of contracting all manner of diseases. Yet, widespread concern over sepsis and hospital attempts at prevention and control in pre- and post-operative wounds not only form an interesting but often neglected part of the story, but also span this hundred-year period as well as recent history with rising antibiotic resistance and hospital mismanagement of infections.[4] While other infections tend to fit more neatly into epidemic periodic cycles, wound sepsis was and still is a continual chronic challenge, one that becomes more important following a serious outbreak or death.

Drawing on hospital ledgers and reports, this chapter pays particular attention to occurrences of wound sepsis among staff at four of Britain's large teaching hospitals, two in England – King's College Hospital (KCH) and St Thomas' Hospital – and two in Scotland – the Royal Infirmary of Edinburgh (RIE) and Glasgow Royal Infirmary (GRI). These hospitals, with their large patient and staff populations and experimental practices aligned with medical instruction, were of course atypical among British medical institutions. General hospitals outnumbered teaching hospitals (of which there were twenty-four in England and Wales by 1911) twenty-five times over.[5] Nonetheless, these four hospitals are important. Not only did these hospitals consistently contain among the largest populations of staff and patients across this long time period, providing great potential for cross infection, but also they were among the first to introduce preventative practices aimed at minimising outbreaks in every different age of infection. For example, RIE, GRI and KCH were associated with the late nineteenth- and early twentieth-century wound sepsis control practices of the surgeon Joseph Lister, while St Thomas' was strongly associated with the hygiene practices of Florence Nightingale.[6] All four of these hospitals were also among the first to institute therapeutic sulphonamide and antibiotic regimes and to establish preventative infection control committees from the 1930s. A more detailed and long-term analysis of these case study hospitals, then, provides us with a clearer insight into the importance of practice on the ground, and enables us to better identify the nuances between hospital management and individual infection management.

Yet, while surgeons like Handfield-Jones and the hospitals in which they worked were keenly aware of the health risks from sepsis across this one-hundred-year period, few historians have explicitly addressed the occupational health of practitioners of medicine and associated work risks. Understandably, historians have tended to focus on the impact of infections on patient health with little attention given to the health of staff.[7] Part of this neglect may be explained by the fact that medicine and nursing were never classed as 'dangerous trades' within the nineteenth and twentieth centuries' occupational health movements, and were unlikely to be considered dangerous while manufacturing and mining were still major employers.[8] Nonetheless, historians are beginning to focus on the medical practitioner as a subject of infection; Thomas Schlich and Ulrich Tröhler have analysed professional risk in relation to the introduction of new medical innovations, particularly surgical gloves.[9] Schlich, in particular, argues that the introduction of gloves into surgical procedures in the 1880s and 1890s was to protect the operator from infection, not the patient, an argument he develops further in this volume.[10] In her book, *Who Cared for the Carers?*

(2014), Debbie Palmer offers a history of the occupational health of nurses within the London Hospital, Cornwall Asylum and South Devon and East Cornwall Hospital, arguing that hospital occupational illness for nurses was tightly bound up with issues of class and gender.[11] Robert Woods provides a brief demographic survey on the health and mortality of Victorian doctors, arguing that members of the Victorian medical profession were not protected by their own 'healing art', and that their life chances were poor when compared with other professional groups and even with the male population as a whole.[12]

By extending this focus on occupational health and risk to specific hospitals during a longer time period and by narrowing the focus to one type of illness, it will become more evident that the introduction and implementation of preventative hospital infection control procedures were not solely for the benefit of patients, but also for the staff who treated them. This chapter builds on Palmer's work on nurses to demonstrate that, in the case of wound sepsis, occupational health was not only reflective of issues of class and gender but was also bound up with professionalism, and prompted a discourse of blame and responsibility across the nursing and medical professions. Failures in infection control (through outbreaks of infection) not only represented a hospital failure, but also meant blame and responsibility was assigned to the individual staff who had contracted the infection. Monitoring the health of the workforce, and differential exposure to risk, was not only used to measure hospital efficiency, but also formed an important yet neglected part of hospital-wide policy to tackle infection. It is, however, worth pointing out that occupational 'risk' is not necessarily a term with which our historic actors would have been familiar; 'risk' is a relatively recent and increasingly applied concept within medical literature and current practice, reflecting in part modern litigation culture and the benchmarked standards of the National Health Service (NHS).[13]

In what follows then, the chapter is divided into two main sections: the first will focus on nurses' health between around 1880 and 1929, when infection control procedures in the form of antisepsis and asepsis were introduced and consolidated and when nursing was becoming professionalised. The second part of this chapter will focus on interactions between doctors and nurses between 1930 and the 1960s, a period in which sulphonamides and antibiotics were successfully used to treat bacterial infections, followed by rising cross infection and the re-emergence of practices of hygiene and surgical cleanliness.

Nurse health, nursing responsibilities, 1880–1929

Towards the end of the nineteenth century, the medical press displayed increasing alarm at the rising mortality and ill health of the profession. Following the reading of a paper on this topic before the Royal Medical and Chirurgical Society in 1886 by Statistical Superintendent at the General Register Office, London, Dr William Ogle (1827–1912), the *Lancet* announced that 'medical mortality is twice, or thrice, or even more times greater than the average'.[14] Drawing on statistics compiled using the most recent census, Ogle argued that there had been a general increase in mortality among the medical profession since 1861 and that the 'mortality of medical men from scarlet fever, typhus, diphtheria, enteric fever, malarial fever, and erysipelas is very largely in excess of the average'.[15] Ogle demonstrated that of men from the 'middle or professional classes' aged between twenty-five and sixty-four for the years 1880, 1881 and 1882, only innkeepers and publicans, brewers, earthenware manufacturers and cutlers had substantially higher death rates than members of the medical profession.

While the medical press began to report the high incidence of disease and mortality rates from the same afflictions among medical practitioners, the governors of hospitals began to monitor the health of their probationer nurses. Probationer nurses not only came into contact with infected patients more regularly than consulting physicians or surgeons, and were thus considered particularly susceptible to illness in their early years of training, but they were also the least experienced in controlling sepsis.[16] Regimes of ward hygiene, personal cleanliness, antisepsis and asepsis were introduced on wards, in operating theatres and into the nursing and medical curricula for the benefit of both patients and staff. Indeed, Florence Nightingale's 1878 report on the sanitary state of the hospital went some way to instigating reform of hygiene practices within St Thomas' Hospital and its associated nurse training school, the Nightingale Training School, established in 1860. The report outlined the 'disastrous

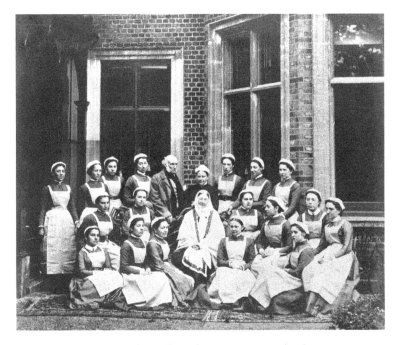

Figure 4.1 F. Nightingale and Sir H. Verney; Claydon House.

practice' of disposing of soiled dressings in buckets rather than laundry chutes before they were washed by a ward maid and boiled in the ward kitchen; the danger of cleaning ward floors only once every six weeks; and the poor ventilation in the wards, particularly at night. Outbreaks of erysipelas, Nightingale stated, rarely led to the closure of wards; bedding often came back from disinfection 'dirtier than when [it] went in', and traces of pus or evacuations could be sometimes seen on 'clean' sheets. These 'uncleanly' practices, Nightingale argued, were not only contributing to the continued ill health of the patients but made probationers sick, especially those working early and late shifts in the wards.[17]

Despite the introduction of hygienic practices that new nurses from the 1870s were expected to carry out and benefit from, a small number of staff still became ill. Extant staff and ward registers from KCH, St Thomas', GRI and RIE provide information about every nurse who entered the hospitals' training schools, including their illness record. These registers highlight the frequency and length of time nurses were 'warded' (i.e. looked after on the ward), and sometimes the reason for their ill health. The earliest of these, from St Thomas' dating from 1871 to 1892, reveals that approximately 9 per cent of the 660 nurses, ward maids and servants listed continued to suffer from ill health, even after hygiene practices were introduced in the 1880s.[18] Around one-third of this 9 per cent were ward maids, who were responsible for cleaning the wards. The fact that many ward maids were ill may suggest that their hygiene practices were still wanting, but the register instead gives the impression that many of them suffered from ill health before the hospital employed them by stating 'health insufficient'. As many of these ward maids were drawn from the local poor communities that the hospital intended to serve – Lambeth and Southwark – the ill health of these workers is perhaps unsurprising; many left after their first bout of illness and never returned.

Nurses constituted the remaining two-thirds of those suffering from ill health recorded in this register, many of whom also resigned on account of their poor health. While this register contains few details about type of illness, it does report that three nurses died, two of typhoid fever in 1873–1874 before systems of sanitation, hygiene and sewerage had become standardised across the hospital. Yet, unlike with ward maids, nurses who became ill were often blamed for their own careless practice. Unlike scarlet fever or similar diseases, sepsis was viewed as entirely preventable in this era of sanitary reform and regarded as an individual's failure to adhere to the new sanitary rules laid out by the hospital. Indeed, Joseph Lister pointed out that post-operative infection after the introduction of antisepsis was no longer due to chance.[19] The provision of Florence Nightingale's 1878 *Memorandum as to Finger Poisoning etc on beginning Ward Work* to every new probationer on their entry to the Nightingale Training School, for example, aimed to provide nurses with strict rules to prevent septic finger.[20] The memorandum rules pointed out that nurses should look upon anything that had soiled their fingers as a possible source of contagion to others and to themselves, and that they should take every care possible to ensure that fingers, hands and nails were scrupulously clean, particularly before putting on new dressings and after touching a patient. The school provided each new probationer with their own carbolic soap in its own soap tin, which they were instructed never to fail to bring to the ward each morning and evening. Also included was the following note: 'No nurse who, being warned, poisons her finger is fit to be a Nurse. If she cannot take care of her own cleanliness, how can she take care of her patient's?'

While the registers for the same period for RIE and for KCH are wanting, the health of staff at these hospitals was sometimes reported in annual reports. The reports of RIE commented that there was a 'good deal of sickness' among staff in the 1880s, three serious cases of illness in 1892–1893 (including one case of erysipelas) and at least one nurse death per year in the 1890s.[21] At KCH, the health of nurses was contained in minutes of the monthly meeting of the nursing committee, and as at St Thomas', an average of between 5 per cent and 9 per cent of nurses were reportedly ill each month.[22] In December 1893, KCH was struck with a particularly bad influenza epidemic, during which 20 per cent of nurses were off sick.[23] Special probationer Collison was so ill during her training that she had 233 days off sick during her two years of training. She left shortly after. Between the 1870s and 1890s then, hospitals recorded up to a 9 per cent illness rate among nurses and were prepared for up to 10 per cent of their nurses to be 'warded' at any one time. Hospitals employed extra nurses and probationers, who could be deployed to any given ward at any given time. In 1891, for example, KCH had twelve extra nurses available in case of illness.[24]

While the records of KCH, St Thomas', GRI and RIE were often vague about the specific diseases from which nurses were suffering before the 1890s, registers from these hospitals began to more clearly distinguish wound sepsis, boils, septicaemia and erysipelas from other ailments towards the end of the nineteenth century. Between 1895 and 1915, the number of probationer nurses at St Thomas' Hospital off duty as the result of ill health remained at approximately 5 per cent, but 'septic finger' and occurrences of wounds sepsis in other parts of the body was recorded in the registers with notable frequency. In her second year of training in 1913, Catherine Duncan was off duty for 128 days for septic foot and left her training at the end of three years. In 1917, charge nurse Irene Guthrie had acute septicaemia affecting a knee joint, returning to her native India to recover. Flora Nairn, a second-year probationer, and Agnes Meade, Jane Spencer and Rosaline Ruddock, all first-year

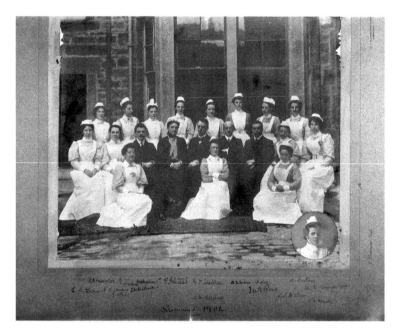

Figure 4.2   Group portrait, Royal Infirmary Edinburgh, 1904.

probationers, caught erysipelas in 1904, 1911 and 1912, respectively, and all were 'warded' for approximately three months.[25] At the RIE in 1918, twenty-one probationers from a cohort of approximately 300 left, sixteen of those for health reasons.[26] Similarly, Dr William Branson's enquiry into the health of nurses at St Bartholomew's Hospital suggested that sepsis was a prominent cause of absence among nurses between 1922 and 1931.[27]

The increased visibility of septic conditions in the hospitals' records from the 1890s were a likely reflection of changing disease categorisations in this period based on a wider acceptance of the existence and nature of microorganisms and the growing importance of bacteriology within medicine, but such visibility also suggested that expanding numbers of nurses were suffering from such conditions. The increased recording of septic conditions converged with new ideas that suggested that a hospital was responsible for the health of its nurses; such ideas challenged but did not overrule the perception that the nurse was to blame for her own ill health. While those at the Nightingale Training School during the 1890s recalled it being a disgrace to acquire a septic finger and were required to report a pricked finger to the ward sister at once, there was now wider public concern over working conditions within new nurse training schools, of which the Nightingale Training School was the first.[28] Concerns over nurse working conditions formed part of the debates of the Select Committee on Metropolitan Hospitals during the same decade. A key aim of such debates was to establish whether individuals or hospitals were responsible for rates of poor health and outbreaks of illness among the nurse workforce.[29] Hospitals were, unsurprisingly, reluctant to accept responsibility for nurse ill health. As histories of nineteenth-century nursing outline, much of this reluctance was bound up with opposition to nursing reform in this period.[30] Opponents to reform often considered inheritable character as more important to nursing than skills and knowledge that one could acquire. Palmer has argued that the formidable Matron Eva Lückes did little to tackle rates of illness among her nursing staff at the London Hospital because she viewed illness as symbolic of their weakness of character and their unsuitability for nursing as a career.[31] Palmer has suggested that Lückes thought the new type of 'lady' middle-class probationer nurse being admitted to the new type of nurse training school was unable to cope with the strenuous workload and thus became ill. In Lückes' view, nurses who became ill needed to be dismissed rather than cared for.[32]

Probationer nurses at St Thomas' and KCH from a middle-class background were seemingly subject to the same disdain from the hospitals' matrons, Louisa Gordon and Katherine Monk, respectively, and claims of ill health due to overwork and poor conditions were often dismissed. Responding to the Select Committee testimony of Isabel Entwisle, a probationer nurse at St Thomas' hospital, who entered the Nightingale School in 1883 and suggested that the seventy-hour working week of a probationer nurse was making many nurses ill, Matron Gordon stated that nurses were not made to work excessively, that most nurses did not break down as Entwisle suggested and that those who found it excessive were not 'cut out' for a career in nursing. Of the ten hours a day that a nurse worked, Gordon said they spent a lot of that time sitting down. She pointed out that only seven probationers out of thirty-four were ill during February 1891.[33] Similarly, Matron Monk defended KCH's treatment of nurses. Responding to the claim that nursing could take ten years off a nurse's life, Monk stated that after sixteen years in nursing, she had never been so well.[34] Gordon and Monk were also quick to point out that illness rates were so low among both patients and staff precisely because the majority of nurses were able to successfully put into practice preventative hygienic systems. Monk claimed that fewer nurses at KCH became ill than at other hospitals due to the 'excellent arrangement for our linen, which, I think, is a great safeguard to them in each ward'. She explained,

> There are circular hermetically sealed drain pipes; one is for infectious linen only, and the moment the linen is removed from the patient's bed it is thrown down this drain-pipe chute and so dropped instantly into carbolic acid; and the other is for ordinary linen, noninfectious; so that the infectious linen is never kept two seconds in the wards after removal from the bed, but simply dropped down this chute into the carbolic acid.[35]

Despite the disdain towards those considered unsuitable for nursing, hospitals did provide care in obvious cases of sepsis, where symptoms of fever and inflammation were manifest; hospital governors understood that they not only had a duty of care to their staff, but that it financially benefited them to do so. After all, it was extremely costly to train up a nurse to the required standard over the course of two or three years, particularly when lodging and board were included, and then to lose their expertise due to illness for any length of time. Many were also paid a wage. The RIE stated in 1890, 'if the health of the Nurses is to be maintained, and if the patients are to receive the adequate and careful nursing so essential to their recovery, the building of the New Home, with increased accommodation, was an urgent necessity and could not be delayed'.[36] The Nightingale Home also had a sickroom for probationers, although many nurses lay in wards when ill and were looked after by resident medical officers.[37] If nurses became too gravely ill or required convalescing, they were sent to convalesce by the sea or in the countryside. St Thomas' nurses were sent to Archer House in Ramsgate on the Kent coast. On their return to St Thomas', recovered nurses took on the role of extra nurse or were given the role of assistant housekeeper, presumably to allow them to get back into work without the responsibility of working with patients straight away. The RIE had a home in Pitlochry 'at the service of invalided nurses', which was supplemented by a rest home in North Berwick and another, Blair House, nearer Edinburgh in 1898.[38] In 1900, the RIE board reported that a timely residence at the house has saved many nurses from a breakdown. It had 242 visits in 1902.[39]

The cost of caring for nurses with some form of sepsis could be particularly high, as nurses were taken off duty as soon as it was reported and did not return until their hospital could be sure they had fully recovered. Nurses with such ailments were perhaps not in as critical a condition as those with scarlet fever but were often incapacitated for a longer period of time. The aforementioned Nurse Duncan was off the wards for 128 days for her septic foot, and nurses were off duty on average for nearly seventy days with a septic finger, while others with scarlet fever and so on were often off duty for approximately sixty days. Indeed, cases at St Thomas' when nurses returned to duty too early were liable to further outbreaks. Bella Dawson Taylor, a probationer in her second year of training, was warded and then sent to Archer House with a poisoned finger in 1911. She returned after two months' sick leave and developed a septic wrist in February 1912, a boil of the chest in August 1912 and a carbuncle on the neck in March 1913.[40] Yet, removing infected staff from wards was considered crucial for preventing the further spread of infection.

Maintaining standards, sharing responsibility, 1930–1965

Some historians have argued that the introduction of antibiotic therapy redefined the role of the British nurse from the 1940s because it undermined traditional nursing techniques, but the evidence I present will show that there was a continued emphasis on hygiene and preventative measures alongside the use of new therapeutics.[41] Hospital records demonstrate that the use of certain therapeutics reduced the incidence of specific diseases like diphtheria and scarlet fever among patients and staff, but staff risk of contracting wound sepsis remained. In fact, the average daily number of nurses off duty annually through illness at the RIE rose in 1937–1938 to 5.4 from an average of 4 in the previous years and decades.[42] Increasing

concerns over hospital-acquired infection, wound-infecting haemolytic *Streptococcus* and the increasingly virulent *Staphylococcus* bacteria and antibiotic resistance meant that the importance of hygiene
and sanitation never went away in this period. It only strengthened
the apparent connection between staff illness and faulty aseptic
practice, and emphasised the hospital's role in providing sufficient
instruction, while broadening the type of staff deemed responsible
for maintaining aseptic standards.

Continued sepsis outbreaks and longstanding emphases on the
importance of hygienic practice on the wards meant that nurses
still bore much of the blame and responsibility for afflictions like
septic finger. Hannah Easson, who began her nurse training at the
RIE in 1939, reported that septic finger 'was terrible … that was
a dreadful thing' because it was considered the nurse's own fault.
Easson recalled nurses getting a 'big telling off' and being sent to
the sick room to get it dressed once they had dutifully reported
it.[43] From the 1930s, the hospitals also more explicitly emphasised
how nurses could minimise their risk of acquiring such infections.
Lecture notes of Mary McLaren Grimwalde (nee Galloway) of
the RIE in 1935, for example, suggest that nurses gave themselves

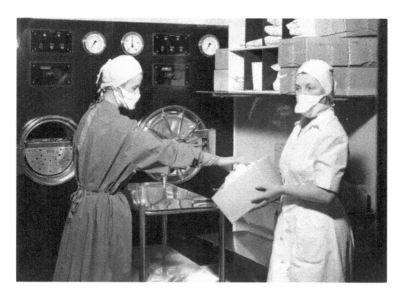

Figure 4.3   Nurses sterilising badges, King's College Hospital, *c.* 1960.

bacteriological examinations, presumably by throat swabbing, while new nurses at the GRI burns unit were required to submit throat swabs, with those testing positive for Streptococci isolated or sent off duty.[44]

Responding to the perceived problem of wound sepsis and increasing cross infection in British hospitals in the interwar period, the Preventive Medicine Committee of the Medical Research Council (MRC) began to publish reports to both influence aseptic practice within the hospital and encourage nurses to take greater responsibility for maintaining disinfection and sterilisation standards. The council's 1941 report, *The Prevention of 'Hospital Infection' of Wounds*, for example, suggested that nurses may be to blame for septic finger: 'among the likely contributory causes of septic fingers are the handling of infected dressings, the over-zealous scrubbing of the hands with a nail brush (sometimes kept in a bowl of disinfectant of dubious activity), and the washing of soiled bandages by hand, to remove discolouring matter before they are boiled'.[45] This report was widely distributed around the KCH nursing cohort; the hospital had at least five copies.[46] The Council's next report of 1944, *The Control of Cross Infection in Hospitals*, continued to emphasise the importance of 'meticulous' aseptic technique for reducing the risk of sepsis, but also argued that hospitals must play a role in sufficiently training their staff to maintain this technique, thus shifting some responsibility from the nurse to the hospital.[47] Again, this report was distributed to staff at KCH. Matron Evie Opie included her own thoughts on the importance of both individual responsibility and nursing instruction in the frontispiece of her personal copy of this report:

> [The] nurse must imaginatively [be] aware of the risks she is avoiding, and this attitude is not learned from memoranda, however carefully drawn up and attentively read. To acquire it, the nurse must have a sound working knowledge of bacteriology and must be taught to 'think aseptically', as the medical student is taught.[48]

The responsibility of hospitals to both adequately educate and take care of their nursing staff was further emphasised with the establishment of the NHS. While individual hospitals had been responsible for these actions previously (typically under the care of dedicated hospital medical officers), care for the health of nurses under the

NHS was increasingly being shifted to general practitioner services. Many found this inadequate. Douglas Hubble of Derby Hospital stated that 'There are no doubt some things which are better done under the National Health Service, but the medical care of nurses in hospitals is certainly not one of them.'[49]

Despite pressure for improvements under the NHS, perceived problems with nursing practice increased and focused more heavily on sterilisation. The Nuffield Provincial Hospitals Trust's 1958 report, *Present Sterilising Practice in Six Hospitals*, again pointed to failures in nursing practice since the Second World War, specifically 'imperfections in sterilizing technique'.[50] While this report did not explicitly address practices at KCH, St Thomas', GRI or RIE, imperfections in sterilising technique were internally identified at these hospitals. At St Thomas' in 1949, bacteriologist Ronald Hare detailed the inadequacy of the hospital's sterilisation technique and maintained that boiling instruments for just three minutes was inefficient, but remained popular with nurses as it 'economised time'.[51] Bacteriological investigations by the subcommittees on cross infection, sterilisation and infection at KCH in 1952 revealed that over 15 per cent of the so-called sterile dishes were unsterile and that nurses were putting equipment such as lumbar puncture outfits and sub-cutaneous infusion sets into the glove steriliser instead of the autoclave.[52] In 1961, A. C. Cunliffe, KCH's Bacteriologist and newly appointed Sepsis Control Officer, reported that one operator at the hospital had even falsified the graph on the manually operated autoclave and removed dressings unsterilised.[53] Such examples of malpractice formed part of Cunliffe's case for the hospital to establish a Central Sterile Supply Department (CSSD), examples of which began to be established at hospitals across the country from the late 1950s.[54] A CSSD, Cunliffe argued, would reduce the risk of human error and thus, patient and staff infection rates, although the hospital only established its department in 1962.

Nurses were also reportedly cross infecting patients. In 1961, Cunliffe traced an outbreak of Staphylococcal infection in Shepherd Ward at KCH's Belgrave Hospital for Children to a nurse sent off sick with septic finger one week earlier.[55] Cunliffe had been able to piece this information together from the wound infection data that the hospital, and indeed other hospitals, had begun to systematically collect in wards from the mid-1950s from both patients and staff.[56] By 1962, KCH sisters across seventeen wards were responsible for collecting data on types of infection (e.g. chest, urine) and methods of investigation (e.g. swab). Wound books from May 1962 to August 1963 suggest that nurses with septic fingers, nails and toes and spots, boils and carbuncles accounted for up to 14 per cent of all Staphylococcal infections tested, over half of which were Tetracycline resistant.[57] However, KCH compared favourably to the London Hospital, which reported a 20 per cent sickness rate from skin and soft tissue sepsis among the nursing staff in 1959, and St Bartholomew's, which reported a rate of 15 per cent.[58]

Of course, economic considerations of nurses being 'warded' or absent from work due to illness continued into this period, too. Sir Wilson Jameson, the Chief Medical Officer of Health, opened the MRC's 1944 *Control of Cross-Infection* report reminding hospital committees and administrators that 'cross-infection is a steady drain on the hospital purse and efficiency'.[59] David Bailey of the Surgical Unit at University College London called Staphylococcal infections in nurses an 'economic burden' and said they have a 'nuisance value out of all proportion to their severity; for, even when a lesion is trivial, the nurse must be removed from contact with patients until it has healed completely'.[60] Again, it was not simply that a septic finger could 'easily impair a man's working capacity for life' but also that it resulted in vast hospital costs in terms of extra staff and care facilities. Figures are wanting for many hospitals, but the London Hospital reported in 1959 that 1,249 days, an average of five to eight days for each nurse, were lost through septic infection.[61]

Yet, it is important to note that responsibility and blame for sepsis outbreaks among hospital staff was also broadened in this period as cross-hospital cooperation became crucial to infection control, and as the expertise of the bacteriologist and their emphasis on hospital ecology began to be taken more seriously by hospital management.[62] Rising rates of sepsis and cross infection in hospitals and reports of the staff deaths, such as that of the unnamed surgeon at St Mary's Hospital that opened this chapter, brought home the importance of such infections to those outside of nursing. Indeed, the aforementioned MRC's 1944 report on control of cross infection emphasised the role of all hospital staff, not just nurses. KCH distributed it to every medical officer and theatre attendant, as well as all nursing staff. The hospital's first cross-infection subcommittee of 1945 comprised of Edward Creed, the Director of the Pathological Department, three pathologists, several surgeons, the sister matron, the sister tutor and the theatre sister, all of whom fed information back to their department or ward. This committee, as well as others like it at other hospitals, recommended the medical examination of all staff via a throat swab before work in wards and operating theatres commenced. A 1939 study of nose and skin swabs from University College Hospital suggested that three out of four theatre staff (including surgeons, theatre and wards nurses, dressers and patients) were nasal carriers of *Staphylococcus*, while Hare's 1949 report for St Thomas' outlined that a high proportion of sepsis in wounds over the past ten years was due to the implantation of organisms on the raw tissues from the nose, throat or hands of the dressers and attendants.[63] These results seemed to correlate with the *Lancet*'s review of the current literature on this topic in 1949 that 40 per cent to 50 per cent of contacts carried coagulase-positive Staphylococci in the nose and upwards of 20 per cent on the hands.[64] In winter 1958/1959, the RIE suggested that 56 per cent of hospital personnel were nasal carriers of *Staphylococcus*.[65] Nasal antibiotic therapy was seen as one solution and given to KCH staff during a 1964 outbreak.[66]

However, while nurses had stringent reporting practices for finger pricks and often felt ashamed of septic finger and errors in practice, some doctors were not quite so diligent or humble. Part of the point of Handfield-Jones's 1936 lecture had been to encourage medical students to take it seriously, albeit with disappointing results. Research conducted in eight hospitals in 1951 by J. W. Goodall, a former member of the team investigating the function and design of hospitals for the Nuffield Provincial Hospitals Trust, found that 'if a doctor is unwell, whether with a cold or anything else, he is a law unto himself'. Unlike nurses who were instantly taken off the ward, Goodall found that the doctor with sepsis generally ignored the complaint and continued to do his ward rounds.[67] Non-medical staff at KCH suggested in 1959 that senior medical staff were among the worst offenders of neglecting aseptic procedures, while Professor William Henry Reid, Head of the hospital's Burns Unit, stated that doctors at GRI were often more casual about these procedures than nurses.[68] Speaking at a conference on hospital infection control in 1963,

R. E. M. Thompson, Bacteriologist to the Middlesex Hospital, warned about the dangers of the senior medics having the worst day-to-day asepsis – 'surgeons lifting the corners of dressings to peep at wounds, operating with their noses outside of their masks etc.' – because they are the very people medical students and nurses imitate.[69] Some doctors' neglect of aseptic hygiene practices for the benefit of their own health, as well as their patients', suggests that they continued to consider this nurses' work, as it had been since the late nineteenth century. Indeed, the *British Medical Journal*'s statement in 1944 that 'the nurse is the most closely concerned in these matters' seems to reflect a wider attitude among the medical profession that there were strict divisions between the nursing and medical professions.[70]

Conclusion

Wound sepsis and related diseases formed part and parcel of the occupational risk taken by nurses and other medical staff in hospitals in Britain between 1870 and 1970. In the first half of this period to the 1930s, up to 10 per cent of hospital nursing staff could be warded at any one time. While few seemingly died from sepsis, it was reportedly a common cause of absence from work, despite the implementation of sanitary measures and regulations to prevent and monitor it. It often took nurses much longer to recover from sepsis-related afflictions than from diseases like scarlet fever. Sepsis was still a prominent cause of nurse illness after the introduction of effective drug therapies in the 1930s. Rising cross infection rates and prominent deaths such as the unnamed surgeon from St Mary's Hospital, led hospitals and the government to take greater steps to reduce the incidence rates of Staphylococcal and Streptococcal infections through the establishment of infection control committees and more stringent standardised preventive practices. Yet, as other chapters in this collection have suggested, the establishment of committees and development of new practices did not necessarily change working cultures; neither did they eradicate incidence rates of staff infection. Throughout this long period, the health of staff was intimately bound up with discussions of working conditions and regimes of staff care. Conditions notwithstanding, hospitals carried the economic burden of looking after their ill staff often because it was in their financial interest to do so.

Yet, the rates of outbreaks are not our only interest here; how these outbreaks were perceived is equally important. Septic infections among staff were among the most feared throughout the period, not just because they could debilitate individuals for a long time, but also because the discourse surrounding hospital-acquired infections embodied a great degree of blame and responsibility. Septic fingers and the like were considered preventable to a large degree, and thus outbreaks signalled carelessness and/or a lack of professionalism and aseptic standards. Among nurses in the first half of the period, illness was not only viewed as carelessness but also as a character weakness, representing their lack of suitability for the new profession of nursing. Such a view was challenged but not overridden by increased calls for hospitals to provide better care for their nurses. After 1930, nurses still bore much of the burden of maintaining aseptic standards, but the sense of responsibility was more widely distributed and included other types of hospital staff, as well as individual hospitals for providing sufficient nurse training and care. However, in reality, not all medical practitioners were willing to adhere to set standards, suggesting that they still viewed aseptic practice as the responsibility of nurses. Nurses and doctors were seen therefore not only to have competing responsibilities within the hospital, but also very different experiences of occupational health.

This chapter has provided only a brief overview of the effect of sepsis on the hospital workforce and is intended as a stimulus for further work in this area, not least in taking seriously the history of medicine and nursing as occupations with fundamental health risks. Research into sepsis in alternative forms of hospitals and in medical spaces beyond the ward and operating may yield very different results. Yet without further research, it is already clear that there is a great more continuity than change in hospital practice across this hundred-year period. The importance placed on preventive aseptic technique and attending to the hospital environment as first established in the late nineteenth century never went away, even after the introduction of drug therapies. In fact, the hospital environment and maintaining standards of hygiene have become more important in the present with the rising threat of methicillin-resistant *Staphylococcus aureus* (MRSA) and antibiotic resistance.[71]

Notes

1 R. M. Handfield-Jones, 'Infections of fingers and hands', *Lancet*, 228 (10 Oct 1936), 833–836.
2 *Ibid.*, 833.
3 T. Schlich, 'Negotiating technologies in surgery: The controversy about surgical gloves in the 1890s', *Bulletin of the History of Medicine*, 87 (2013), 170–97, 177; T. H. Pennington, 'Listerism, its decline and its persistence: The introduction of aseptic surgical techniques in three British teaching hospitals, 1890–99', *Medical History*, 39 (1995), 35–60, 56.
4 The Mid Staffs NHS Foundation Trust Public inquiry, Independent Inquiry into Care provided by Mid Staffs NHS Foundation Trust January 2005–March 2009, chaired by Robert Francis QC House of Commons 375-1, www.midstaffspublicinquiry.com. Accessed 6 October 2017.
5 R. Pinker, *English hospital statistics, 1861–1938* (London: Heinemann, 1966), 57.
6 M. A. Crowther and M. W. Dupree, *Medical lives in the age of surgical revolution* (Cambridge: Cambridge University Press, 2007); M. E. Baly, *Florence Nightingale and the nursing legacy* (London: Wiley, 2nd edition 1998); and M. Worboys, *Spreading germs* (Cambridge: Cambridge University Press, 2000).
7 For example, G. J. Ayliffe and M. P. English, *Hospital infection: From miasmas to MRSA* (Cambridge: Cambridge University Press, 2003); F. Condrau, 'Standardising infection control: antibiotics and hospital governance in Britain, 1948–1960', in C. Bonah *et al.* (eds), *Harmonizing 20th century drugs: Standards in pharmaceutical history* (Paris: Editions Glyphe, 2009), 327–39; F. Condrau and R. Kirk, 'Negotiating hospital infections: The debate between ecological balance and eradication strategies in British hospitals, 1947–1969', *Dynamis*, 31, 385–405; Pennington, 'Listerism, its decline and its persistence', 35–60.
8 On the nineteenth-century occupational health movement, see, for example, B. Harrison, *'Not only the dangerous trades': Women's work and health in Britain, 1880–1914* (London: Taylor & Francis, 1996).
9 T. Schlich and U. Tröhler (eds), *The risks of medical innovation: Risk perception and assessment in historical context* (London, New York: Routledge, 2006).
10 Schlich, 'Negotiating technologies in surgery'.
11 D. Palmer, *Who cared for the carers?: A history of the occupational health of nurses, 1880–1948* (Manchester: Manchester University Press, 2014); See also D. Palmer, '"To help a million sick, you must

kill a few nurses"': Nurses' occupational health, 1890–1914', *Nursing History Review*, 20 (2012), 14–45.

12 R. Woods, 'Physician, heal thyself: The health and mortality of Victorian doctors', *Social History of Medicine*, 9 (1996), 1–30.

13 P. Griffiths, A. Renz, J. Hughes and A. M. Rafferty, 'Impact of organisation and management factors on infection control in hospitals: A scoping review', *Journal of Hospital Infection*, 73 (2009), 1–14.

14 Tapetum Lucidum, 'Mortality in the medical profession', *Lancet*, 127 (30 Jan 1886), 201; 'Royal Medical and Chirurgical Society', *Lancet*, 127 (30 Jan 1886), 201–4; A. Mantle, 'Mortality from infectious diseases in the medical profession', *Lancet*, 127 (20 Feb 1886), 374.

15 William Ogle, 'Statistics of mortality in the medical profession', *Medico-Chirurgical Transactions*, 69 (1886), 217–237.

16 For the education of nurses in wound sepsis, see C. L. Jones, M. Dupree, I. Hutchison *et al.*, 'Personalities, preferences and practicalities: Educating nurses in wound sepsis in the British Hospital, 1870–1920', *Social History of Medicine*, 31 (2018), 577–604.

17 London Metropolitan Archives (hereafter LMA), Nightingale Collection, A/NFC84/002, F. Nightingale, 'Report of the committee appointed to inquire into the sanitary state of St Thomas'', 1878; LMA, Nightingale Collection, A/FNC84/2, 'Remarks on spread of disease', 1878.

18 LMA, St Thomas' Hospital Archive (hereafter StTH), HO1/ST/C/02/003, 'Ward register 1871–1892, includes ward maids, servants and staff'.

19 Schlich, 'Negotiating technologies in surgery'.

20 LMA, StTH, H01/ST/NTS/C/16/001, F. Nightingale, 'Memorandum for probationers as to finger poisoning etc. on beginning ward work', 1878.

21 Lothian Health Board Archives, Edinburgh (hereafter LHB), 1 4/89–92 Royal Infirmary of Edinburgh, Annual Report, 1889/1890; Royal Infirmary of Edinburgh, Annual Report, 1892/1893; LHB1 4/93–96, Royal Infirmary of Edinburgh, Annual Report, 1893/4; Royal Infirmary of Edinburgh, Annual Report, 1896/1897. Palmer also notes that eight nurses died at the London Hospital between 1888 and 1889. Palmer, *Who cared for the carers?*, 1.

22 King's College Archives, London (hereafter KCHA), KC/N/M1-7, Minutes of the Nursing Committee, 1886–1968.

23 KCHA, KH/G/M1, Annual court of the corporation of the president, vice-president and governor of King's College Hospital, 24 Feb 1892.

24 KCHA, KH/G/M1, Annual Report of King's College Hospital, 1891.

25 StTH, HO1/ST/C3/1, Ledger of probationers who were admitted to posts at St Thomas'.

26 LHB1 4/116–121, Royal Infirmary of Edinburgh, Annual Report, 1918/1919, 29–31.

27 W. Branson, 'The health of nurses', *Lancet* (13 Jan 1934), 91–92.
28 StTH, H01/ST/NTS/Y22, 'Recollections: Miss Izod', 1900. The Nightingale Training School at St Thomas' Hospital was shortly followed by schools at the twelve London teaching hospitals. Carol Helmstadter and Judith Godden, *Nursing before Nightingale, 1815–1899* (Surrey: Ashgate, 2011).
29 See, for example, *Report on the Select Committee of the House of Lords on Metropolitan Hospitals, etc. with the Proceedings of the Committee* (London: HMSO, 1890); *Third Report from the Select Committee of the House of Lords on Metropolitan Hospitals, etc.* (London: HMSO, 1890).
30 B. Abel-Smith, *A history of the nursing profession* (London: Heinemann, 1960 reprinted by Ashgate, 1992); A. M. Rafferty, *The politics of nursing knowledge* (London: Routledge, 1996).
31 Palmer, *Who cared for the carers?* See also K. Waddington, *Charity and the London hospitals, 1850–1898* (Rochester, NY: Royal Historical Society, 2000), 129.
32 Helmstadter and Godden, *Nursing before Nightingale.*
33 StTH, H01/ST/A/053/001, Evidence to the Select Committee on Metropolitan Hospitals, 'Extracts re St. Thomas' Hospital 1891 Feb', 83–92.
34 'Second Report of the Select Committee of the House of Lords on Metropolitan Hospitals, 1890–1. King's College Hospital', *Hansard*, 18924.
35 'Second Report of the Select Committee of the House of Lords on Metropolitan Hospitals, 1890–1. King's College Hospital', *Hansard*, 18912.
36 LHB1 4/89, Royal Infirmary of Edinburgh, Annual Report, 1889/1890, 23.
37 R. Wake, *The Nightingale Training School 1860–1996* (London: Haggerston Press, 1998).
38 LHB1 4/79, Royal Infirmary of Edinburgh, Annual Report, 1879/1880, p. 15; LHB1 4/97, Royal Infirmary of Edinburgh, Annual Report, 1897/1898, p. 53; LHB1 4/98, Royal Infirmary of Edinburgh, Annual Report, 1898/1899.
39 Royal Infirmary of Edinburgh, Annual Report, 1901/1902, 22.
40 StTH, H01/ST/C/03/001, Register of Nightingale probationers who were appointed to posts on the staff of St. Thomas' Hospital, with details of service in the hospital and subsequent appointments, 125.
41 M. E. Baly, *Nursing and social change* (London: Routledge, 1995) 178–192; P. Starns, *Nurses at war: Women on the frontline 1939–45* (Stroud: Sutton Publishing, 2000), 73.
42 Royal Infirmary of Edinburgh, Annual Report, 1937/1938, 34.

43 Royal College of Nursing Archives, T/49, Susan McGann, interview with Hannah Easson, 11 Aug 1992.

44 Royal College of Nursing Archives, C625/2, Mary McLaren Grimwade, nee Galloway, lecture notes, 1935. 'General Nursing lecture 10', 29 Jul 1935; L. Colebrook *et al.*, *Studies of burns and scalds: Reports of the Burns Unit, Royal Infirmary, Glasgow, 1942–43* (London: HMSO, 1944), 35.

45 *The prevention of 'hospital infection' of wounds* (London: Medical Research Council, War Wounds Committee and Committee of London Sector Pathologists, HMSO, 1941).

46 See KCHA, KH/NL/PUB4/10, Publications and personal papers; Ministry of Health and other government reports (HMSO), 1948.

47 *The control of cross infection in hospitals* (London: The Cross Infection in Hospitals Committee of the Medical Research Council, HMSO, 1944).

48 *Ibid.*, KH/NL/PUB4/10, KCHA.

49 D. Hubble, 'The health of nurses in hospitals', *Lancet* (26 Nov 1949), 1110.

50 *Present sterilising practice in six hospitals* (London: The Nuffield Provincial Hospitals Trust, 1958).

51 StTH, H01/ST/A/129/001, General purpose and finance committee minutes and papers', August 1948–1949, report by R. Hare, 'Report to the Board of Governors on the sterilisation procedures used in the hospital and the measures designed to prevent bacterial infection following wounds or the injection of therapeutic substances', 7 Jul 1949.

52 KCHA, KH/MBS/M1, Reports of cross infection subcommittee, 1945–1952, 30 Sep 1952.

53 KCHA, KH/MBS/M2, Reports of the medical committee, including reports of sterilisation and infection subcommittee, 1958–1966, A. C. Cunliffe, 'The case for central sterile supply department', 'Reports of cross infection subcommittee, 1945–52', 27 Sep 1961.

54 *Central sterile supply: principles and practice* (London: The Nuffield Provincial Hospitals Trust, 1963).

55 KCHA, KH/MBS/M2, Reports of the medical committee, including reports of sterilisation and infection subcommittee, 1958–1966, A. C. Cunliffe, 'Report on Belgrave Hospital for Children', 12 Nov 1962.

56 Ayliffe and English, *Hospital infection*, 186.

57 KCHA, KH/MBS/M2, Reports of the medical committee, including reports of sterilisation and infection subcommittee, 1958–1966, '*Staphylococcal* infections', May 1962–Aug 1963.

58 D. M. Davies, '*Staphylococcal* infection in nurses', *Lancet*, 275 (19 Mar 1960), 644–645.

59 *The control of cross infection in hospitals*, 4.
60 D. Bailey, 'Acute infections of the fingers and hand', *Lancet* (26 Jan 1952), 167–171.
61 Davies, '*Staphylococcal* infection in nurses'.
62 K. Hillier, 'Babies and bacteria: phage typing, bacteriologists, and the birth of infection control', *Bulletin of the History of Medicine*, 80 (2006), 733–761.
63 E. A. Devenish and A. A. Miles, 'Control of *Staphylococcus aureus* in an operating theatre', *Lancet* (13 May 1939), 1088–94; Hare, 'Report to the Board of Governors'.
64 '*Staphylococcal* cross-infection', *Lancet* (17 Sep 1949), 518–519.
65 LHB1/80/61, J. Murdoch, Memorandum on *Staphylococcal* infection in the Royal Infirmary, Edinburgh, 1959.
66 KCHA, KH/MBS/M2, Reports of the medical committee, including reports of sterilisation and infection subcommittee, 1958–1966, Cunliffe, 'Sepsis Report', 16 Jun 1965.
67 J. W. D. Goodall, 'Cross-infection in hospital wards: its incidence and prevention', *Lancet*, 259 (19 Apr 1952), 807–809.
68 KCHA, KH/MBS/M2, Reports of the medical committee, including reports of sterilisation and infection subcommittee, 1958–1966, Cunliffe, 'Report of the Cross-Infection Committee', 18 Dec 1959. William Henry Reid, interview with Susan Gardiner, 26 Feb 2015.
69 KCHA, KH/MBS/M2, Reports of the medical committee, including reports of sterilisation and infection subcommittee, 1958–1966, 'Conference on the Personal factor in Hospital infection', 26 Jun 1963.
70 'Cross-infection in hospitals', *British Medical Journal*, 4344 (8 Apr 1944), 497.
71 J. M. M. Boyce and D. M. Pittet, 'Guideline for hand hygiene in health-care settings: Recommendations of the Healthcare Infection Control Practices Advisory Committee and the HICPAC/SHEA/APIC/IDSA Hand Hygiene Task Force', *Infection Control and Hospital Epidemiology*, 23 (S12) (2002), S3–S40; P. Washer and H. Joffe, 'The "Hospital Superbug": Social representations of MRSA', *Social Science & Medicine*, 63 (2006), 2141–2152.

5

Learning the art and science of infection prevention and control: a practical application

Susan Macqueen

This chapter reflects on my experiences and memories of infection control through my nurse training and career. When I started training in the early 1960s, we were required to live in hospital accommodation for the first year. There were no male nurses and no male toilets. We had to be in by 10.30 p.m. and could request a late pass from the warden each month. Too many requests would be reported to matron. Luckily, we were provided with free meals, as my first monthly pay packet gave me £11 in my pocket. Matron had to give permission if you wanted to get married, but this was frowned upon whilst you were training. I undertook my general nurse training at Addenbrooke's Hospital, Cambridge, United Kingdom (1962–1966) and was taught microbiology, common infectious diseases and how to prevent the spread of infection. These themes appeared to be an important part of nursing, though in retrospect the teaching was ritualistic, with little understanding of the application of theory to practice. What was often taught in the nursing school was different to ward practice. The culture on the ward was set by the ward sister who would often have 'her own way of doing things' which may or may not have been influenced by the individual consultant. This, in turn, influenced the behaviour of trained staff who often took delight in confusing you with their knowledge, which in hindsight, was not always correct. For example, different antiseptics and wound dressing changes for the same type of wound, or when to wash your hands during the process. The names and actions of microorganisms were complex, and I could not associate the theory with the practice of nursing: I just knew that if I did not keep things clean, I would be in trouble!

From 1966 to 1968, I spent time as a staff nurse on the children's ward, where babies and young people were admitted with medical and surgical conditions including infectious diseases, such as pertussis, gastro-enteritis, chest infections, chickenpox and measles. I do not remember thinking about the epidemiology of these diseases, let alone whether they were hospital-acquired infections. All babies were nursed in single cubicles at the top end of the ward near sister's desk, and there was one isolation room at the bottom end of the ward by the entrance. Staff wore cotton gowns and a mask when attending the babies or children with contagious infections. Cleaning equipment was on the daily list of duties. I interspersed this tutelage with six months' training in Part 1 Midwifery at Southmead Hospital, Bristol. And from 1968–1969, I went on to the Hospital for Sick Children, Great Ormond Street, London, to do my Paediatric Nurse Training (thirteen months). I became a night sister there in 1969 for one year, during which time I remember overhearing a junior nurse on the Infectious Disease Ward say, 'If that sister asks me one more time where the infection came from, I will scream. How should I know?' I then took up a ward sister's post at the Whittington Hospital, London from 1970–1972, returning to Great Ormond Street Hospital (GOSH) in 1972 as a ward sister on the Medical and Infectious Diseases Ward (Cohen). I became an infection control nurse (ICN) in 1980 and retired in 2011.

As part of nurses' training, my cohort was taught about the history and impact of notable British and European experts who had influenced the identification of infectious diseases and their control. These included the English physician Edward Jenner (1749–1823), who pioneered the use of vaccination; the Hungarian physician Ignaz Semmelweis (1818–1865), who advocated handwashing to prevent puerperal fever in childbirth (caused by the transmission of bacteria from corpses to living bodies); the Victorian nurse and hospital reformer Florence Nightingale (1820–1910), who influenced the implementation of wide-ranging sanitary procedures in hospitals on the basis of her experience in the Crimea; the French physician Louis Pasteur (1822–1895), who formulated the process of pasteurisation, linked bacteria with disease and developed a vaccination for rabies; Joseph Lister (1827–1912), the English physician who founded the aseptic barrier technique in surgery; and Robert

Koch (1843–1910), the German physician widely known for formulating criteria to establish a causal relationship between a causal microbe and a disease (Koch's postulate).[1]

This historical context surrounding cleanliness and the need for good order and system was useful in understanding how and why infection control processes had emerged, but it was not always reflected by good practice. I remember on ward rounds during the 1960s, doctors in their long-sleeved white coats sometimes washing their hands, but junior doctors did not have time to do so before the consultant asked questions about the patients. They certainly did not wash their hands between each patient activity. And it was not until 2010 that the National Patient Safety Agency developed its 'Clean Your Hands' campaign, along with the World Health Organization (WHO) 'First Patient Safety Challenge – Clean Care is Safer Care' campaign on hand hygiene.[2] Up to 6 February 2017, the WHO succeeded in recruiting 19,217 hospitals and healthcare facilities in 177 countries to register their commitment to hand hygiene as part of the global campaign. At GOSH, the staff were slightly more motivated to wash their hands, as they were working with babies and young children. However, there was room for improvement, and consistent compliance took a while for clinical staff to achieve. The results of hand hygiene audits in April 2009 found that in twenty-four out of forty-eight wards and departments (2,659 observations of various staff groups) there was a 92 per cent compliance rate. Of this total, nurses were 99 per cent compliant (959 observations) and doctors 76 per cent (640 observations).[3] A German study of hand hygiene compliance in 2016 confirmed this increase in compliance among paediatric healthcare workers. It demonstrated only small differences between adult and non-adult intensive care units (ICUs), with neonatal ICUs and paediatric non-ICUs maintaining higher compliance than adult care units. Performance among nurses was better than among physicians, and overall rates of hand hygiene performance were significantly higher after patient contact than before.[4] I recollect that when I was a ward sister on the paediatric infectious disease ward, the consultant was very strict about hand-washing and was a good role model. However, I noted on many other wards that any audit results on hand hygiene were generally glossed over by medical staff as 'not done properly, not very scientific or I do not have to wash my hands every time you say so'. The emphasis was on the 'you', not the evidence-based information used in the audit tool.

My training in the history of infection and my experience on the ward gave me an intense interest in communicable diseases and later infection prevention and control (IPC). It also made me aware of my own role as part of the history of infection control. As a student nurse in 1962, I remember giving my first intravenous injection of penicillin to a male patient on a surgical ward (supervised by the ward sister, of course), and I was only told the injection was necessary because of an infection. I did not realise, at the time, that only thirty-four years earlier Sir Alexander Fleming had discovered the value of penicillin in destroying the bacteria *Staphylococcus*. As we know, the prescribing of penicillin and other antibiotics subsequently became commonplace, with many clinicians complacent about their use. During the 1950s, outbreaks of serious *Staphylococcus aureus* infections were spreading in neonatal nurseries, and penicillin-resistant *S. aureus* became a common hospital pathogen.[5] Over the next few decades other antibiotics were developed, and they became a necessary support for advances in medicine. Transplantation, anti-cancer therapy, major surgery and increasing use of indwelling devices would not be so successful today, without antibiotics.

Previously clinicians, including nurses, have been slow in acknowledging or have been unaware of the steady rise in serious antibiotic resistance. Until I became an ICN I thought only of the action of the antibiotic on the individual patient, not what effect it might have on the larger population. To change behaviour in administering these drugs requires a global strategy. The lack of political and economic consensus in many parts of the world makes this an almost impossible task. Yet, the medical fraternity, politicians and economists are now working to slow the trend of resistance, and highlighting the need for funding and research into developing antimicrobials and diagnostics.[6] In the 1950s, when *S. aureus* infections were becoming more commonplace, Dr Brendan Moore, a microbiologist at Torbay Hospital, Devon, decided that nurses might have more influence than doctors in controlling outbreaks. This was the first hospital to appoint an ICN, in April 1959; her name was Miss E. M. Cottrell and she worked full time in the role.[7] Following the establishment of infection control as a specialty in the 1960s, the

Infection Control Nurses Association (ICNA) was founded in 1970, and Brendan Moore became its first president. The appointment of an ICN in the United States followed in 1963.

I was recruited as the first ICN at GOSH in 1980, after an outbreak of *Salmonella* had occurred among the children. I later wondered if this was a pseudo-outbreak culminating from a laboratory contamination, but I had no proof since little epidemiological detail was recorded. In the early 1960s, Addenbrooke's Hospital was a pilot site for a new government initiative for Central Sterilising Service Departments. Therefore, during my general training I had only used sterile packs and instruments that were delivered and returned to the wards daily. My experience of GOSH was rather different. My first assignment at the hospital was the cardiac ward, with an age range from newborns to sixteen years. Most of the children had congenital heart diseases, and many had a tracheostomy and/or were ventilated. Those with an artificial airway were assigned at least one nurse for twenty-four-hour care, depending on the complexity of their ministration. After cardiac bypass surgery, they were allocated two nurses for at least twenty-four to forty-eight hours. The 'runner' nurse had the duty of ensuring that all equipment was 'sterilised' and replenished, and that clean laundry and nappies were in abundance. This was more than a full-time job, however, as the runner also had to relieve the nurses for meal breaks.

What happened in practice was that the word 'sterile' was often used in the wrong context, such as 'sterilising' bedpans, potties, metal trays and gallipots along with red rubber suction tubes, when they were only disinfected. The contemporary definition of 'sterilisation' is 'a validated process used to render a product free from viable microorganisms'. [8] Cleaning of equipment was haphazard. Every four hours, the 'tracheostomy suction trays' and 'mouth and eye care trays' were briefly rinsed in warm soapy water by hand (automated cleaning being the best method prior to the disinfection or sterilisation process today). Everything was then boiled for five minutes in the treatment room 'steriliser'. This was a large metal container with a lid and a tap for the water supply. There was an electrical heating mechanism to heat the water to boiling point. Every ward had one of these in the sluice (for metal bedpans, metal potties, glass urinals and vomit bowls), and some had one in the treatment room (for surgical instruments). However, because of time restraints and lack of space in the 'steriliser', the equipment was often not totally immersed in the water and had to be done in several batches. On average, the amount of equipment on the cardiac ward to be 'sterilised' every four hours would be ten to fourteen tracheostomy trays, ten to fourteen mouth and eye care trays and three vomit bowls. Red rubber suction catheters (sixteen catheters per tray) were cleaned in soapy water on the ward, and the patency of them was checked by running tap water through the lumen. There was no way of identifying the cleanliness inside the catheters, which were tied in bunches with cotton tape. The trays were then re-assembled and distributed back to the child's bedside. The same trays did not go back to the same child. And there was no documentation of this process. When I became an ICN, I cut several of the catheters open to find blood and sputum encrusted in the 'clean' lumen – which is a good source of cross infection. As Chair of the Clinical Practice Committee (1988–2006), I had many heated discussions with anaesthetists in order to change this practice. We worked with manufacturers to ensure that small, soft-ended disposable suction tubes would be appropriate for newborn babies, and eventually these were manufactured a few years later to everyone's satisfaction.

Part of the night nurse's duties was to pack the sterilising drums with cotton wool balls, gauze and cotton tapes along with hand-made cotton buds on the end of wooden sticks (for mouth care). Metal instruments such as Spencer Well's artery forceps or dressing and chest drain forceps were packed in separate drums. The drums were labelled with the ward and date and sent for autoclaving every twenty-four hours. When needed on the ward, the contents were removed from the sterilised drums with Cheatle forceps and the lids kept closed. These forceps were kept in a clean metal kidney dish with a lid and boiled every twenty-four hours. This was a practice that needed changing, as once the drums were opened or the forceps handled and exposed to the air, they could no longer be considered sterile. Leaving them for twenty-four hours would allow any microorganisms to multiply and increase the risk of infection.

Before disposable nappies came on the market in the early 1960s, terry towelling and muslin nappies were used at GOSH. The nurses had to rinse the soiled nappies in the sluice on the ward before soaking them in a bucket of Hycolin. This was a soluble phenolic disinfectant, withdrawn in the 1970s as a result of the European Biocidal Products Directive. The nappies were then rinsed out again before being sent to the on-site hospital laundry. In addition to wearing a terry towelling and muslin nappy, which was kept in place with a safety pin, each baby would have a red rubber sheet placed beneath its bottom, on which was placed another terry towelling and muslin nappy to prevent soiling of the sheets. There were no rubber panties in the early years. On average, each baby would go through twenty-four nappies in twenty-four hours. This process of use and recycling was a good source of *Pseudomonas* and gastro-intestinal pathogens, especially viruses.

When I worked on the Observation Ward (an isolation unit) at Queen Elizabeth Children's Hospital, Hackney, London, as part of my paediatric training, I was astounded to see reusable intravenous giving sets with red rubber tubing and metal mesh filters. All the children had intravenous drips, due to dehydration from gastroenteritis, and all were on antibiotics. I remember being told the antibiotics were given because of the drip as there was a risk of infection. I remember thinking that we did not do this routinely at Addenbrooke's Hospital or at GOSH, and I thought it slightly 'old fashioned'. I was told that the consultant was doing research into gastro-enteritis and this was part of the protocol. I never saw the research protocol and did not feel I could ask about it as I was only a junior nurse. The maintenance of equipment was poor, and coverings on chairs and couches were often cracked or torn (as they were at GOSH), leaving sources of microorganisms. I do not remember any discussions of whether infections were hospital- or community-acquired, as such terms were not part of the contemporary vocabulary.

One of my first tasks as an ICN was to explore the reasons why most children in the cardiac ward became colonised with *Pseudomonas aeruginosa* within twenty-four hours of being admitted. It was known at the time that respiratory equipment was a common cause of cross infection. While I was working on the cardiac ward as a student, I was aware of the end cubicle being used as the ventilator disinfection room, which was under the domain of the ventilator technician. At the time, I was unaware of the process and did not question practices, as I was too busy learning how to

care for sick children. Whilst investigating the process as ICN, I
noted that the technician had soaked the rose bushes he had been
given at work in the sink used for decontaminating equipment; I
also found that clean and dirty equipment was held in the same
small cubicle. None of it was labelled 'clean' or 'dirty'. The ventilator tubes and connections were rinsed in the sink and then soaked
in Cidex (a glutaraldehyde solution withdrawn in 2002 due to tox-
icity), in a large plastic bin with a lid. They were then rinsed under
the tap and hung up to dry on a tape line along the window. 'Clean'
tubes were taken haphazardly before they were dry (*Pseudomonas*
thrives well in moist areas) and attached to ventilators for the next
child. Elastoplast marks left on the tubes were not washed off,
and the tubes were not always totally submerged in the disinfectant. There was no documentation of how long the equipment had
been soaking, thus allowing flaws in the process of decontamination. Everyone had been too busy to note that basic cleaning and
disinfection of the equipment had been overridden by the greater
need to use that equipment for the patients. After reporting this
to the Infection Control Committee, the Chief Executive charged
the microbiologist and me with looking for equipment that would
decontaminate the items safely. In the interim, we arranged for the
equipment to be decontaminated at University College Hospital
nearby, as a matter of urgency. We identified a hospital in Hamburg,
Germany, which appeared to have the same daily respiratory equipment workload as at GOSH. It had an automated washer/disinfec-
tor machine installed. We visited the hospital to see the equipment
in use and then went on to the factory where these machines were
made. The manufacturers were very helpful and were able to supply
our specific needs. The visit to Germany, the buying and installation
of up-to-date automated equipment away from the ward, the separation of clean and dirty articles at ward level and a review of the
educational needs of the staff resolved the problem.

Before I took up the post as ICN, I was a ward sister on the
Infectious Disease and Dermatology unit for nine years. To prevent
cross infection, after discharge of a child, we would fumigate each
cubicle with a formaldehyde spray. All equipment would be laid
out to ensure contact with the chemical to kill any microorganism. When this was completed, the fumigation machine would be
removed and the doors to the cubicle sealed for two hours. After

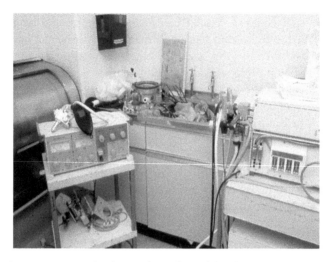

Figure 5.1   Rose bushes in the sink used for decontamination of respiratory equipment on the cardiac ward at GOSH in 1980.

this we would run in, holding our breath, and open the windows to air the room and get rid of the smell. The chemical made you cough as well as stinging your eyes. Only then did we clean the equipment and prepare the room for the next patient. We are now taught to clean equipment first, before disinfection, as organic matter may inhibit the action of the chemical. I thought I knew about infection control. When I became part of the Infection Control Team (ICT) and worked alongside the microbiologist and laboratory scientific staff, however, it was like a new language to me. I had moved to a different specialist area with different understanding and practices. I realised that infection control and epidemiology had not been taught in a systematic, scientific manner, or at least I had not applied in my thinking the significance of the chain of infection (microorganism, source, exit point, method of spread, entry point, person at risk). Networking with other departments and my colleagues in their specialist disciplines, I noted also their lack of knowledge to applied microbiology. I had to learn and re-learn the components and rationale of an infection control programme. This included studying the environment and its cleanliness, catering and laundry, disinfection and sterilisation methods for equipment, microbiology and virology laboratory methods and epidemiological

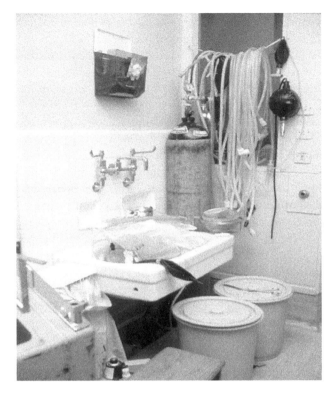

Figure 5.2   Cubicle for decontamination of ventilator tubing on the cardiac ward at GOSH in 1980.

surveillance in hospital-acquired infection, the action of antimicrobials, employee health, leadership and management, especially communication and education, absorbing the research literature and looking at practice and patient outcomes.

Changing people's attitudes through education was no easy feat. I sought education from my colleagues in the ICNA (now the Infection Prevention Society), the Hospital Infection Society and the Hospital Infection Research Laboratory in Dudley Road Hospital, Birmingham, along with my microbiology and virology teammates. At the time, there were few courses. In 1983, the Nurses, Midwives and Health Visitors Act (1979) came into force, and the English National Board (ENB) inherited the legal responsibility for approving institutions in England where professional nursing and allied courses were provided. The only available course in England was the ENB 329 'Foundation in Infection Control' in Birmingham.

In the late 1980s, I became interested in medical anthropology,[9] which helped towards my understanding of the cultural beliefs and ritualistic behaviour exhibited by staff despite their scientific medical and nurse training.[10] Link nurse programmes had been around in the 1980s and successfully implemented to support education in ward-based staff whilst introducing new urinary catheter care guidelines.[11] At GOSH, we introduced a full infection control link nurse (ICLN) programme in 1994, and then expanded it to include other healthcare workers, so that all wards and departments had a representative. This included the chaplains. This measure helped promote the message of good infection prevention practices.

During the early 1980s, two major public enquiry reports were published. The first was the report on the Stanley Royd Hospital food poisoning outbreak, which affected 355 patients (nineteen of whom died) and 106 staff.[12] The cause was identified as cross contamination of raw chicken and cooked beef in the kitchens, and poor hygiene practices in general. Regarding the hygiene practices, the report committee determined, 'it was the practice for the metal topped kitchen tables to be cleaned with a high pressure disinfectant jet, to be scrubbed and then wiped off with the same squeegees as were used on the floors'.[13] The second report followed the outbreak of legionnaires' disease at Stafford District General Hospital, where there were 175 cases, including twenty-eight fatalities.[14] The cause of the outbreak was traced to the air-conditioning cooling tower on the roof of the hospital. Unfortunately, the microbiologist came out badly in the report. The hospital admitted twelve patients with pneumonia over a weekend (two of whom died), and a further sixteen cases were admitted over the next twenty-four hours. The report noted that 'there was no sense of urgency by the microbiologist and specimens, sent in the routine post, went to the wrong laboratory'.[15]

In 1986, the Study on the Efficacy of Nosocomial Infection Control (SENIC) provided evidence that if you target infection control, hospital-acquired infections could be reduced by up to 50 per cent.[16] SENIC was widely used as an educational tool at the time. And in 1988, the 'Cooke Report' on Hospital Infection Control was the first official document supported by the government to cite the ICN as an essential part of the ICT.[17] During these early years as an ICN, I learned quickly and became increasingly politically aware, joining a number of national working parties. In 1995, I was involved in an outbreak concerning wooden tongue depressors, which was to influence national practices in paediatrics.[18] Between September 1995 and April 1996, *Rhizopus microsporus* was isolated in twenty-three patient surveillance stool samples, in four different wards at GOSH. Despite the high number of immune-suppressed children at GOSH and the increased risk of fungal infections, no child had been infected with this organism. However, in 1995, four cases of cutaneous infection with *R. microsporus* were reported in vulnerable preterm infants in one neonatal nursery in the West Midlands.[19] We found the source to be wooden tongue depressors from a specific new NHS supplier. The wood had come from unmanaged forests in China and had not been treated in a hot kiln before being put on the production line. The heat in the kiln would have killed these environmental microorganisms. At the time, there were no standards for the production of wooden tongue depressors, as they were not designed to be used as splints. The spatulas at GOSH were used to collect stool samples, hence the findings. Yet, it was common practice in neonatal care to use these wooden spatulas as intravenous splints to support the indwelling devices on very small limbs. This is what led to the serious infection in babies in the West Midlands.[20] By changing suppliers, it had been estimated, GOSH would have saved £220 per annum. Yet, the laboratory materials in the investigation alone cost the hospital £530. We reported our findings to the Medical Devices Agency, and they issued a national warning.[21] The pressure was on for manufacturers to produce a cost-effective splint that was small enough for the job. This they achieved, and helped to change the practice.

During the 2000s, there were many guidelines issued by the government which required re-thinking of the management of IPC.[22] These guidelines were helpful for reinforcing the economic and clinical message and directing the chief executive and director of finance to work more closely with the ICT. I discovered that in the US there was a legal claim directed at the Infection Control Committee and the Infection Control Practitioner because of responsibilities the ICT have in preventing infections such as

Aspergillus (a fungal infection) during building work.[23] At GOSH, about 80 per cent of the children were immuno-suppressed and therefore susceptible to infection. Finding the definitive proof that hospitals were responsible for giving their patients infections was notoriously difficult. However, lawyers were focusing on compliance with health-and-safety guidelines and good practices.[24] Having previously attended a legal course on what evidence a lawyer is looking for when a patient makes a claim of a hospital-acquired infection, I was concerned to ensure that GOSH did not become liable. At the time, GOSH was constantly undergoing major building work and from the late 1980s, the ICT was involved in infection control protective guidelines, including the installation of clean air systems. Specialist scientific advice had been sought, as this was a new and costly area of expertise. In the event, no cases of GOSH hospital-acquired aspergillosis were identified, despite close monitoring.

The importance of the environment became an interest which helped me investigate other types of outbreaks. A methicillin-resistant *S. aureus* (MRSA) outbreak occurred at GOSH from September 2004 to January 2005, involving six wards. There were ten cases: eight patients (three with bacteraemia) and two staff were affected. The source was the dermatology ward which housed many children with major desquamating (or peeling) skin diseases. There were three main causes: first, a lack of total compliance with universal precautions, especially hand hygiene practices. Secondly, environmental cleaning standards were not maintained. Staff who had nursed children with MRSA had picked up skin scales on their shoes and walked to the nurse's station to sit at the computer. Handbags and boxes of equipment had been left under the nurse's station on the floor, and not moved for cleaning. Dust collected, and consequently the environment outside the cubicles became heavily contaminated with MRSA. The MRSA was transferred from shoes to boxes and handbags, and then to hands which further contaminated a wider environment before hands were washed. And thirdly, a cubicle with an air handling unit had not been commissioned correctly, and the ongoing monitoring system had failed. Many children with MRSA had been nursed in this cubicle, and skin scales carrying MRSA had accumulated within the false ceiling. Some of the air had been re-circulated and dispersed into the ward. With the constant move of both patients and staff, the microorganism had spread to other wards.

The cost to GOSH of controlling this outbreak was over £434,632. There is nothing like an outbreak to educate colleagues about adherence to infection control guidelines, the prevention of hospital-acquired infections and how to save money and reduce unnecessary suffering to the patient and their family. However, it takes time for changes in practice to become embedded in everyday behaviour. A good microbiology and virology laboratory can help to collect evidence to inform staff of problems and advise how they can change practices. Seasonal outbreaks of viral diarrhoea and vomiting (D&V) are common and are mostly due to Rotavirus and Norovirus in a children's hospital. With the introduction of molecular biology methods in routine laboratories, we were able to be more specific in identifying hospital-acquired cases. Previously, using a case definition, we had to assume most cases were acquired in hospital, meaning wards were closed, causing disruption to patients, staff and the finance department:

GOSH statistics on ward closures due to viral D&V

April 2004–March 2005: 17 wards were closed (time range 3–9 days).

April 2005–March 2006: 11 wards were closed (time range 3–7 days).

April 2006–March 2007: 9 wards closed (time range 3–10 days).

April 2007–March 2008: 6 wards closed (time range 3–33 days).

Working closely with research colleagues, GOSH's virology department was able to obtain capsid sequencing on strains of Norovirus during an outbreak in 2002, which demonstrated that there was more than one strain and more than one outbreak in the hospital at the same time.[25] At Christmas 2007, staff were also astounded to learn that over 100,000 genomes of Norovirus were found on the lid of a box of biscuits in sister's office, where the staff helped themselves frequently. The infectious dose is only ten virions, so this caused a sudden compliance with handwashing.[26] Unfortunately this reaction was short-lived. Nevertheless, this type of information enabled the ICT to target specific education and speed up the reaction of ward staff to disinfecting the immediate environment in probable cases as soon as symptoms started. It also encouraged staff to report incidences earlier. And this more focused approach helped reduce the number of ward closures.

When I became Chair of the ICNA in 1997, I was more involved in national and international work.[27] This gave me a wider perspective of the work of government and other agencies and how this influenced infection control guidelines and legislation. The 'Health Act 2006: Code of Practice for the prevention and control of healthcare-associated infections and its successor under the Health and Social Care Act (2008) gave credence to IPC, and forced managers and clinicians to comply, and thus give a higher profile to IPC.[28] This legislation reinforced a Department of Health document from 2003 called *Winning Ways*, which stated that 'a Director of Infection Prevention and Control (DIPC) will be designated within each organisation' who would have corporate responsibility, on behalf of the Chief Executive, for executing and monitoring the IPC strategy. The DIPC would also 'have the authority to challenge inappropriate clinical hygiene practice as well as antibiotic prescribing decisions'.[29] Nationally, most appointees were microbiologists or nursing or medical directors, with a few ICNs. I was a member of the working party which produced a national job description to help cement the role.[30] The post holder would be responsible for the ICT, reporting directly to the chief executive and the board. An annual report, open to the public, would be produced that included the state of healthcare-acquired infection (HCAI) and reduction rates for MRSA. The DIPCs were cautious at first about revealing a negative message to the public, but it was important to educate professionals and the public in risk management and indicate what action should be taken when things go wrong. The code stated that NHS organisations must audit key policies and procedures for infection prevention. The production of an operational policy laid down the structure and function of an IPC framework, on which to drive a strategy forward. At GOSH, and in most other large, acute hospitals, the trust had to assure the DIPC that IPC was in the clinical governance structure, and on the risk register; that senior IPC leads were in all clinical areas and had a strategic plan to reduce HCAIs in their area; that modern matrons had authority to call people to account over IPC issues; that there was an effective Link IPC Programme; that IPC surveillance, policies, training and audit were adhered to; that additional resources were provided (both in personnel and financial terms) in outbreaks; and that core dimensions in IPC were in all staff development plans.

The more practical initiative from the Department of Health 'Saving Lives: reducing infection, delivering clean and safe care' was introduced in 2005 and revised in 2007.[31] The high impact intervention (HII) or bundles of care approach helped trusts achieve infection control targets by providing a focus on evidenced-based elements of the care process, and a method for measuring the implementation of policies and procedures. One of the first bundles was Central Venous Catheter Care, a priority for implementation at GOSH, because there were many children with central venous catheters. The hospital intranet system was developed to capture GOSH-acquired central venous line infections for every 1,000 line days. The data was controlled by the ICT, and each ward had its own data as well as hospital-wide data, so the wards could compare their results. The ICLNs were charged with providing ward education, and using the data to remind medical staff to chart whether a line infection was hospital-acquired or not. This took two or three years to establish, but became embedded once the infection rates had been reduced.[32] The pride in achieving 'avoidable infections' was evident in the medical and nursing staff who shared the information with parents on the ward. Other published care bundles were Peripheral Intravenous Cannula Care; Renal and Urinary Catheter Care; Care for Ventilated Patients; Surgical Site Infections; Reducing the Risk from *Clostridium difficile*; and Cleaning and Decontamination of Clinical Equipment. There was also guidance on Antimicrobial Prescribing, MRSA Screening and Taking Blood Cultures. These were helpful initiatives, and staff were motivated to reduce HCAI, becoming more compliant when audit results were available, and made open to the public. Transparency with hospital-acquired infections was slowly developing.

Looking back on my experiences, and the changes that have occurred in IPC, one thing is clear: it takes a long time to change practice. When I started nursing, I felt very subservient to the system. Most ward sisters instilled fear in the nurses and junior doctors and ruled with an unquestionable strictness. I felt my discipline of infection control was ruled by the anxiety of being told off by sister or senior staff nurses rather than any detailed microbiological knowledge. When we socialised in the hospital or discussed our day's work it would only be with someone in our set, as it was an unwritten rule that you did not mix with someone above you. As my career progressed and I became more knowledgeable and vocal, I realised how much you can learn from your colleagues but also how resistant to change they can be. However, where there is a political will, there is a way. There is no doubt that the focus on the national direction by the Department of Health has helped guide healthcare workers and managers through the maze of information, and sometimes contradictory advice. The use of information technology has integrated data collection, helping evidence-based healthcare to move forward. Systems of working are more integrated, and there is now a more organised provision of care in the speciality of IPC. Hopefully, with international collaboration, this will help combat the increasing problem of antimicrobial resistance.

Notes

1 For an introduction, see S. W. B. Newson, *Infections and their control: A historic perspective* (London: Sage, 2009).
2 World Health Organization, *WHO Guidelines on hand hygiene in health care: First global patient safety challenge clean care is safer care* (Geneva: World Health Organization, 2009), www.who.int/gpsc/5may/registration_update/en/ (accessed 12 May 2017); National Patient Safety Agency, 'Clean-Your-Hands campaign' (2010), www.npsa.nhs.uk/cleanyourhands/resource-area/ (accessed 13 May 2017).
3 C. Fuller, J. McAteer, R. Slade *et al.*, 'Short summary of the hand hygiene observation tool (HHOT): Feedback intervention trial' (London: Royal Free and University College Medical School, 2007), npsa.nhs.uk/EasySite Web/GatewayLink.aspx?alId=7022 (accessed 15 May 2017).
4 W. Wetzker, K. Bunte-Schönberger, J. Walter, G. Pilarski *et al.*, 'Compliance with hand hygiene: reference data from the national hand hygiene campaign in Germany', *Journal of Hospital Infection*, 92 (2016), 328–331.
5 Anon, 'Penicillinase-resistant penicillins', *Lancet*, 2 (1960), 585–586.
6 J. O'Neill, 'Tackling drug-resistant infections globally: final report and recommendations', *The review on antimicrobial resistance* (2016), https://amr-review.org/sites/default/files/160518_Final%20paper_with %20cover.pdf (accessed 12 December 2020).
7 A. M. N. Gardener, M. Stamp, J. A. Bowgen, B. Moore, 'The infection control sister: A new member of the control of infection team in general hospitals', *Lancet*, 280 (1962), 710–711.

8 International Standards Organisation (ISO), EN. '14937:2009. Sterilization of health care products – General requirements for characterization of a sterilizing agent and the development, validation and routine control of a sterilization process for medical devices' (revised ISO 14937:2000).

'It is important to note that in a sterilisation process, the nature of microbial inactivation is exponential, and the survival of a microorganism on an individual item can thus be expressed in terms of probability. While this probability can be reduced to a very low number, it can never be reduced to zero'. See Medicines and Healthcare Products Regulatory Agency, 'MHRA: Sterilization, disinfection and cleaning of medical equipment: guidance on decontamination from the Microbiology Advisory Committee (the MAC manual)'. Part 1 Principles. (2010), www. mhra.gov.uk/Publications/Safetyguidance/Otherdevicesafetyguidance/CON007438 (accessed 9 April 2017).

9 C. G. Helman, *Culture, health and illness* (London: Hodder Arnold, 1984); M. Douglas, *Purity and danger: An analysis of the concepts of pollution and taboo* (London: Routledge, 1984); M. C. Doughty and T. Tripp-Reimer, 'Interface of nursing and anthropology', *Annual Review of Anthropology*, 14 (1985), 219–241; P. Holden and J. Littlewood, *Anthropology and nursing* (London: Routledge, 1991).

10 S. Macqueen, 'Anthropology and germ theory', *Journal of Hospital Infection*, 30 (1995), 116–126.

11 R. Horton, 'Linking the chain', *Nursing Times*, 84 (1988), 44–46; Y. T. Ching and W. H. Seto, 'Evaluating the efficacy of the infection control liaison nurse in the hospital', *Journal of Advanced Nursing*, 15 (1990), 1128–1131.

12 J. Hugill, *The Report of the committee of inquiry into an outbreak of food poisoning at Stanley Royd Hospital* (London: HM Stationery Office, 1986).

13 *Ibid.*, 64.

14 J. Badenoch, *First report of the committee of inquiry into the outbreak of Legionnaires' Disease in Stafford in April 1985* (London: HM Stationery Office, 1986).

15 *Ibid.*

16 R. W. Haley, D. Quade, H. E. Freeman, J. V. Bennett, 'CDC SENIC Planning committee. Study on the Efficacy of Nosocomial Infection Control (SENIC Project): Summary of study design', *American Journal of Epidemiology*, 111 (1980), 472–485.

17 Department of Health and Social Security, 'Guidance on the control of infection in hospitals prepared by the joint DHSS/PHLS hospital

infection working group (The Cooke Report)' (London: Department of Health and Social Security, 1988).

18 H. Holzel, S. Macqueen, A. MacDonald *et al.*, '*Rhizopus microsporus* in wooden tongue depressors: A major threat or minor inconvenience?', *Journal of Hospital Infection*, 38 (1998), 113–118.

19 S. J. Mitchell, J. Gray, M. E. Morgan *et al.*, 'Nosocomial infection with Rhizopus microsporus in preterm infants: Association with wooden tongue depressors', *Lancet*, 348 (1996), 441–443.

20 *Ibid.*

21 Medical Device Agency 1996 Hazard MDA: HN 9604. Not electronically archived.

22 R. J. Pratt, C. M. Pellowe, H. Loveday and N. Robinson, 'The EPIC project: Developing national evidence-based guidelines for preventing healthcare associated infections. Phase 1: Guidelines for preventing hospital-acquired infections – Department of Health (England)', *Journal of Hospital Infection*, 47 (2001), S3–82; Chief Medical Officer, *Getting ahead of the curve: a strategy for infectious diseases (including other aspects of health protection)* (London: Department of Health, 2002); Chief Medical Officer, *Winning ways: Working together to reduce healthcare associated infection in England* (London: Department of Health, 2003); Department of Health, *Towards cleaner hospitals and lower rates of infection: A summary of action* (London: Department of Health, 2004); Department of Health, *Going further faster: Implementing the saving lives delivery programme* (London: Department of Health, 2006); Department of Health, *Essential steps to safe, clean care: Reducing healthcare-associated infections* (London: Department of Health, 2006); Department of Health, *Saving lives: Reducing infection, delivering clean and safe care including MRSA* (London: Department of Health, 2007); R. J. Pratt, C. M. Pellowe, J. A. Wilson *et al.*, 'The epic2 project: national evidence-based guidelines for preventing healthcare-associated infections in NHS hospitals in England', *Journal of Hospital Infection*, 65 (2007), S1–64.

23 S. M. Cheng and A. J. Streifel, 'Infection control considerations during construction activities: Land excavation and demolition', *American Journal of Infection Control*, 29 (2001), 321–328.

24 Health and Safety Executive, 'Control of substances hazardous to Health Regulations 2000 (as amended in 2004), General enforcement guidelines and advice' (2002), www.hse.gov.uk/foi/internalops/ocs/200–299/273_20/ (accessed 15 May 2017).

25 C. I. Gallimore, D. W. Cubitt, A. F. Richards and J. J. Gray, 'Diversity of enteric viruses detected in patients with gastroenteritis in a tertiary referral paediatric hospital', *Journal of Medical Virology*, 73 (2004), 443–449.

26 Public Health Agency of Canada, 'Norovirus – Pathogen Safety Data Sheet' (2017), www.phac-aspc.gc.ca/lab-bio/res/psds-ftss/msds112e-eng. php (accessed 12 April 2017).

27 These include 1998 Member of the Expert Advisory Panel to the National Audit Office on the Management and Control of Hospital Acquired Infection in Acute Trusts in England; 1998 Member of the Expert Advisory Panel on the DOH Communicable Disease Strategy; 1998–2000 Member of the Project Advisory Group of the National Guidelines for the Prevention of Hospital-acquired Infection (Pratt *et al.*, 'The epic2 project'), 2000–2003 Member of Hospitals in Europe Link for Infection Control through Surveillance (HELICS – 3) project.

28 Department of Health, 'Health and Social Care Act 2008: Code of practice on the prevention and control of infections and related guidance' (2008), www.gov.uk/government/uploads/system/uploads/attachment_data/file/449049/Code_of_practice_280715_acc.pdf (accessed 20 April 2017).

29 Chief Medical Officer, *Winning ways*, 21.

30 Role Specification of Director of Infection Prevention and Control (2011), http://Webarchive.Nationalarchives.Gov.Uk/20120118164404/ Hcai.Dh.Gov.Uk/Files/2011/03/Document_Dipc_Role_Final_100810. Pdf (accessed 8 May 2017).

31 Department of Health, *Saving lives*.

32 J. S. Soothill, K. Bravery, A. Ho *et al.*, 'A fall in bloodstream infections followed a change to 2% chlorhexidine in 70% isopropanol for catheter connection antisepsis: a paediatric single centre before/after study on a hemopoietic stem cell transplant unit', *American Journal of Infection Control*, 37 (2009), 626–630.

Part III

Practice and infection control:
Focus on gloves

6

Wax paste and vaccination: alternatives to surgical gloves for infection control, 1880–1945

Thomas Schlich

In this chapter, I discuss the history of various technologies for infection control in surgical operations. My account starts with the uptake of surgical gloves by practitioners in the late nineteenth century, which was a protracted process, and explains the relative disinterest of many surgeons in this particular technology by situating it in the context of other contemporary strategies of infection control. Exploring such alternative innovations shows that technological change in surgery and infection control does not happen in a vacuum. There are always multiple technological solutions to a problem. This chapter explores the alternatives to surgical gloves that were not taken up, arguing that this historical awareness provides a deeper understanding of the evolution of modern surgery and infection control.[1]

William Halsted and surgical gloves

Today, rubber gloves represent an important part of infection control in hospitals. In surgical operations, it is inconceivable for surgeons and nurses to work with their bare hands. Gloves were first used by operators during surgery in the 1880s. At the time, their introduction caused considerable controversy among surgeons, who only gradually adopted the innovation.[2] If we look at the historical literature, we can see that many authors have been quite impatient about surgeons' hesitation to use surgical gloves. This impatience results from a teleological perspective on the history of medicine. From such a perspective, historians judge events and developments in the past according to whether they lead up to how things are now.

In our case, it means that anything that was conducive to the use of surgical gloves is considered rational. Anything that went towards a different solution of the problem is judged to be irrational. For example, Justine Randers-Pehrson, in her historical account for the introduction of gloves, found it 'curious that it took lively minds so long to come around with the notion of an impermeable glove in surgery'. It was 'even more curious', she wrote, that, 'when the proposal was finally made in the eighteen-nineties, it required more than a decade of passionate argument before final universal acceptance could be achieved', explaining that 'the human mind does not always dart straight to the obvious'.[3] However, a closer investigation of the discussions at the time can show that surgeons had good reason to be sceptical about wearing gloves, including the loss of manual dexterity against the yet unproven benefits of gloves for infection control.[4]

There is one example in the history of surgical gloves that demonstrates how historians can benefit from a broader perspective when trying to understand why new techniques for infection control were accepted or rejected. It is the relatively well-known story of the first introduction of rubber gloves into the operating room (OR). This event happened in 1889 at the Johns Hopkins Hospital Department of Surgery, then headed by the famous William Halsted. As Halsted recalled it later, the nurse in charge of his OR 'complained that the solution of mercuric chloride [the antiseptic substance that he used at the time] produced a dermatitis of her arms and hands'. Halsted wanted to keep this 'unusually efficient woman' in his OR, so he 'one day in New York requested the Goodyear Rubber Company to make as an experiment two pair of thin rubber gloves with gauntlets'.[5] The fact that this nurse was Halsted's later wife makes for a popular medical history anecdote. But the story has a less sanguine part: for a long time, it was only the nurses who used the gloves, rather than the operators. It took seven years until the operating surgeons wore them on a routine basis too.[6] Indeed, as publications from the 1880s and 1890s show, gloves were used for the purpose of maintaining sterility in all kinds of procedures around an operation, but they were not worn for the operation itself. Thus, Halsted's gynaecological colleague Hunter Robb wrote in 1894 about the routine at Johns Hopkins: 'After the patient is well arranged and all is ready, we remove the gloves, and after washing our hands once more in the bichloride solution ..., we can proceed with our work'.[7] It was only in December 1896 that surgeons started wearing gloves during their operations as a rule, and it was not even Halsted who started this new practice but his assistant, Joseph Bloodgood.[8] This 'delay' has been a puzzle for historians of medicine ever since. Even Halsted himself wondered in retrospect how he 'could have been so blind as not to have perceived the necessity for wearing them invariably at the operating table'.[9]

Halsted's 'blindness' to the virtue of gloves was not the result of any sloppiness; Halsted was fastidious in all things related to germ-free surgery.[10] There is another possible reason for his relative disinterest in gloves, namely that he was busy working at a different strategy of preventing wound infection. Intriguingly, Halsted had developed his alternative strategy not because he was indifferent to germ theory and bacteriology, but because he had a special interest in it. The standard method of infection control at the time was Joseph Lister's system of antisepsis. In his system, Lister aimed at eliminating all germs in and around the wound by the use of carbolic acid. Halsted was sceptical about its efficiency and put it to the test by using the latest bacteriological methods developed by Robert Koch in Germany. As a result, he found that with antiseptic substances such as carbolic acid, it was impossible to eliminate all bacteria that could be found in and around surgical wounds. In reaction, Halsted tried to figure out some better way of preventing wound infection. His strategy was to create conditions in the patient's wound and tissues that would prevent bacteria already present from causing an infection.

To determine these conditions, Halsted performed a series of experiments. In one of these experiments he introduced bacteria into the peritoneal cavity of dogs, and he noticed that no harm occurred as long he carefully avoided any mechanical injury to the tissues. But if he bruised the tissue or cut off some small part of it from its blood supply beforehand, 'a single bacterium ... was able to multiply and cause a fatal peritonitis'.[11] Consequently, Halsted put his main focus on careful and gentle operating techniques to avoid any such injury. He wrote in 1891 that 'the obstruction to the circulation produced by sutures and ligatures is often the immediate cause of suppuration in infected

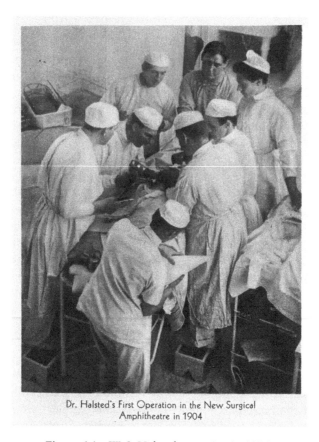

Dr. Halsted's First Operation in the New Surgical
Amphitheatre in 1904

Figure 6.1   W. S. Halsted operating in 1904.

wounds.'[12] Halsted's first biographer, William MacCallum, characterised his procedures to be 'of mathematical precision, with
healing almost as precisely ensured'.[13] Much of Halsted's infection prophylaxis was embodied in his surgical technique rather
than in preventing contamination from the outside. For this reason, gloves were not high on his agenda. The example of Halsted
shows how a narrow focus on the simple acceptance or rejection of a surgical technology can obscure the broader context
of technological change. Moreover, Halsted's careful operating
style was not the only proposed alternative to the use of surgical
gloves, as discussed next.

Living as a surgeon: strategies of preventing wound infection through touch

A wide range of techniques of hand disinfection were used in the 1880s. On this subject, an 1888 publication by Paul Fürbringer (1849–1930) acquired canonical status. Fürbringer, who was not a surgeon, but Head of the Department of Internal Medicine of the Friedrichshain Hospital in Berlin, came up with a standardised procedure, in which he first washed his hands with soap, then with alcohol and finally with an antiseptic substance. Fürbringer's procedure was based on a series of bacteriological laboratory tests, and it was quickly adopted as the gold standard of hand disinfection in surgery. It is apparent from the scientific literature of the time that any new suggestions, such as the later use of gloves, had to be measured against the baseline of the Fürbringer method. The procedure was widely adopted in numerous variations, for example in Kurt Schimmelbusch's *Guide to Aseptic Wound Treatment*. Schimmelbusch's textbook on aseptic surgery was first published in 1892 and quickly became the authoritative reference work for the new technology, integrating and standardising the various elements of aseptic surgery into a formalised system based on Kochian bacteriology.[14] Any criticism of the method or any modification had to satisfy the new laboratory-based standards – standards that demanded 'an experimental arrangement that was transparent and controllable at any time', something that required a high investment in time and effort for anybody who wanted to criticise them, as Fürbringer himself pointed out in one of his papers.[15]

Another strategy that was focused on the operator's hands consisted of keeping them clean between operations. The surgeon had to avoid any contact with potentially infectious material, even when not on the job. This included keeping fingernails extremely short and required constant vigilance about what was touched by the surgeon's hands. With some authors, for example Theodor Kocher, this approach amounted to a whole regime of living as a surgeon.[16] In the context of the hospital standardisation project of the American College of Surgeons, the Chicago surgeon Albert Ochsner described in 1904 how things should be done: For keeping the surgeon's hands away from any possibility of contamination, 'in dressing suppurating wounds, forceps and rubber gloves are used to prevent the hands from touching pus ... Both of the assistants and the surgical nurse wear rubber gloves during all operations, while I wear gloves only in operations in the presence of pus.'[17] The operator wore gloves only 'in operations upon suppurating cases', not when working on clean wounds. The gloves were thus used not to protect the patient's wound but to avoid contamination of the surgeon's hand via the patient's pus.[18]

Catching an infection from a patient was a very real danger. The German pioneer of asepsis, Kurt Schimmelbusch, for example, died at age thirty-five due to a septic infection caught in the OR, and he was not an isolated case. In Britain, Charles B. Lockwood (1856–1914) also died from an infection he had contracted in an operation on a patient with peritonitis.[19]

The strict segregation between septic and aseptic cases, rooms and operators was another common strategy. It was, for example, a central technique of Gustav Adolf Neuber in Kiel, the first practitioner who claimed to introduce asepsis as an alternative to antisepsis.[20] Neuber rejected the use of antiseptic substances, particularly in wounds and dressings, and advocated a strict regime of anti-contamination instead. He called this strategy 'asepsis' to distance himself from Lister and his use of antiseptic chemicals. His system focused completely on keeping infectious cases and material away from clean environments and wounds, by spatial, temporal and personal separation. Neuber never gained much influence among his colleagues. He first developed his system in a professionally subordinated position as assistant surgeon to the eminent Friedrich von Esmarch at the University Hospital in Kiel. Subsequently, he set up his own private hospital in the city, where he put his ideas into practice. Others developed the approach into a formalised aseptic regime that aimed at preventing any contamination with germs in the first place, instead of killing germs that were already present in the wound. The method was based on Robert Koch's new bacteriology and the methods of bacteriological testing that were characteristic of his scientific approach.[21] Its development into a generally usable method was a collective accomplishment, in which Ernst von Bergmann and his student Schimmelbusch played prominent roles.[22] In any case, the concept of the separation of septic and aseptic cases was maintained in modern surgery, for example by Ochsner, who instructed surgeons to make sure that 'aseptic cases are always operated first and later those containing pus'.[23] The Chicago surgeon likewise postulated that 'the assistant who has charge of the patients who are primarily aseptic has nothing to do with the patients who are not aseptic primarily from the character of their disease and *vice versa*'.[24]

Other surgeons kept the germs at a distance by developing no-touch techniques for their operations. The best-known instance of this approach is the set of instruments designed by the flamboyant William Arbuthnot Lane in London. These special instruments had long handles to use for operative treatment of bone fractures. He instructed his readers that 'not only must you not touch the interior of the wound with your hands nor permit the patient's skin to do so either, but you must never let any portion of an instrument which has been in contact with your skin or with that of the patient touch the raw surface. All swabs must be held in forceps and applied to the wound in that manner … After an instrument has been used for a length of time, or forcibly, it should be re-boiled or placed in a germicidal solution.'[25] Antiseptics were not to be applied: 'No germicidal or other liquid should be introduced into the wound', he wrote.[26] This method has mockingly been called 'the knife and fork method of operating',[27] but the no-touch approach has been used in various later contexts too.

Still another strategy consisted of coating the surgeon's hands with a layer of some substance to prevent contamination of the wound by hand-borne germs and at the same time avoid the 'inconveniences' associated with gloves. As with gloves, at this stage, the goal was to protect the patient from being infected through the surgeon's hand. For this purpose, some surgeons suggested covering the skin with a coating of soap. The problem was that the soap layer would dissolve during the operation. Others therefore suggested filling the pores of the skin and the irregularities of the epidermis with paraffin, which was more durable. Another idea was to mix paraffin with xylol, douse the surgeon's hands with the mixture, and let the xylol evaporate so that a water-repellent layer of paraffin stayed behind on the hand.[28] Carl Haegler in Basel came up with a special paste using gutta-percha (a latex product) that he rubbed into his hands in a low concentration. Washing in cold water took care of the initial stickiness. However, as soon as the concentration of the substance was high enough to coat the whole hand in one layer it became too brittle and was easily removed through rubbing.[29]

Carl Ludwig Schleich in 1900 proposed using a coating of insoluble wax paste. The so-called Schleich paste was a preparation of wax, which was brought into an emulsion with water. The paste was to be applied in a thin layer and the water would evaporate, leaving a thin layer of pure beeswax on the surgeon's hands, which, as Schleich wrote, was like a 'soft skin of collodium, but more elastic and not cracking'. If rubbed it looked shiny, smooth and polished and behaved towards watery solutions like a glass surface. According to Schleich, the paste would enclose the bacteria in the pores of the skin so that they could not get into the wound. The surgeon explained that this approach imitated that natural process of the production of fat through the sebaceous glands of the skin which, in nature, also served to protect it from bacteria. In this way, he claimed to have created an aseptic 'microscopic glove', which was 'impermeable for water, blood juices, and bacteria'. Moreover, the layer could be removed at any time by washing one's hands with a special marble dust soap, and it could be re-created at will as needed.[30] Schleich also claimed that the use of his marble dust soap on a regular basis, forty to fifty times per day, would render the surgeon's hands sterile, equalling a continuous aseptification.[31]

The Schleich paste was suitable to be combined with chemical disinfection because the smooth surface made antiseptic substances more effective. The skin of the hand became as easily sterilisable as a smooth glass surface.[32] But Schleich's method remained controversial. In his bacteriological studies, Haegler found that the application of Schleich's wax paste did not make hands aseptic at all. In addition, the lightly alkaline serum of the blood in the surgical wound would dissolve the layer and thus quickly wash it off during the operation.[33] Schimmelbusch claimed that there was no paste that was sufficiently elastic and strong to withstand all the movements of the hand. The paste coating would get fissures and flake off. Greasing one's hands would be beneficial under certain conditions, though not for protecting the patient from contamination from the hands; rather, for protecting the hand from contamination.[34]

None of these methods was taken up on a large scale, mainly, it seems, because the coatings were not durable enough to last through a surgical intervention. But the theme persisted. A later version of this approach was published in 1943, when three researchers at the University of Chicago reported their observation that 'cationic detergents deposit an invisible, non-perceptible film on the hands which retains bacteria under it'. This film was quite durable, they reported, one could use one's hands for three hours without disrupting it and its outer surface possessed considerable 'bactericidal power'.[35] The researchers tried the technique in abdominal operations on animals, in which they used it instead of gloves and found a striking reduction in the number of microorganisms from the treated hands, as compared to the untreated control subjects. The researchers believed 'that these results point the way for improved methods of hand hygiene, e.g., for surgeons, medical personnel dealing with contagious cases, food-handlers, etc. In instances when surgical gloves are not available, it might be feasible to perform a reasonably sterile operation by protecting the hands with frequent dips in a solution of one percent cationic soap.' They expressed their hope 'to encourage others to search for ... a detergent which will deposit a film with greater resistance to solution in water'.[36]

Attempts at the systemic prevention of surgical infection

Vaccination served as the model for a very different approach to dealing with wound infection. It followed 'the idea of strengthening and supporting the organism in its struggle against potential infections prophylactically', as the German surgeon Erwin Payr characterised it.[37] There were various ways to pursue this approach. Some researchers tried to create specific immunity against the agents of wound infection, while others aimed at boosting the body's immune defence more generally before surgical operations.

One important publication on this topic came from Johannes Mikulicz, Chair of Surgery at the University of Breslau. Mikulicz was a leading surgeon of his time, who in the last decades of the nineteenth century played a decisive role in perfecting the system of aseptic surgery. He was one of the pioneers of glove use and had, among other things, added the face mask to the list of surgical standard equipment. However, Mikulicz was also interested in following an alternative path to prevent surgical infection. He wanted, as he wrote in 1904, to follow the example of the current treatment of infectious diseases and add to the strategy proposed by Lord Lister – the one suggested by Edward Jenner, namely, 'specific preventive inoculation' for rendering 'individuals more capable of resisting infection'. This approach had not been used very often by surgeons because of the multitude of different germs involved in wound infection and because the alternative of antisepsis was quite efficient: 'there is not so great practical necessity as in the case of general infectious diseases because the majority of wounds are efficiently guarded from infection by antiseptic treatment', he explained.

But there was one condition that had eluded the aseptic system. This exception concerned the operations on those organs which in themselves contained pathogenic organisms, such as the intestines or the stomach. If such an organ were opened up during an operation, 'the natural power of resistance of the peritoneum in the individual is not sufficient to overpower the mass of bacteria introduced'.[38] Doctors should therefore tip the balance and increase the peritoneum's power of resistance against the intestinal bacteria. The way to do that was by 'producing an artificial hyperleucocytosis' – an increase of the white cells circulating in the patient's bloodstream. Mikulicz knew that other researchers had already worked in this direction and had used protein substances, 'albumoses, especially spermin', to stimulate white cell production to fight infections of pneumococci in laboratory animals. This kind of experiment, he thought, had shown 'that during the stage of hypercytosis the blood of humans and dogs possessed a higher bactericidal value than normal blood'.[39]

In his own experiments, Mikulicz tried to mobilise 'great masses of leucocytes' which 'may overcome the bacteria. The animal experiments were carried out by 'Dr. [Hiyaki] Miyake of Japan, who recently worked in my clinic', 'in the Breslau Hygienic Institute under the control of Professor Flügge'.[40] Carl Flügge was the local hygienist at Breslau. He was an expert concerning Robert Koch's bacteriology and cooperated with Mikulicz, who had judged it to be 'indispensable to get in touch with a professional bacteriologist, who in all these things sees clearer and less biased than we surgeons'. At this point, Mikulicz and Flügge had already conducted multiple experimental studies on wound infection control. These studies were performed in both Flügge's bacteriological laboratory and Mikulicz's ORs.[41] It was a relationship that nicely illustrated the alignment of laboratory science and surgery, in which surgeons and bacteriologists worked side by side, chose particular problems from surgical practice and translated them into laboratory models, solved them in the lab and took the solutions back to the OR by adjusting surgical practices in accord with their experimental findings. One of the results of this cooperation had been the surgical face mask.[42] Now this model of cooperation was applied to the question of immunological infection control.

Mikulicz mentioned that similar experiments had been carried out by others in 1902 'to increase the resistance of the peritoneum against *Bacillus coli* infection', using 'small quantities of normal saline solution'. Through this stimulation 'the natural resistance in guinea-pigs' had been increased 'sevenfold to sixteenfold', he reported. There were even three experiments of this kind that had been performed on humans 'in cases of laparotomy' with an injection 'from 30 to 60 cubic centimeters of saline solution' into the patient's abdominal cavity with a possible positive result. Other investigators had stuck to the laboratory and produced hyperleuco-cytosis in guinea pigs with various substances. In addition to saline solution, bouillon, nucleic acid and tuberculin were used as stimulants. One of the previous researchers had 'injected virulent cholera vibrios' into the animals' abdominal cavities at the peak of the artificial hyperleucocytosis and had noted 'a more or less marked increase in the resistance of the peritoneum to the injected cholera bacilli'. The most powerful reaction had been obtained with nucleic acid. Mikulicz tried to do the same in his experiments and achieve specific immunity against *Bacilli coli* – a bacteria species he had chosen because it was pathogenic for the guinea pig, which he could easily use as an experimental animal. He even measured and quantified the dosage of the stimulant by using as a measure the loop that was used in bacteriological testing to pick up the (killed) bacteria in comparable amounts: 'Between half a loopful to two loopfuls of a sterilized culture were injected into the peritoneum from a strain of *Bacillus coli*', he wrote. He waited for 'a definite interval, which was different in different experiments' and then infected the rodents with living cultures, following a typical Kochian trajectory. He observed that 'the animals tolerated the introduction of five loopfuls of living virulent culture'. These animals then also survived the escape of the contents of the intestine into the abdominal cavity in an experimental operation. He concluded that 'the active immunization with a strain of *Bacillus coli* (derived from man) was ... able to protect against other *Bacillus coli* strains that were accidentally present in the contents of the intestine'. Mikulicz thus interpreted his observation as evidence of an active and specific immunisation to the killed bacteria that he had injected into his guinea pigs.[43]

However, the Breslau surgeon subsequently dropped the strategy of active and specific immunisation. The diversity of the strains of bacteria in the gastrointestinal tract was just too high to make sure that every possible infectious agent was included in the immunogenic solution to be injected pre-operatively. Instead, the research group focused on the enhancement of general resistance through hyperleucocytosis. They tested injections of various fluids into the peritoneum and found that normal saline produced marked hyperleucocytosis in the peritoneal fluid. Even better results, they found, were obtained with nucleic acid. When they injected a 5 per cent solution of nucleic acid, the animals reacted by showing a temporary decrease of white blood cells that was, however, followed by the desired hyperleucocytosis in the peritoneum as well as in the blood. The researchers continued by infecting the guinea pigs with a strain of virulent bacterium coli to test their immune status. For this purpose, they had established in preliminary experiments that the minimum lethal dose was a quarter of a loopful of the living bacteria. They then used this measure to quantify the effect of the immunisation and injected the treated animals with multiples of the lethal dose. Thus, they found that those animals which had received a single injection into the peritoneum of one cubic centimetre of normal saline solution for stimulating their immune system now had their 'power of resistance doubled', which meant they survived the administration of two lethal doses. However, Mikulicz found that to be a 'relatively weak' effect. Nucleic acid worked better: after intraperitoneal injection of this substance the power of resistance of the peritoneum was raised between sixteen and twenty times. The same effect was produced by injecting a 0.5 per cent solution of neutralised nucleic acid subcutaneously. If the subcutaneous injections were repeated, the resistance could be raised to up to thirty-two times the normal measurement.[44]

The researchers complemented these rather abstract experiments by a scenario that was more similar to the conditions that occurred in surgical practice. In a series of tests, they 'simulated

the natural conditions' occurring in peritonitis due to a perfora-
tion of the gastrointestinal tract. The experiments consisted of
performing a laparotomy, making an incision in the stomach or
intestine and pushing its content into the abdominal cavity. The
researchers then examined the animals: 'of five control animals
which had not been previously prepared, four died from peritonitis'. However, as Mikulicz continued in his paper, 'ten animals had been prepared. These recovered without exception.
The preparation consisted in three intraperitoneal injections of
nucleic acid, two injections of sterilised bacteria coli, three more
injections of nucleic acid into to the peritoneum, and two sub-
cutaneous injections of nucleic acid. In each case laparotomy
was performed seven hours after the injection.' This result, he
thought, opened 'up a new field for the surgeon in preventing
post-operative peritonitis'.[45]

Encouraged by the outcomes of his animal experiments, Mikulicz
'felt justified in beginning similar experiments … upon man'. He
injected nucleic acid solution under the skin of fifty-eight of his
patients. Fifty-five of them underwent different operations 'upon
the stomach, intestine or other abdominal viscera, and in three
cases for extra-abdominal disease'. All of them were found to have
hyperleucocytosis in their blood. However, it was not clear if this
translated into a better surgical outcome or not. The problem was
that the method did not provide 'absolute certainty like a specific
immunization', which was the obvious gold standard for Mikulicz.
The treatment only increased 'the natural immunity', which 'may
in certain circumstances, even when increased thirty-fold, nevertheless be insufficient'. However, he had the 'impression that the
cases hitherto treated have given more favourable results, not only
in numbers of cases recovered but also in the progress of individual
cases, than the analogous cases of earlier date where the operation
was performed without the preparation'.[46] Of the fifty-five oper-
ated-upon patients, forty-five were found to have an 'abdominal
cavity [that] was exposed to infection by the contents of the stomach or intestines or by some other infectious secretion. Thirty-eight
of these cases recovered, and in none of the seven fatal ones was
peritonitis the cause of death.' However, ultimately, Mikulicz set
more trust in the intraperitoneal infusion of normal saline solution,
which he thought would also increase the power of resistance of the

peritoneum, and which he now used 'in all laparotomies in which the peritoneum runs some risk of infection'.[47]

Even though to us today such attempts might look bizarre, at the time, Mikulicz's considerations were not seen as marginal. Thus, a commentator in the *Journal of the American Medical Association* wrote in 1904 concerning Mikulicz's irrigation of the abdominal cavity with saline solution: 'The procedure is so simple and so entirely free from danger and the results to be anticipated are so promising that it would seem a mistake not to adopt the measure whenever it appears to be indicated.'[48]

Alternative innovation

As the previous examples suggest, there was a whole landscape of alternative innovations developed to deal with wound infection, but these are not discussed in mainstream medical histories. The history of antisepsis is another example that shows the neglect of alternatives in traditional historiography. For a long time, the history of antisepsis has been told as a story of innovative spirit versus conservative stubbornness. In this narrative, surgeons who accepted Lister's antisepsis early on were seen as avant-garde. Those who did not were thought to be resistant to innovation. This was a teleological discussion, in that it presumed the adoption of antisepsis was the natural outcome of historical events. In the past two decades, new historical work has resulted in a different perspective: historians have shown that many contemporary surgeons were not particularly interested in Lister's ideas and practices. They have also shown that this was not because these surgeons were conservative or stubborn, but that they were busy developing their own innovations. They were finding other ways and strategies for preventing wound disease.

There was, for example, a group of doctors, scientists and administrators in the 1860s, who, as Michael Worboys writes, 'transferred the rhetoric and prescriptions of the sanitary movement from the urban environment ... to urban hospitals and their patients'.[49] Examples include James Young Simpson and Florence Nightingale. For the proponents of sanitation, Lister's focus on applying one chemical substance, carbolic acid, was a distraction from what really needed to be done, namely reforming the hospitals.[50] Seen from that perspective, antisepsis was a more conservative approach to solving the problem at hand, and it was Lister who thus 'resisted' substantial change. But even at the more technical level, there were many alternatives to Lister's antisepsis. As Worboys also states, 'each surgeon had his own ideas and techniques',[51] and each of these surgeons, 'in their different ways, made wounds clean, halted sepsis, controlled inflammation and improved the healing power of the patient's constitution'.[52]

One of the most influential alternatives to antisepsis was the 'cleanliness and cold water school'. Its protagonist, Thomas Spencer Wells, who was subsequently often portrayed as stubbornly resisting Lister's innovation, 'emphasized the role of general sanitary principles and scrupulous cleanliness and purity'.[53] Wells performed and documented thousands of invasive interventions – in particular ovariotomies – with minimal complications, without using antisepsis.[54] Wells is only one example. Historians can find many more creative and rational innovations by contemporary surgeons, such as George Callender and Lawson Tait.[55] But the historiography of surgery lost sight of this diversity once Lister had been declared the founding figure of antisepsis and the avoidance of wound infection in the late nineteenth century.

Exploring the history of alternatives to surgical glove use shows the extent to which the historiography of surgery has been shaped by underlying teleological principles, which take the present state of things as the quasi-natural outcome of history. One of the problems with this perspective is that it makes the fluidity and contingency of technical change invisible. It sanitises and streamlines the diversity of new and old surgical technologies and the technical creativity that went into these technologies. Historians should take a broader perspective and follow the advice that John Pickstone gave in 1992 to study 'the real, messy, contested and complex debates by which, over time, some procedures were accepted in preference to others'.[56] It is worth looking at how surgical technologies have existed in the setting of multiple and heterogeneous agents and structures, including doctors, patients, manufacturers, objects, germs, wounds, institutions, regulations and so on, and how specific technologies and their uses emerged in such settings and how they were shaped by the settings and, in turn, reconfigured them.[57] Within such a scenario, the context of change is as variable and fluid as is the technologies themselves.

There are a couple of ways of broadening one's historical perspective. One of these is to not only look at techniques that were new at the time, but also to include the use of old techniques, as the historian of technology David Edgerton recommends.[58] This is particularly suitable if one considers that newness itself varies according to perspective, context and rhetoric. To be sure, for the historical actors discussed in this chapter, it was often important to claim novelty for the techniques they proposed. In science and medicine, credit, priority and intellectual property have always been closely linked to originality.[59] However, historians cannot simply accept such claims at face value. 'What constitutes an innovation was very much a matter of perspective, and often a matter of conflicting perspectives', as Ilana Löwy has written.[60] As Sally Frampton notes in her study of ovariotomy, fundamentally, 'the "new" is very much a representation', it is 'fixed to a specific time period'. In the second half of the nineteenth century, ovariotomy could be presented as new or as old, according to the needs of the historical actors in particular contexts. 'Thus', Frampton concludes, 'notions of "newness" are to be seen as constructed rather than necessarily pertaining to a linear temporality'.[61] Historicising newness in this way also makes it possible for the historian to escape the conscription into the retrospective adjudication of priority claims.[62]

Going beyond the awareness of the historically constructed nature of novelty, other authors have criticised the exclusive interest in the new in an 'innovation-centric history'. In his monograph *The Shock of the Old*, Edgerton observes a widespread assumption 'that the new is much superior to older methods'. In reality, he argues, this judgement is often not well-founded. It is a widespread, but often erroneous, belief 'that the new would be better in the longer run'[63] – a belief that, importantly, can even become a self-fulfilling prophecy. As he further points out, the unreflecting assumption of the superiority of the new has a significant historiographical corollary. If we accept it, we need to explain why some historical actors did not take on the new, why they put up 'resistance', as it is called. 'Resistance to new technology' becomes a puzzle to be solved with the help of psychological and sociological factors.[64]

Therefore, the adherence to the simple dichotomy of acceptance versus rejection of new techniques is problematic. Issues are more complex and such a dichotomy obscures what choices existed at particular times and how the historical actors dealt with them. Recognising these complexities will make it easier to avoid anachronistic explanations such as resistance, inertia, blindness and so on to explain why certain new technologies were not taken up by historical actors. We can instead try to understand the rationales that were motivating contemporaries, such as Halsted's attempts to prevent surgical infection by optimising the condition of the wound.

As we have seen, at closer examination, alternative options emerge wherever one looks in the history of surgery. Multiple versions of modern surgery emerge, among which dealing with the problem of wound infection through the surgeon's hands is just one example. Alternative technologies could be old or new, surgical or non-surgical. Taking them into account helps explain the choices and decisions that were made by historical actors. It is highly interesting, to express it with a metaphor, to explore the 'paths not taken' in surgical infection control, to look at the multiple parallel roads, the narrow trails and dirt tracks, as well the main highways. Such a broader perspective makes it possible to appreciate also the diversity of technologies today. It puts us in a better position to take notice of alternative forms of understanding and solving problems, and to beware, as David Edgerton has put it, of 'overblown claims of a one best way' of dealing with technical, surgical and medical challenges.[65]

Notes

1 For this line of argument, see also T. Schlich and C. Crenner, 'Technological change in surgery: An introductory essay', in T. Schlich and C. Crenner (eds), *Technological change in modern surgery: Historical perspectives on innovation* (Rochester, NY: University of Rochester Press, 2017), 1–20.

2 T. Schlich, 'Negotiating technologies in surgery: The controversy about surgical gloves in the 1890s', *Bulletin for the History of Medicine*, 87 (2013), 170–197.

3 J. Randers-Pehrson, *The surgeon's glove* (Springfield, IL: Charles C. Thomas, 1960): 3, 14, 30. See also T. Schlich, 'Why were surgical gloves not used earlier? History of medicine and alternative paths of innovation', *Lancet*, 386 (2015), 1234–1235.

4 Schlich, 'Negotiating technologies in surgery', 170–197.

5 W. S. Halsted, 'Ligature and suture material', *Journal of the American Medical Association*, 60 (1913), 1119–1126, 1123.

6 J. M. T. Finney, *A surgeon's life: The autobiography of J. M. T. Finney* (New York: G. P. Putnam's Sons, 1940), 90.

7 H. Robb, *Aseptic surgical technique. With especial reference to gynaecological operations, together with notes on the technique employed in certain supplementary procedures* (Philadelphia: Lippincott, 1894), 57.

8 Halsted, 'Ligature', 1124; S. J. Crowe, *Halsted of Johns Hopkins: The man and his men* (Springfield, IL: Thomas, 1957), reports that Joseph Bloodgood was the first surgeon at Johns Hopkins who wore gloves for every operation and that he started doing that in 1896; J. C. Bloodgood, 'Halsted thirty-six years ago', *American Journal of Surgery*, 14 (1931), 89–148, see 93.

9 Halsted, 'Ligature', 1124.

10 Randers-Pehrson, *Surgeon's glove*, 58.

11 W. G. MacCallum, *William Stuart Halsted, surgeon* (Baltimore: Johns Hopkins, 1930), 233, also 86–87.

12 W. S. Halsted, 'The treatment of wounds', *The Johns Hopkins Hospital Reports*, 2:5 (March 1891), 304–313, see 305.

13 MacCallum, as cited by M. Bliss, *Harvey Cushing: A life in surgery* (New York: Oxford University Press, 2005), 101.

14 C. Schimmelbusch, *Anleitung zur aseptischen Wundbehandlung* (Berlin: Hirschwald, 1892), 49–51; E. von Bergmann, 'Nachruf an Dr. Kurt Schimmelbusch', *Berliner klinische Wochenschrift*, 32 (1895), 730–731.

15 P. Fürbringer, *Untersuchungen und Vorschriften über die Desinfektion der Hände des Arztes nebst Bemerkungen über den bakteriologischen Charakter des Nagelschmutzes* (Wiesbaden: J. F. Bergmann, 1888), 3; P. Fürbringer, 'Zur Desinfection der Hände des Arztes', *Deutsche medizinische Wochenschrift*, 14 (1888), 985–987, P. Fürbringer and Dr Freyhan in Berlin, 'Neue Untersuchungen über die Desinfection der Hände', *Deutsche medizinische Wochenschrift*, 23 (1897), 81–85. On Fürbringer, see Pagel in *Biographisches Lexikon hervorragender Ärzte des neunzehnten Jahrhunderts* (Berlin: Wien 1901), 567–568.

16 C. L. Schleich, *Neue Methoden der Wundheilung, ihre Bedingungen und Vereinfachung für die Praxis* (Berlin: Springer, 1899), 106–109. See, for example, T. Kocher, 'On some conditions of healing by first

intention, with special references to disinfection of hands', *Transactions of the American Surgical Association*, 17 (1899), 116–142.

17 A. J. Ochsner, 'Aseptic surgical technique: Minimum requirements for aseptic surgical operating in a hospital in which the personnel of the operation room is permanent', *Annals of Surgery*, 40 (1904), 453–463, 457.

18 *Ibid.*, see 456. See also P. Kernahan, 'Franklin Martin and the standardization of American Surgery, 1890–1940' (unpublished PhD thesis: University of Minnesota, 2010).

19 von Bergmann, 'Nachruf an Dr. Kurt Schimmelbusch', 730–731. For Lockwood, see T. H. Pennington, 'Listerism, its decline and its persistence: The introduction of aseptic surgical techniques in three British teaching hospitals, 1890–99', *Medical History*, 39 (1995), 35–60, see 56.

20 G. Neuber, *Die aseptische Wundbehandlung in meinen Privat-Hospitälern* (Kiel: Lipius & Tischler, 1886); G. E. Konjetzny and E. Heits, *Gustav Adolf Neuber und die Asepsis* (Stuttgart: Enke, 1950).

21 T. Schlich, 'Asepsis and bacteriology: A realignment of surgery and laboratory science', *Medical History*, 56 (2012), 308–343.

22 J. Mikulicz, 'Ueber der neuesten Bestrebungen, die aseptische Wundbehandlung zu vervollkommnen', *Verhandlungen der deutschen Gesellschaft für Chirurgie*, 27 (1898), 1–37, 1–2. For more context, see Schlich, 'Asepsis'.

23 Ochsner, 'Aseptic surgical technique', 456.

24 *Ibid.*

25 W. A. Lane, *The operative treatment of fractures*, 2nd edition (London: Medical Publishing Company, 1914), 138.

26 *Ibid.*, 139.

27 Anon, '"Knife and fork" surgery', *The Star* (Lyttleton, New Zealand), 7696 (4 May 1903), 3.

28 All these methods are mentioned in C. S. Haegler, *Händereinigung, Händedesinfektion und Händeschutz* (Basel: Schwabe, 1900), 170–174.

29 Haegler, *Händereinigung*, 167.

30 Schleich, *Neue Methoden*, 106–109, 'collodium', see 106, 'microscopic glove', 108.

31 *Ibid.*, 111–113.

32 *Ibid.*, 108–109.

33 Haegler, *Händereinigung*, 170.

34 Schimmelbusch, *Anleitung zur aseptischen Wundbehandlung*.

35 B. F. Miller, R. Abrams, D. A. Huber *et al.*, 'Formation of invisible, nonperceptible films on hands by cationic soaps', *Proceedings of the Society for Experimental Biology and Medicine*, 54 (1943), 174–176, see 175.

36 *Ibid.*, see 176.
37 E. Payr, *Die physiologisch-biologische Richtung der modernen Chirurgie*, inaugural lecture held on 11 Dec 1912, in the auditorium of the University of Leipzig (Leipzig: Hirzel, 1913), see 29, more in fn. 9, 50–51.
38 J. von Mikulicz-Radecki, 'Experiments on the immunization against infection of operation wounds, especially of the peritoneum', *Lancet*, 2 (July 2, 1904), 1–4, see 1.
39 *Ibid.*, 1.
40 *Ibid.* H. Miyake joined Mikulicz during a two-year long stay in Germany, see S. Hiki and Y. Hiki, 'Professor von Mikulicz-Radecki: Breslau, 100 years since his death', *Langenbeck's Archives for Surgery*, 390 (2005), 182–185. Miyake worked with Mikulicz in 1898–1900 and again in 1903–1904, E. Kraas, Y. Hiki and I. Umhauer (eds), *300 Jahre deutsch-japanische Beziehungen in der Medizin* (Berlin: Springer, 1992), 79.
41 J. Mikulicz, 'Ueber Versuche, die "aseptische" Wundbehandlung zu einer wirklich keimfreien Methode zu vervollkommen', *Deutsche medizinische Wochenschrift*, 33 (1897), 409–413, 412; Mikulicz, 'Bestrebungen', 3. On Flügge, see S. Berger, *Bakterien in Krieg und Frieden. Eine Geschichte der medizinischen Bakteriologie in Deutschland 1890–1933* (Göttingen: Wallstein, 2009), 45–46. Flügge's compendium, Dr C. Flügge, *Grundriss der Hygiene für Studierende und Praktische Ärzte, Medicinal- und Verwaltungsbeamte* (Leipzig: Veit, 1889), was completely based on Kochian bacteriology.
42 On this relationship, see Schlich, 'Asepsis'.
43 Mikulicz, 'Experiments', all quotations 1.
44 *Ibid.*, 2.
45 *Ibid.*, 2.
46 *Ibid.*, 3.
47 *Ibid.*, 4.
48 Anon, 'Immunization against surgical infection', *Journal of the American Medical Association*, July 30 (1904), 332–333, see 333.
49 M. Worboys, *Spreading germs* (Cambridge: Cambridge University Press, 2000), 77.
50 *Ibid.*, 84.
51 *Ibid.*, 76.
52 *Ibid.*, 102.
53 *Ibid.*, 80.
54 *Ibid.*, 186.
55 P. J. Kernahan, 'Causation and cleanliness: George Callender, wounds, and the debates over Listerism', *Journal of the History of Medicine and*

Allied Sciences, 64 (2008), 1–36; and A. Greenwood, 'Lawson Tait and opposition to germ theory: Defining science in surgical practice', *Journal of the History of Medicine and Allied Sciences*, 53 (1998), 99–131.

56 J. V. Pickstone, 'Introduction', in J. V. Pickstone (ed.), *Medical innovations in historical perspective* (Basingstoke: MacMillan Press, 1992), 1–16, see 16.

57 T. Schlich, *Surgery, science and industry: A revolution in fracture care, 1950s–1990s* (Basingstoke: Palgrave, 2002), 241.

58 D. Edgerton, *The shock of the old: Technology and global history since 1900* (London: Profile, 2006).

59 R. K. Merton, *The sociology of science* (Chicago: Chicago University Press, 1973), 293, as discussed in S. Frampton, '"The most startling innovation": Ovarian surgery in Britain, c. 1740–1939' (PhD thesis: University College London, 2013), 138–139.

60 I. Löwy, 'Medicine and change', in I. Löwy *et al.* (eds), *Medicine and change: Historical and sociological studies of medical innovation* (Paris: INSERM, 1993), 1–4, see 3.

61 Frampton, 'Ovarian surgery', 271.

62 Merton, *Sociology of science*, 301–303.

63 Edgerton, *The shock*, 8.

64 *Ibid.*, 9; Pickstone, 'Introduction', 1; and Frampton, 'Ovarian surgery', 134.

65 D. Edgerton, 'From innovation to use: Ten eclectic theses on the historiography of technology', *History and Technology*, 16 (1999): 111–136, see 129.

7

The evolving role of gloves in healthcare

Jennie Wilson

The hands of healthcare workers have been acknowledged as a key vehicle for the transmission of healthcare-associated infections (HAI). There is evidence that they acquire transient microorganisms through touch and that these are readily transferred to other surfaces and to patients.[1] Hand hygiene has been perceived as a cornerstone of infection prevention and control in protecting patients from HAI, but since the mid-1980s, non-sterile clinical gloves (NSCG) have come into widespread use. Attitudes to both hand hygiene and the use of gloves have evolved over time, and this chapter explores how changes in perceptions in recent decades have influenced clinical practice.

The role of hands in the transmission of healthcare-associated infection

In 1847, Ignaz Semmelweis developed a theory that 'cadaveric particles', acquired on the hands of medical students, were responsible for causing puerperal fever in women in labour in the obstetric clinic. The mortality rate from puerperal fever fell from 18 per cent to 2 per cent once he instituted the policy that required medical students to wash their hands with a solution of chlorinated lime between performing autopsies and examining patients in the clinic. Although the work of Semmelweis provided critical evidence for the role of hand hygiene in preventing the transmission of infection, the significance of the findings was not widely recognised until Louis Pasteur developed the germ theory of disease. Moreover, as Thomas Schlich argues in his chapter in this volume, the take-up of surgical gloves in the nineteenth century was not a foregone conclusion. And although we now consider hand hygiene an essential infection control measure in all healthcare situations, until relatively recently it was seen primarily as an infection control measure in high-risk situations such as surgery.

This is illustrated in a study by Mortimer *et al.*, conducted in 1966, which set out to determine the extent to which *Staphylococcus aureus* was transmitted by the airborne route.[2] Modern ethics of clinical research were not well developed, and the study was undertaken in a newborn nursery. As part of the methodology, nurses were required to not wash their hands between contact with different babies. Whilst such a study would be considered unethical now, its design provides important data on the role of hands in the transmission of pathogens between patients. The nursery was divided into two areas marked by a red line on the floor. In area one there were two babies with a typable strain of *S. aureus* and two other babies admitted from the delivery suite. In area two, there were four babies admitted from the delivery suite. In area one, the nurses were not to wash their hands before and after contact with the babies; babies with the typable strain were also to be handled and their nappy changed directly before contact with the other babies. In area two, the nurses were to wash their hands before and after all contact with the babies. All the babies were then swabbed to determine which had acquired the typable *S. aureus*. As might be

Table 7.1   Evidence for role of hands in transmission of *Staphylococcus aureus* in a newborn nursery

Acquisition rates of Staphylococci from index baby			
Group	*No. exposed*	*Acquisitions*	
		No.	%
Airborne	158	16*	10
Physical contact (Total)	126	49	38
- *handwashing*	*21*	*3*	*14*
- *no handwashing*	*105*	*46*	*43*

* 9 = 'definite' (no other source of the strain identified); 7 = 'possible' (strain identified in neighbouring baby for up to two days before)

Source: Mortimer *et al.*, 1966

expected, given what we now know about transmission on hands, the study showed that in cases where the nurses did not wash their hands, a high proportion of babies acquired the typable *S. aureus*. There was also some presumed airborne transmission to babies in area two (Table 7.1).

The emergence of non-sterile gloves in the delivery of routine clinical practice

Whilst sterile latex gloves were widely used in surgery to protect the patient from microorganisms on the hands of the surgeon, prior to the 1980s gloves were rarely used in other clinical settings. Then, the main type of NSCG in use was polythene – flimsy and of limited value in protecting the hands, as they ripped or came off easily. Although some latex gloves were available, they were considered expensive and unnecessary. In the mid-1980s, concerns about transmission of the human immunodeficiency virus (HIV) in healthcare settings through contact with body fluids resulted in the advice from the Centers for Disease Control for healthcare workers to apply Universal Precautions (UP) in the care of all patients.[3] This advice was predicated on evidence that HIV and other blood-borne viruses were present in blood and a range of other body fluids, and that healthcare workers should use protective clothing to minimise the risk of infection. The UP advice also acknowledged that it was not possible to know which patients carried infection, and therefore the precautions should be applied in the care of all patients.

Over the next decade, it was recognised that using gloves for contact with body fluids had wider benefits in terms of other pathogens found in high concentrations in body fluids. In 1987, an approach called Body Substance Isolation (BSI) was proposed.[4] This recommended the use of gloves for contact with all moist and potentially infectious body substances (e.g. blood, faeces, urine, sputum, wound drainage etc.) from all patients, regardless of their presumed infection status. In the Guidelines for Isolation Precautions in the US, the Hospitals Hospital Infection Control Advisory Committee amalgamated BSI and UP as Standard Precautions (SP). These were described as a single set of precautions to be used for the care of all patients in hospitals, regardless of their presumed infection status;

this measure was designed to reduce the risk of transmission of blood-borne and other pathogens in hospitals. Similar guidance was adopted in the UK with national guidelines on preventing HAI in both acute and non-acute care settings.[5] Key to SP was the concept of risk assessment, requiring healthcare workers to judge the risk of exposure to blood and body fluids and to use gloves and other protective clothing when direct contact was anticipated.[6] In addition, it was considered that wearing gloves did not replace the need for handwashing, since gloves may have defects or may be torn during use, and hands can become contaminated during removal of gloves. As indicated by the World Health Organization (WHO) guidelines on hand hygiene, gloves should be used for discreet procedures and changed immediately after use and between patients, and hands should be washed after removal.[7] Over time, these policies have resulted in NSCG becoming widely available. Initially, cheaper vinyl gloves were preferred, but now more conformable nitrile gloves provide a better fit, are offered in a range of attractive colours and are cost-effective compared to vinyl. The drive to make gloves readily available has seen the widespread use of glove dispensers located throughout clinical areas.

Evidence of problems with the use of non-sterile clinical gloves

From the early days of UP, there was evidence of non-adherence to guidance on their use, in terms of both underuse and overuse. In a 2004 study, staff caring for patients who were in isolation were observed not to change gloves between procedures.[8] In the case of gloves, Girou *et al.* demonstrated that 100 per cent of gloves sampled grew bacteria, and almost all grew the same pathogens as those on the patient. This result showed that gloves acquire pathogens in the same way as hands, and hence act to transfer organisms from surface to surface by contact. Scholars in the 1980s had previously demonstrated in laboratory experiments that microorganisms acquired by touch are readily transferred to the next thing touched; thus hands, gloved or otherwise, are efficient vectors of microorganisms between patients and their environment in healthcare settings.[9]

In the framework for 'five moments of hand hygiene' proposed in the WHO guideline, it is suggested that non-sterile gloves should be perceived as 'a second skin' to prevent exposure of hands to body fluid, and that 'glove removal should be a strong cue for hand hygiene'.[10] The WHO guidance also makes clear recommendations for situations when non-sterile gloves are not required. These include procedures such as taking blood pressure or temperature, subcutaneous and intramuscular injections, mouth/eye care and washing and dressing patients.[11] However, there is an emerging body of evidence that the use of NSCG has extended widely beyond the recommended intention of direct contact with blood and body fluid, with gloves routinely used for a range of low- or no-risk activities. In a study on the impact of the national 'Clean Your Hands' campaign instigated by the National Patient Safety Agency in the UK, researchers observed that NSCG were worn for more than a quarter of episodes, and that they were commonly worn for procedures not associated with contact with blood and body fluids. In addition, if the healthcare worker wore gloves, they were also less likely to wash their hands after the procedure.[12]

The remainder of this chapter will focus on our case study findings. We have explored hand hygiene behaviour in the context of NSCG use, using the 'five moments of hand hygiene' as a guide as to when gloves should be changed (see Figure 7.1). This work has involved both auditing use of NSCG to determine when and how they are used, and interviews with staff to determine their attitudes to gloves and drivers of their behaviour.[13] Table 7.2 illustrates the risk of cross contamination observed in two acute hospitals during seventy-eight episodes of care where NSCG were used, comprising a total of 295 procedures. The finding that a series of tasks are commonly performed together during an episode of care indicates the real risk in everyday clinical practice of cross transmission between dirty and clean procedures on the same patient or between patients. Analysis of these episodes demonstrated an overall compliance rate of only 50 per cent of the five moments of hand hygiene. The most commonly missed moments were 1 (before contact with the patient) and 4 (after contact with the patient), which accounted for 21 per cent and 30 per cent of hand hygiene breaches. However, in 69 per cent (54/78) of episodes of care, more than one moment of hand hygiene was breached.[14] In addition, in almost 60 per cent of occasions where gloves were used, the procedure did not involve direct contact with blood and body fluid, mucous membranes, isolation

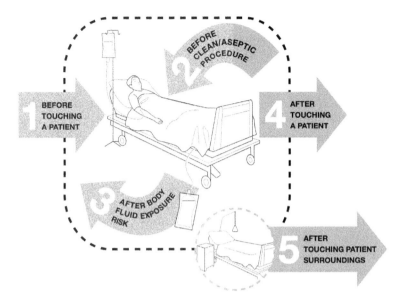

Figure 7.1   Clinical situations where gloves should or should not be worn.

Table 7.2   Risk of cross contamination and appropriateness of glove use. Data from observation of clinical practice in two hospitals in England

	No. episodes	% Cross contamination	No. procedures	% Use inappropriate
Hospital A	69	58%	104	38%
Hospital B	109	43%	191	68%
OVERALL	178	49%	295	57%

Source: Wilson, Bak and Loveday, 'Applying human factors and ergonomics'

precautions or hazardous substances, and gloves were therefore not required (see Table 7.2). Hand hygiene was not performed after glove removal for 41 per cent of care episodes, despite evidence derived from Ebola studies that hands are vulnerable to contamination from gloves when they are removed.

The most common procedures for which gloves were observed being worn were in helping a patient move from one place to another, bed making, cleaning surfaces and manipulation of intravenous (IV) devices. The routine use of gloves for handling of IV devices is interesting because it illustrates the common perception that somehow gloves are needed to protect these 'high-risk' devices. Yet, clean gloves are no less contaminated with transient microorganisms than hands themselves, and therefore confer no additional protection. This suggests that gloves have been incorporated into routine practice and are not being used according to the principles of existing infection control policy and guidance. One of the advantages of capturing data on the sequence of items touched during an episode of care is that it demonstrates the reality of practice and provides very powerful data on the potential for cross contamination. Such data is not generally captured through routine audits of hand hygiene, as these tend to focus on single 'moments' rather than the sequence of events between 'moments.' Table 7.3 illustrates examples of touch sequences observed whilst staff were wearing gloves.

Table 7.3   Examples of touch sequences during observed episodes of care

Sequence of items touched by same pair of non-sterile gloves during a procedure to add an IV drug to a fluid bag	Sequence of items touched by same pair of non-sterile gloves when attending to an IV pump	Sequence of procedures undertaken wearing same pair of non-sterile gloves
Syringe	Linen on trolley	Empty urine catheter bag
Injection water	Bed (Patient 1)	Give patient mouth care
Medication for reconstitution	Chart (Patient 1)	Check blood sugar with BM stick
Medication injected into fluid bag	Chart (Patient 2)	
Labels	IV pump (Patient 1)	
Watch	Chart (Patient 1)	
Trolley	Patient 1	
IV administration set in other patient zone		
IV administration set		
IV bag in kidney bowl		

Source: Author's unpublished data

Drivers of glove use behaviour

These observations show that the overuse and misuse of gloves is so embedded in patterns of behaviour that education alone is unlikely to improve practice. A second component of our research has therefore focused on attempting to understand the drivers of glove use behaviour in order to design successful intervention strategies. We have interviewed healthcare workers across a range of professional groups at two acute hospitals about their attitudes to the use of NSCG.[15] These interviews highlight some key beliefs and attitudes underpinning glove use behaviour, which can be summarised under themes of emotion and socialisation, both professional and organisational (Figure 7.2).

Emotion is a key influence on glove use behaviour, and healthcare worker decisions about using them are strongly personal. Whilst from an infection prevention perspective the primary purpose of NSCG is to minimise the risk of transfer of pathogens between patients, interviews with healthcare workers suggest that, for them, the main purpose of gloves is to increase their own safety. They use them to avoid contact with things they perceive as 'dirty' or 'unpleasant' and to give them confidence when dealing with patients (see Figure 7.3). This thin layer of latex provided by gloves

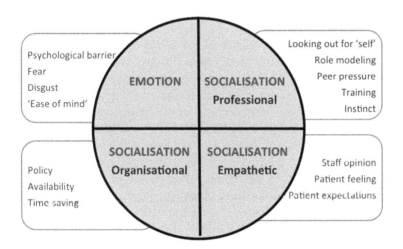

Figure 7.2   Drivers of glove use behaviour.

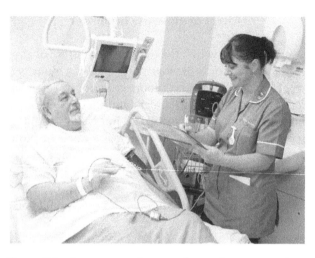

Figure 7.3   A nurse carrying out observations on a patient.

confers a huge sense of safety to protect from perceived, but mostly non-specific, risks, commonly expressed as 'dirt' or 'bad stuff'. They act as a barrier that means the healthcare worker does not need to 'worry about what they are touching'.[16]

Other studies have also suggested that emotion plays an important role in healthcare worker attitudes to infection prevention, and Pamela Wood has shown in her contribution to this volume how important emotional concepts of 'dirt' can be to actual practice.[17] A 2014 study found that student nurses disliked touching sweaty skin and worn clothes.[18] Another account showed that nurses had their own social construct of 'dirt', which was a key driver in determining whether they applied infection control precautions but was not informed by a scientific analysis of infection risk. Precautions were also moderated by familiarity with the patient.[19] This finding resonates with work that has identified hand hygiene behaviour as being strongly influenced by perceptions of exposure to 'dirt' or 'germs', with family sources considered much less harmful than non-family and public sources. Whitby *et al.* suggest that these perceptions of dirt are acquired early in childhood and have an important influence on the decision to wash hands.[20] Our research indicates that healthcare workers use gloves to avoid contact with sources of 'dirt'. This has the perverse consequence of neutralising the trigger that would normally induce hand hygiene, which contributes to the risk of cross contamination and lack of hand hygiene at appropriate points during care that we observed in association with gloves (Table 7.4).

There is also a perception that even if you wash your hands, you cannot guarantee they are totally clean. This may be an adverse effect of the common practice of using fluorescent dye and 'globoxes' as a training tool to reinforce hand hygiene among healthcare workers. They may actually transmit the message that 'even though I've washed my hands, I've still got fluorescent dye on them so hand hygiene can't be relied on and I'm better to use gloves'.[21] Other mixed messages appear to have arisen from the concepts of contact and standard precautions. Contact precautions are widely used for patients colonised or infected with multi-drug resistant pathogens, and confer the strong message that gloves should be put on before entering the room and removed on leaving, but with little emphasis on changing them between dirty and clean tasks performed in the room. On the other hand, standard precautions suggest that since we cannot tell who is harbouring harmful pathogens, protective clothing should be worn for contact with all patients. By combining these two concepts, staff draw the logical conclusion that since they don't know who has got what infections, then they should treat everyone the same, and wear gloves for contact with all patients.

The second key influence is socialisation, primarily reflecting organisational and professional drivers but with empathy for the viewpoint of patients also playing a role. Organisational factors include the accepted standards of practice disseminated in policies and procedures. Staff cite these as being an important influence on their practice, although evidence from observations of how gloves are used suggests that perhaps it is more the perception of policy than the reality of the actual guidance they contain that underpin practice.[22]

In an exploration of the attitudes of third-year student nurses, we found that 90 per cent would routinely wear gloves for washing an adult patient and 80 per cent for taking a methicillin-resistant *S. aureus* screening nasal swab, despite gloves not being a requirement for these tasks in infection prevention and control policy.[23] Other

Table 7.4   Examples of attitudes towards the use of non-sterile clinical gloves. Participants number in brackets

Theme	Examples from interviews
Emotion	I'm putting these on because there's something I don't want to touch or catch, yes, my own cleanliness, the hygiene (386)
	We have people with lots of different infections that I wouldn't want to catch (386)
	And you feel like you don't want to take their shoes off without wearing gloves because you know you will wash your hands but just like feels like you know you don't want to touch it (175)
	To make sure that you are safe because if something were to happen and we were accused of mistreating somebody, like if they got sick or something and we weren't shown to be wearing gloves ... then they could say well you're liable for it because we've not taken proper care (184)
	We were told not to use them at all but then it [made?] the patient uncomfortable and so I'd be doing all sorts of disgusting dirty tasks you can't imagine without wearing gloves (174)
	I feel a lot safer wearing gloves which means I feel more confident (184)
Socialisation –organisational	If the gloves are around everywhere people tend to use them more, whereas I remember back in those days in nursing home setting[s] you would have to go all the way round to the main nursing station to get a pair of gloves so people won't be using gloves as often (175)
	You get told on the ward and when you're doing your training when and where to wear the gloves ... it's just something you do rather than something you overly think about (176)
	And it's a bit like Chinese whispers in a way and no-one's ever quite sure where the information originally came from (181)
	[my decision to wear gloves] I think it's a mixture of policy and your personal [influence] (386)

(*Continued*)

Table 7.4 (Continued)

Theme	Examples from interviews
Socialisation – professional	Even if they were a senior [and] said to me oh you're not to wear gloves any more than if they couldn't show me something to support that then I would still continue wearing gloves (173)
	It's a personal decision as to whether you feel you want to wear gloves for ... because you don't want to touch that skin, that's a completely personal point of view (387)
	Sometimes I do think you don't need to wear gloves for that [task/procedure] but I guess that's personal choice isn't it that they don't feel quite right not to wear gloves (172)
	I think perhaps the public perception about health, hygiene in hospital and cleanliness I think they expect that nurses wear gloves because that would be better but I'm not sure that it is always better (182)
	It's a barrier between nurse and patient and I think if you are washing someone ... student nurses come and they put gloves on to do a bed bath and I think that's really inappropriate ... if someone was going to wash my face and put gloves on I would find that quite insulting (182)

Source: Author's unpublished data

aspects of this survey of student nurses suggest that staff do not construct a logical analysis of potential contact with body fluid and associated risk of infection. For example, only 25 per cent said they would wear gloves for washing a baby, as they apparently perceive a baby to be less dirty than an adult – which is ironic given that babies have a high density of *S. aureus* on their skin.[24] Similarly, whilst only 60 per cent said they would wear gloves routinely for changing a nappy, 99 per cent would wear them routinely for changing an incontinence pad.[25] A significant proportion of student nurses reported routinely using gloves to undertake a wide range of tasks for which gloves are not recommended, and where there is no risk of contact with body fluids, for example injections, handling unsoiled bed linen and dressing patients. Other researchers have highlighted this lack of scientific basis for decisions made about infection control precautions, and inconsistent attitudes by nurses to the use of gloves.[26] An online survey combined with focus groups of student nurses identified similar inappropriate use of gloves for tasks associated with no risk of exposure to blood and body fluids, their use apparently driven by the culture of the clinical environment rather than hospital policy.[27]

However, some policies drive inappropriate glove use. For example, gloves appear to be widely worn for preparing IV drugs, despite there being no risk of exposure to blood and only a risk of contact with hazardous chemicals when handling cytotoxic drugs. There appears to be a universal notion that handling antibiotics is somehow dangerous, with beliefs that it is particularly hazardous if healthcare workers are allergic to penicillin. These risks are unfounded, and although commonly cited by guidance, the use of gloves is unnecessary for preparing and delivering IV medications.

Organisational drivers also include strong 'messaging' that endorses the use of gloves, for example their location throughout the clinical area and the sense that it is quicker to put on a pair of gloves than perform hand hygiene. Since gloves are commonly placed outside rooms or bays, they drive the tendency to put on gloves early, increase the risk they will become contaminated by touching the environment outside the patient area and reduce opportunities for changing gloves between procedures. A range of 'professional' drivers then influence glove use, including role modelling from respected peers or acquiring practice habits that fit in with the professional 'norm'. Our interviews with staff and survey of student nurses indicated a very strong perception that decisions about when and where to wear gloves were considered personal judgements and not open to challenge by other professionals.[28]

Empathy-related drivers are expressed in comments about negative associations with gloves, for example that they act as a barrier to touch and might convey the impression to the patient that they are considered 'dirty'. In contrast, staff also identified positive connotations of glove use; they believed that gloves conveyed a sense of 'being hygienic' (although our observations of practice suggest that the opposite is true) and that patients, whose perceptions of healthcare are informed by television and films, expect healthcare worker to wear gloves. Staff also identified gloves as a 'psychological barrier' that could make patients feel more comfortable about intimate tasks being performed by 'strangers'. This particularly relates to contact with the genitals, where the attitudes expressed reflect a concept of 'I'm not really touching that person if I've got gloves on'. The latex enables staff to cover up that emotional awkwardness about touching people in private areas and extends to helping them to manage their disgust at touching things they perceive to be unpleasant or dirty. However, they also report responding to cues from the patient, recognising that the patient might see gloves as providing a psychological barrier for them also. This perception appears to be valid. In a survey of 142 members of the public, we found that 94 per cent indicated that they would prefer healthcare workers to wear gloves for washing their genital area. The public were also perceptive about where gloves were required, indicting a high preference for their use for tasks involving contact with blood or body fluid but not for low-risk tasks such as 'assisting to the toilet' or 'feeding'.[29] As patients, respondents demonstrated that they were passive observers of poor practice by healthcare workers. One commented, 'they [the staff] were wearing gloves for the whole of my consultation; they didn't wash their hands yet touched a large number of items in the room including a keyboard and phone'. However, it is difficult for patients to be sufficiently empowered to challenge behaviour that is so embedded amongst healthcare workers; 25 per cent had challenged the practice of staff in relation to gloves but had not experienced a positive response as a result.

Why does the misuse of gloves matter?

The evidence emerging from our research and that of others demonstrates that gloves are now widely used to protect the wearer from things they perceive to be 'dirty', and that guidance about the use of gloves is confused and not based on sound infection control principles. Risk assessment to support decision making about when to wear gloves is ill-defined, and staff lack competence. Gloves are perceived as the default position to prevent transmission of infection, although in reality because of the way they are used they are likely to increase the risk of transmission. Emotion related to disgust is recognised as a key driver of hand hygiene, but we have found that this emotion *triggers* glove use, and if gloves are worn, the drive for hand hygiene is reduced.[30] This combination of behaviour patterns, widespread use of gloves in situations where their use is not indicated and the tendency for healthcare workers to put them on too early and take them off too late presents real hazards in terms of cross transmission of pathogens in healthcare settings. Such associations are difficult to prove, but a recent report on an outbreak of group A *Streptococcus* found the organism on a third of the curtains, a finding readily explained by the patterns of glove use we have observed.[31]

Reflections on changing patterns of glove use

Our observations on current patterns of use of NSCG can be set in the context of important changes to both nursing roles and attitudes to risk in modern industrial societies. The eminent sociologist Anthony Giddens coined the term the 'risk society' in the 1980s, as a way of describing a society preoccupied with the hazards and insecurities of modernisation.[32] Prior to the 1980s, most healthcare workers did not perceive contact with patients to be intrinsically risky, and did not routinely wear protective clothing. In the past, healthcare operated with strong 'command and control' structure. The sister or 'matron' had ultimate control over all aspects of care and the decisions about how it was delivered. As these structures have eroded, staff have more autonomy to make their own decisions and have developed a greater sense of personal risk. This preoccupation with the perceived hazards of touching patients underpins current glove use behaviour. The sense of personal autonomy to makes decisions about protecting the self is also evidence in the student nurses' responses that their own judgement was the primary driver of their glove use behaviour.

Whilst clear policy is important for communicating best practice, it is evident that staff often do not know about or follow what is written in policies, or perhaps adapt those policies to fit their own perceptions of risk. This is illustrated by the emergence and adaption of UP, which we have shown has been modified to encompass a concept that gloves are required for contact with all patients, because the ones who present a risk cannot be distinguished. Similarly, perhaps the frequent demonstration of the inadequate of hand hygiene using fluorescent dye and a 'glo-box' has led healthcare workers to believe that hand hygiene is not effective, and that therefore it is safer to wear gloves. In the past, an aseptic technique required the use of forceps and careful consideration of the 'clean' and 'dirty' areas of a sterile field. Today, the procedure has been greatly simplified by the replacement of forceps by gloves, but perhaps this too has diluted the sense of asepsis and created the idea that gloves render the hands sterile.

Protection of healthcare workers is clearly highly desirable, but currently there is a significant gap between policy and practice in relation to glove use that increases the risk to patients of acquiring HAI. Changing practice will be hugely complex but essential in addressing the future challenges of HAI.[33] Interventions will need to embrace the notion of human factors, and take account of the influence of the organisation, the staff and patients and what they think and believe, the ergonomics of care delivery, and how gloves and hand hygiene can be safely and efficiently integrated into everyday clinical tasks.

Notes

1 C. A. Mackintosh and P. N. Hoffman, 'An extended model for transfer of micro-organisms via the hands: Differences between organisms and the effect of alcohol disinfection', *Epidemiology and Infection*, 92 (1984), 345–355.

2 E. A. Mortimer Jr E. Wolinsky, A. J. Gonzaga and C. H. Rammelkamp Jr, 'Role of airborne transmission in Staphylococcal infections', *British Medical Journal*, 1 (1966), 319.

3 Centers for Disease Control, 'Perspectives in disease prevention and health promotion update: universal precautions for prevention of transmission of Human Immunodeficiency Virus, Hepatitis B Virus, and other bloodborne pathogens in health-care settings', *MMWR*, 37 (1988), 377–388, www.cdc.gov/mmwr/preview/mmwrhtml/00000039.htm.

4 P. Lynch, M. M. Jackson, M. J. Cummings and W. E. Stamm, 'Rethinking the role of isolation practices in the prevention of nosocomial infections', *Annals of Internal Medicine*, 107 (1987), 245–246.

5 R. J. Pratt, C. Pellowe, H. Loveday *et al.*, 'The epic project: Developing national evidence-based guidelines for preventing healthcare associated

infections. Phase 1: Guidelines for preventing hospital-acquired infections', *Journal of Hospital Infection*, 47, supplement (2001), S1–S82; C. M. Pellowe, R. Pratt, H. Loveday *et al.*, 'The epic project. Updating the evidence-base for national evidence-based guidelines for preventing healthcare-associated infections in NHS hospitals in England: A report with recommendations', *British Journal of Infection Control*, 5 (2004), 10–15.

6 Pratt *et al.*, 'The epic project'.

7 World Health Organization, *WHO guidelines on hand hygiene in health care* (Geneva: World Health Organization, 2009).

8 E. Girou, S. H. T. Chai, F. Oppein *et al.*, 'Misuse of gloves: The foundation for poor compliance with hand hygiene and potential for microbial transmission?', *Journal of Hospital Infection*, 57 (2004), 162–169.

9 Mackintosh and Hoffman, 'An extended model'.

10 H. Sax, B. Allegranzi, I. Uçkay *et al.*, '"My five moments for hand hygiene": A user-centred design approach to understand, train, monitor and report hand hygiene', *Journal of Hospital Infection*, 67 (2007), 9e21.

11 World Health Organization, *WHO guidelines on hand hygiene*.

12 C. Fuller, J. Savage, S. J. Besser and A. Hayward, '"The dirty hand in the latex glove": A study of hand hygiene compliance when gloves are worn', *Infection Control and Hospital Epidemiology*, 32 (2012), 1194–1199.

13 H. Loveday, S. Lynam, J. Singleton and J. Wilson, 'Clinical glove use: Healthcare workers' actions and perceptions', *Journal of Hospital Infection*, 86 (2014), 110–116; J. Wilson, J. Prieto, J. Singleton *et al.*, 'The misuse and overuse of non-sterile gloves: Application of an audit tool to define the problem', *Journal of Infection Prevention*, 16 (2015), 24–31; J. Wilson, A. Bak, A. Whitfield *et al.*, 'Public perceptions of the use of gloves by healthcare workers and comparison with perceptions of student nurses', *Journal of Infection Prevention*, 18 (2017), 123–132; J. Wilson, A. Bak and H. Loveday, 'Applying human factors and ergonomics to the misuse of non-sterile clinical gloves in acute care', *American Journal of Infection Control* (in press).

14 Wilson, Bak and Loveday, 'Applying human factors and ergonomics'.

15 Loveday *et al.*, 'Clinical glove use', and Wilson, Bak and Loveday, 'Applying human factors and ergonomics'.

16 *Ibid.*

17 See Chapter 3 in this volume.

18 S. Ratcliffe and J. Smith, 'Factors influencing glove use in student nurses', *Nursing Times*, 110 (2014), 18–21.

19 C. Jackson and P. Griffiths, 'Dirt and disgust as key drivers in nurses' infection control behaviours: An interpretative, qualitative study', *Journal of Hospital Infection*, 87 (2014), 71–76.

20 M. Whitby, M. McLaws and M. Ross, 'Why healthcare workers don't wash their hands: A behavioral explanation', *Infection Control and Hospital Epidemiology*, 27 (2006), 484–492.

21 Wilson, Bak and Loveday, 'Applying human factors and ergonomics'.

22 Wilson *et al.*, 'Public perceptions of the use of gloves', and Wilson, Bak and Loveday, 'Applying human factors and ergonomics'.

23 Wilson *et al.*, 'Public perceptions of the use of gloves'.

24 T. Oranges, V. Dini and M. Romanelli, 'Skin physiology of the neonate and infant: Clinical implications', *Advances in Wound Care*, 4 (2015), 587–595.

25 Wilson *et al.*, 'Public perceptions of the use of gloves'.

26 Jackson and Griffiths, 'Dirt and disgust as key drivers', and K. Lee, 'Student and infection prevention and control nurses' hand hygiene decision making in simulated clinical scenarios: A qualitative research study of hand washing, gel and glove use choices', *Journal of Infection Prevention*, 14 (2013), 96–103.

27 Ratcliffe and Smith, 'Factors influencing glove use in student nurses'.

28 Wilson *et al.*, 'Public perceptions of the use of gloves', and Wilson, Bak and Loveday, 'Applying human factors and ergonomics'.

29 Wilson *et al.*, 'Public perceptions of the use of gloves'.

30 Whitby, McLaws and Ross, 'Why healthcare workers don't wash their hands'.

31 N. Mahida, A. Beal, D. Trigg *et al.*, 'Outbreak of invasive group A Streptococcus infection: Contaminated patient curtains and cross-infection on an ear, nose and throat ward', *Journal of Hospital Infection*, 87 (2014), 141–144.

32 A. Giddens, *Modernity and self-identity: Self and society in the late modern age* (Cambridge: Polity, 1991).

33 Wilson, Bak and Loveday, 'Applying human factors and ergonomics'.

Part IV

Practice and infection control:
In the laboratory

8

Constructing the 'Sanitary Officer': the Pathologist's role in infection prevention and control at St Bartholomew's Hospital, London, 1892–1939

Rosemary Cresswell

In 1892, the role of Sanitary Officer was created at St Bartholomew's Hospital (Barts), London. The successful candidate was required to be qualified in medicine and to hold a diploma in public health. The job included receiving reports about cases of infectious disease from doctors and nurses at the hospital, notifying the Local Sanitary Authority about the patients involved, and investigating the cause, looking after the condition of sanitary appliances and inspecting the sanitary circumstances of the hospital. Frederick Andrewes, the Demonstrator in Practical Medicine at Barts, was the first Sanitary Officer to be recruited. Andrewes continued to undertake this role alongside his appointment as the Pathologist to the Hospital in 1897 and maintained both responsibilities until his retirement in 1928. Although Andrewes was appointed Sanitary Officer first, and Pathologist to the Hospital five years later, his successors in the 1920s and 1930s inherited both roles simultaneously, as the activities had become entwined.

Historians have perceived the cleanliness of hospitals to be the responsibility of the Matron. Therefore, although this chapter focuses on the appointment of a doctor to act upon risks of infection at the hospital, the second half of the chapter examines the roles of Matrons at Barts in managing and reporting issues relating to cleanliness, and innovations in sanitation, in contrast with the tasks carried out by the Sanitary Officer, to understand the difference in the work of the leaders in infection prevention and control. By contrasting the role of the Pathologist with that of the Matron, this chapter demonstrates that pathologists were involved in hospital management, patient care and infection control at a much earlier stage than has been suggested by the existing historiography of infection prevention and control. The chapter highlights the shifting boundaries and division of labour between the Sanitary Officer and Matron during this period, a time in which, as the role of the Sanitary Officer expanded, the scope of the Matron's jurisdiction contracted. What it highlights is a more systematic and scientific approach being taken to infection prevention and control, adopted by a very energetic Sanitary Officer investigating sources of infection within an institutional setting. Barts, in this case, seems to have been an 'early adopter' of this practice, shaking off the conservative image it is sometimes associated with.

Although there are several historical studies on the role of Matrons, an understanding of their everyday roles requires further research. Stuart Wildman and Alistair Hewison have critiqued golden-age views of the Matron as 'all powerful, all knowing' with regard to infection control and cleaning.[1] They have claimed that, by the beginning of the twentieth century, the Matron was established as in charge of the nursing service, and of cleaning, catering, linen and laundry, only to lose control of this role prior to the Second World War when these services became centralised.[2] Peter Ardern has similarly argued that before penicillin, 'the only way to prevent cross-infection was by scrupulous cleanliness, carefully supervised by the Matron. Matron, as the head of nursing care, was the key figure in the fight against infection, and cleanliness was her primary weapon.' Ardern uses interviews from the 1930s and 1940s which emphasise cleaning equipment, sterilisation and care to avoid cross infection with clothing.[3]

Responsibilities like those of Frederick Andrewes at Barts have not been discussed by historians and microbiologists, perhaps because Barts, the oldest continually open hospital in the country, was unusual and pioneering in creating the position of the Sanitary Officer. Bacteriologists' roles in showing that bacteria caused wound infection from the early 1880s have been recognised by Hugh Pennington, Graham Ayliffe and Mary English.[4] Kathryn Hillier has discussed the practice of bacteriologists in infection control from the early twentieth century, using serological typing for streptococci and later staphylococci, with phage typing complicating and extending their work in the 1950s. She claims

that prior to this period, bacteriologists were regarded as technical staff not involved in patient care, only asserting themselves in
the wards and meeting rooms of hospitals from the 1950s.[5] Ayliffe
and English acknowledge that microbiologists were involved in
rounds on surgical wards in the 1950s.[6] By the 1960s and 1970s,
they note that infection-control committees and infection-control
officers (or hospital epidemiologists) were created, stimulated by
the crisis of the post-war Staphylococcal infections. The National
Health Service (NHS) Subcommittee on Control of Staphylococcal
Infections in Hospitals recommended these appointments in 1959.
The roles were taken first by surgeons and physicians and were usually later held by medical bacteriologists.[7] Indeed, Hillier adds that
the Ministry of Health suggested that 'one person on the [infection
control] committee be made the "Control of Infection Officer" and
that "the hospital bacteriologist is often the person of choice"'.[8] Yet
the situation was rather different at Barts, where preventing and
controlling infection risks was a role for medical bacteriologists as
early as the 1890s.

This chapter demonstrates Barts' pioneering appointment of
pathologists as Sanitary Officers, further contesting the hospital's
conventional reputation as being a traditional and conservative
institution. I have already disputed this charge elsewhere, in my
work that compares doctors' use of bacteriological knowledge,
specialists and techniques at Barts and at Addenbrooke's Hospital,
Cambridge, in the late nineteenth and early twentieth centuries.
Bacteriological methods were initially used more regularly at Barts,
and the hospital provided a higher level of funding for its laboratory
at an earlier stage, despite Addenbrooke's Hospital's connections
with the University of Cambridge and links with scientific research.[9]

Creating the role of the Sanitary Officer

Keir Waddington's and Hugh Pennington's research into surgeons
at Barts provides important context about the decision to appoint
a Sanitary Officer, as, typically for the time, surgeons at Barts did
not have uniform ideas about infection prevention.[10] In the 1880s,
two of the five full surgeons were 'antipathetic' towards antiseptic
methods, and others had a mixed antiseptic-aseptic methodology,

combining practices which aimed to destroy germs with ones that would provide a sterile operating environment.[11] Frederick Andrewes reminisced that most of his surgical training at Barts in the 1870s and 1880s was carried out as though Joseph Lister did not exist.[12] Waddington cites Barts surgeons William Morrant Baker, George Callender and William Savory as opponents of Listerism, although Savory acknowledged the danger of sepsis before opting for the simpler approach of cleanliness, and Michael Worboys refers to Savory as the 'first champion' of the 'Cleanliness School of surgeons'.[13]

Barts has a broad and diverse history of approaches to infection control and prevention, largely down to the attitudes of individual surgeons. Holmes Coote argued in 1870 that 'simplicity and cleanliness of dressing ha[d] prevailed for several generations' at Barts, and the surgeon William Lawrence taught him about 'disinfecting applications' if wounds or discharge became foul.[14] Coote was concerned that using carbolic acid might be problematic, resulting in doctors being less concerned about hygienic practices.[15] Callender published statistics to show how cleanliness was significantly improving surgical mortality rates, developing his own methods of cleaning and dressing wounds, tube drainage for amputated limbs (a technique used by French surgeons Joseph François Malgaigne and Édouard Chassaignac in Paris), cotton wool bandages, carbolic lotion for washing and healing, and the isolation of patients from others with diseases.[16] Sir James Paget, Assistant Surgeon at the hospital from 1847, and full Surgeon from 1861–1871, claimed that mortality rates dropped from 15 per cent in 1847–1857, to 10 per cent in 1857–1867, and to 2 per cent between 1867 and 1877, with historian Lindsay Granshaw arguing the decline was in line with the timing of the adoption of Callender's rather than Lister's methods.[17]

The younger surgeons working at the hospital – Henry Butlin, Harrison Cripps, Thomas Smith and Alfred Willett – used mixed antiseptic/aseptic methods.[18] Smith had visited Edinburgh to learn Lister's practices, and his House Surgeon had also learnt directly from Lister. He undertook a study over three years to test the effectiveness of the methods, arguing for practitioners to be patient, and likened working with the human body to a chemical laboratory, where it was a challenge to replicate methods for 'beginners like ourselves'. Methods should not be condemned, he argued, if surgeons found there to be limitations in treating contaminated wounds, with his study revealing that children suffered from toxic effects of carbolic acid, and there were difficulties in detecting secondary haemorrhages under the layers of gauze.[19] Cripps even personally paid for an operating theatre to be rebuilt in marble and alabaster in 1896.[20] Henry Butlin used the latest medical products, including a microscope to study carcinomas in the 1870s, ahead of many other practitioners, and he developed his own appliance designs.[21] Charles Barrett Lockwood became a Demonstrator in Anatomy at the Medical College in 1881 and full Surgeon from 1903, and had experience of working in Emanuel Klein's laboratory at Barts and setting up his own small laboratory. He had also observed Lister in Edinburgh, and his partnership with Butlin became known as the 'Aseptic Firm'.[22] Lockwood taught extra classes in bacteriology and wrote the textbook *Aseptic Surgery* in 1896; Thomas Schlich refers to Lockwood as the 'British champion of asepsis', and Michael Worboys has characterised him as the 'leading theorist of the new aseptic surgery in Britain'.[23] In his textbook, Lockwood argued that an operation was a 'bacteriological experiment'.[24] He developed a hand disinfection method, 'the Lockwood system', which has recently been explained by Laura Newman. This included scrubbing the hands and forearms in hot water and soap for three minutes, and soaking them in 'binionide of mercury'. This technique was discussed in the *British Medical Journal* in 1901 and at the annual meeting of the British Medical Association in 1904. Yet, Lockwood was sceptical about gloves, not only because they could tear, but also because he believed they impaired the surgeon's sense of touch. He tragically died at the age of fifty-eight from a septic finger after pricking himself during an operation for a case of appendicular peritonitis.[25] These examples show, therefore, that despite a mixed reception amongst surgeons, the relevance of microbiological techniques and practices was enthusiastically embraced by some practitioners at Barts, and the hospital was a ripe environment for the development of further expertise in infection prevention and control.

In June 1891, the Medical Council recommended that a Sanitary Officer should be appointed. Noting they had first heard the suggestion in March of that year, the Treasurer and Almoners' Committee finally discussed this proposal in February 1892. The Medical

Council decided that the Sanitary Officer should be responsible 'for seeing that all cases of infectious disease, either arising, or admitted for treatment, in the Hospital, are duly notified to the Local Sanitary Authority as required by Act of Parliament'. Reflecting the training which the Officer was expected to have received and the work involved, there was the assumption this role would be held by a 'Medical man', with a diploma in public health, rather than being a nursing post for a woman, indicating the expertise in knowledge of disease transmission which was required. He should maintain 'such relations with the Medical and Surgical Staff of the Hospital and with other members of the Hospital Staff as will tend to the efficient performance of his duties'. All medical staff suspecting infectious disease should notify the Clerk who would notify the Sanitary Officer. The Sanitary Officer also needed to be aware of the condition of sanitary appliances and inspect the sanitary circumstances of the hospital. Every three months he would submit a report to the Treasurer and Almoners. For these tasks, he should receive a salary of £100.[26] In light of this new appointment, in April it was decided that a clause needed to be added to the job descriptions of the charges of all physicians, surgeons, the Matron and Assistant Matron, and sisters, stating they must report suspected cases of infectious disease or any insanitary conditions to the Clerk of the Hospital, who would inform the Sanitary Officer.[27]

Frederick Andrewes submitted his first reports as Sanitary Officer in 1892.[28] He combined this role with work as an Assistant Physician at the Royal Free Hospital and as Demonstrator in Practical Medicine at Barts.[29] Meanwhile, Alfredo Kanthack was appointed a Lecturer in Pathology in 1893. The Medical Council campaigned for the role of hospital pathologist in 1894–1895, asking for him to be paid £600, even though, as the Treasurer pointed out, the highest salary for anyone on the medical staff was 100 guineas (£105). Despite the doctors offering to contribute to a fund for the Pathologist, if the Governors also did so, the request was declined, and the role was created with a salary of £100, only the same payment which had been agreed for the Sanitary Officer a few years before, even though the doctors stressed how time-consuming the job of Pathologist would be. Indeed, when the issue of this low salary was raised again in 1902, representatives of the Medical Council complained. Barts physician William Church argued that

£100 did not reflect the 'importance' of the work which was necessary for the treatment of patients, and that a higher wage was needed as the Pathologist did not have the time to undertake the private work from which consulting physicians and surgeons earnt their living. Kanthack was appointed, but he soon left for the post of Professor of Pathology at the University of Cambridge in 1897, with Andrewes becoming the Pathologist to St Bartholomew's Hospital and Lecturer in Pathology. In 1902, Church claimed that Kanthack was lost to Cambridge because of the poor salary, although the Treasurer replied that there were other reasons for his resignation. Although his colleagues had argued that the role of the Pathologist was very demanding, Andrewes carried on in the part-time role of Sanitary Officer until his retirement in 1928, and his successors as pathologists and bacteriologists to the hospital, Ronald Canti and Lawrence Garrod, also took on this additional task.[30] Despite the pressure of these jobs, Andrewes also managed to find time for research, ranging from being the first to classify different streptococci, to furthering knowledge regarding lymphadenoma and arteriosclerosis. His work gained wide recognition, and he was invited to give the Dobell and Croonian lectures to the Royal College of Physicians in 1906 and 1910, and the Harveian Oration in 1920. He was made a Fellow of the Royal Society in 1915, he was awarded the OBE in recognition for work in the First World War in 1919, and was knighted in 1920.[31]

Andrewes' early work in the role of Sanitary Officer combined routine investigations and reporting with recommendations for practical and innovative methods to manage infection in the wards and the operating theatre. These ranged from a report on the methods of disinfecting bedding, linen and clothing to the Treasurer and Almoners' Committee, to the purchase, in 1892, of the Washington Lyon patent steam disinfector, which had been patented in 1880 and widely available since the mid-1880s. The hospital's architect and surveyor Edward B. I'Anson was charged with costing up the apparatus and conversion of the former Treasurer's stables to house the device. Although Figure 8.1 is from a slightly later date, it is useful in showing the scale of the apparatus which might have been installed; the original 1880s disinfector was on wheels and had to be moved by a horse.[32] Acquisition of the disinfector was a lengthy process, as subsequent discussions with the Medical Council compared

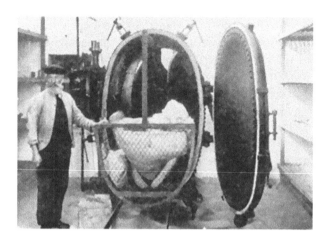

Figure 8.1   The 'Washington-Lyon Steam Disinfector' as depicted in
W. Robertson and C. Porter, *Sanitary Law and Practice: A Handbook for
Students* (1905).

the benefits of the Washington Lyon and Nottingham patent steam
disinfectors. When the Nottingham device and its many accessories
were ordered, the purchase was unsuccessful, as the manufacturers
were being sued by the makers of the Washington Lyon disinfector. Presumably the apparatus was finally ready by January 1894
when a disinfector attendant was appointed.[33] During the 1890s,
medical instrument makers were capitalising on a 'market opportunity to promote a wider range of aseptic products', emphasising
the need to buy 'sterilising apparatus and suitable furniture'.[34] In
keeping with this trend, Barts' expenditure increased by 70 per cent
between 1860 and 1895, with expenses including the purchase of
three sterilisers, and a theatre with a brass and glass operating table
for Cripps.[35]

Pennington has argued that Barts lacked a central policy for
sterilising, with Lockwood's team being held as exceptional.[36]
However, the work of the Sanitary Officer indicates that there *was*
coordination at Barts. For example, as well as suggesting sterilising equipment, Andrewes was asked for his opinion on methods
of improving cleanliness. A report was requested regarding a chute
for ward refuse and dirty linen in 1901, since such equipment was
already in use at the East London Hospital (a hospital for children
in Shadwell) and at King's College Hospital. The chute would be

used for infected linen and cast-off dressings and poultices that would be sent down the shoot in watertight receptacles. After working through his ideas, Andrewes thought this system could be improved with an external hand-operated lift, as the room was already filled with lavatories, sinks, pipes and closets.[37] In 1905, Andrewes reported on the disinfectant Cyllin, which he thought should be used to replace carbolic acid as it was cheaper. It was also apparently eleven times more powerful against the typhoid bacilli than carbolic acid.[38] In 1917, Andrewes was inspired by a wartime military innovation in 'extensive' use in military camps to propose that there was the 'opportunity' to obtain a new technology for preventing the spread of infection at Barts; 'disinfection of the naso-pharynx by means of a steam spray conveying a finely atomized disinfectant' was in the experimental stage in treating meningococcus carriers and for 'checking the spread of other respiratory infections'. He wanted to test the 'value of the method in checking the spread of measles, influenza + amongst nurses + others'.[39]

More mundane tasks involved investigating the provision and functioning of toilets in the Medical College in 1904, in response to complaints from the Warden.[40] Andrewes continued to report on lavatories which needed replacing around the hospital.[41] Another role was to check the drains up to three times per quarter – indeed, he commented in 1907, for example, 'I have inspected the drains at the usual monthly intervals and found them in good general condition', indicating that he undertook these routine tasks personally. Usually these were kept clean, but occasionally there were hazards to solve, such as an accumulation of human teeth from the dental department in one small drain in 1910. Problems with staff shortages during the First World War also meant that the manholes were not kept thoroughly clean.[42] Other measures undertaken by Andrewes included re-vaccinating the female staff in order to prevent smallpox.[43]

As I have explored in my previous research, the number of cases of infectious disease at Barts challenges the idea which has prevailed since Brian Abel-Smith's book *The Hospitals*: that general hospitals began to reject cases of infectious disease from the 1860s. Barts had isolation wards and, between 1880 and 1920, over eighteen patients with diphtheria were admitted to the hospital per year, with seventy or more patients treated for the disease between 1888–1890 and 1893–1897, with a peak of 148 in 1890.[44] 'Diphtheria wards' were still referred to in the Sanitary Officer's Reports in 1915, and as late as 1928, two cases of the infectious disease were admitted, one 'in error' (diphtheria was not suspected) and the other because an urgent tracheotomy was needed.[45]

Despite diphtheria cases being treated in an isolation ward, there were constant problems, with cross infection being an ongoing concern. For example, in 1902, there was an inconclusive investigation regarding a patient possibly contracting diphtheria from a nurse who may still have been infectious following her discharge from Radcliffe, the isolation ward.[46] In 1903, Andrewes came to the conclusion that the only method of transmission of diphtheria could be via contaminated eating utensils, and he ordered them all to be disinfected by heat.[47] A patient developed diphtheria on 4 July 1908, after being admitted with hip disease on 21 June, but Andrewes could not find a reason for the infection; there was no other case on her ward, the House Surgeon had not been in contact with a patient with diphtheria and the forceps had been sterilised before she had a tooth extracted.[48] In 1910, a patient was admitted to Kenton Ward with cancer of the stomach in February and died in March in Radcliffe Ward. An advanced carcinoma was revealed by the autopsy, with diphtheria probably contributing to his death. However, the patient's daughter had suffered from diphtheria four months earlier, so it is possible he may not have contracted diphtheria as a result of his hospital admission.[49]

From the very early twentieth century, much of the Sanitary Officer's quarterly reports consisted of documenting the search for the sources of hospital cross infection, usually regarding diphtheria or scarlet fever, but sometimes erysipelas. In 1913, at least six cases of scarlet fever resulted from an 'inadvertent' admission of a patient on Mary Ward – in other words, the patient would not have been admitted to Barts if there had been a suspicion of scarlet fever on admission.[50] In 1907, twenty-four cases of cross infection occurred in four months, and Andrewes' summer stand-in, demonstrator Hugh Thursfield, exclaimed 'there is no reason to suppose that there has been any relaxation of the rules of asepsis in the theatre or in the ward'. He recommended the ward and theatre be closed for thorough disinfection, including fumigation with sulphur, washing of the walls with disinfecting solution, whitewashing of the ceilings and more. Thursfield also recommended that the operating table needed to be replaced as it had already been condemned, that the boxes in which soiled linen was placed were very hard to clean and they smelt, and that the bins were also occasionally evil-smelling, although they were of good design and cleaned with perchloride of lime. He suggested some disinfectant powder should also be used.[51]

Barts was not alone as a general hospital experiencing transmission of highly infectious diseases. Diphtheria cases were clearly treated at The London Hospital, too. As Debbie Palmer has explored, seven nurses died at The London Hospital between 1888 and 1890 as a result of infectious diseases, including two from scarlet fever and one from diphtheria. Matron Eva Lückes instructed nurses to be careful with patients suffering from diphtheria, including using Lysol solution to wash their hands, not eating in the patients' rooms and gargling twice a day. There was a particular outbreak of these two diseases in October 1888 which affected six nurses.[52]

As the example of diphtheria demonstrates, it was not only patients who suffered from cross infection, but also staff. Perhaps referring to Andrewes' attempts to examine staff as vectors of infection, in 1898 surgeons Walsham and Cripps noted that portions of the skin of fingers of the surgeon, dressers (medical students on surgical wards), nurses and patients had been snipped off for bacteriological tests.[53] A persistent problem was the infestation with the fungal infection ringworm amongst the junior medical staff. Despite sterilisation of the toilet seats, towels and bedding, the infection continued. Nearly all the new residents arriving in April 1903 were infected within three months, and so the whole quarters were evacuated while the accommodation was cleansed and disinfected.[54] In 1907 and 1910, the infection briefly returned, even though the medical staff had been relocated to new quarters.[55]

From the 1890s, pathologists recognised that people who had suffered from typhoid could transmit the typhoid bacilli in stools and urine for weeks or months after suffering from the disease, and Robert Koch argued that more attention needed to be paid to this risk.[56] In 1904, a patient was 'carbolised' and considered to be non-infectious, but probably transmitted typhoid to a patient and a nurse. Andrewes questioned this 'rite', which he put in inverted commas, because although it was 'commendable', infection came from inside the patient, and therefore stools should be disinfected during the entire time that a patient was within the hospital.[57] After the proof of the concept of carriers from 1905–1906, the Sanitary Officer's reports from 1911 increasingly reveal the search for carriers of diphtheria, typhoid and potentially scarlet fever, amongst staff as well as patients.[58] The following extract shows the procedure for preventing further cases:

> [O]n October 18 1911, a patient, aged 3, was admitted to Isolation Ward with diphtheria. … having given a negative result on throat culture, he was transferred to Luke on Nov 30. He remained in bed in Luke till early in March when he began to get up + perambulate the ward. During the time he was in bed no case of diphtheria arose. At the end of March [a nurse] who was on duty in Luke developed diphtheria + a few days later a child in the ward … also developed it: both were transferred to Isolation. A bacteriological examination of the throats of all children in the ward now revealed the fact that [the patient] still harboured diphtheria bacilli. He had presumably been a 'carrier' since October, but only began to do harm when he got up + mixed with other patients. He was sent to a fever hospital; no children were for a time admitted to Luke + no further cases occurred.[59]

There are many more examples, including that of a House Physician, who was found to be a carrier of diphtheria in 1918, being removed to a Fever Hospital.[60] After an outbreak of diphtheria in 1922, three nurses remained carriers – one nurse was sent away but the other two nurses had their tonsils removed and their condition was cured. Apparently, this method was usually successful for those carrying the bacilli in their throats, but curing nasal carriers was much more difficult.[61] From 1922, Andrewes mentions occasionally carrying out experiments with animals to test the virulence of the bacteria transmitted by carriers.[62] Therefore, there was a turn in this area of infection control from the collective 'inclusive' measures of 'swamps, streets and sewers', to the individual 'exclusive' measures in the early twentieth century.[63] A recognition of accountability for cross infection also increased during this period. In 1939, one of the doctors wrote, 'As you are aware the public are now so sensitive to the question of puerperal sepsis that if an epidemic occurred and every precaution had not been taken, the Hospital's reputation would suffer severely.' It was considered 'extremely unsatisfactory' that 'suspect cases' were kept so close to the maternity ward, but this was unavoidable within the contemporary hospital buildings.[64]

Despite Andrewes' attention to bacteriological methods, he continued to use sanitarian theories of cleanliness for controlling infection, including preventing atmospheric pollution. Charles Murchison coined the 'pythogenic theory' to refer to diseases generated from filth in the early 1860s, and the term 'miasmatic' also continued to be used for germs which appeared to stem from environmental nuisances.[65] Sanitarian practices to prevent disease in the 1860s included removing privies from wards, whitewashing walls and preventing contaminated air entering wards and ventilation systems, together with disinfecting wards and beds.[66] The danger of 'sewer gas' was discussed in the records for Addenbrooke's Hospital, Cambridge, in the 1880s, for example, in relation to 'odorous test smoke' revealing how the drains were permitting the gas to enter the building.[67] As late as 1907, Andrewes tested the lavatories in the Nurses' Home at Barts with a smoke test to see if sewer air was leaking from the closets.[68]

As Nancy Tomes has explored for the US, sanitarians became particularly concerned about household plumbing in the mid-nineteenth century. 'Sewer traps' were fitted because of a concern that deadly gases could be emitted from the public sewers which had a direct route through toilets and washbasins into homes.[69] In a similar way to Andrewes' smoke test, the 'peppermint test' was recommended in 1884 in an American publication by Roger S. Tracy. This household handbook proposed dropping peppermint oil in the toilet to see if the odour could be smelt elsewhere in the home. If it could, this would indicate that sewer gas and germs could be escaping from the pipes.[70] Although Tomes argues that public health experts in the US no longer believed 'airborne bacteria from sewer and toilet' were a serious threat by the early 1900s, especially following experiments which attempted to prove this, the American public remained concerned, demonstrated by continued sales of products to prevent sewer gas in the home.[71]

In Britain, there is evidence that there was continuing concern about sewers transmitting disease in hospitals in the early 1900s. Palmer's research on nurses' health at the South Devon and East Cornwall Hospital has revealed that the 'dreadful stench from the sewer ventilator' was cited as a factor in causing ill health as late as 1909.[72] It is possible that when, in 1907, Andrewes tried to solve the problem of foul smells which he thought were resulting from the removal of valves from overused toilets, for which he had used smoke tests a year or two before, he may have been attempting to remove unpleasant odours at Barts, rather than prevent disease.[73] Yet in 1911, he also approached four cases of erysipelas in President Ward with sanitarian methods and decided that there should not be builders' rubbish and Corporation carts for the removal of rubbish near the wards. However, he was clearly conflicted about the reason for doing so. He commented,

> I must admit that I cannot understand how builder's rubbish can cause erysipelas, but I am satisfied that it ought not to be allowed to accumulate in proximity to the wards. Should the present measures not suffice, I consider that it will be necessary to find accommodation for the disinfecting apparatus at some spot further from the wards.[74]

Andrewes' reluctance to dismiss the idea of airborne transmission of this illness supports Worboys' argument for continuity in germ theories. Worboys has explained that the continuing concept of miasma, and its ability to cause diseases such as typhoid, cholera and malaria to be transmitted by airborne germs, persisted into the 1890s.[75] As late as 1939, Lawrence Garrod, by then the hospital's Sanitary Officer and Bacteriologist, reported the foul smells emitted by the emptying of the grease traps on Friday mornings, and the need to close the windows and move patients from the balconies, although he may just have been concerned that this was an unpleasant experience for the patients.[76]

By the late nineteenth century, then, overlapping sanitarian- and bacteriologically informed practices reinforced the need for cleanliness. Alison Bashford has argued that sanitarian practices were not 'replaced' but 'displaced largely into a female domain of work'.[77] Published in 1911, Herbert Macleod's textbook, *Hygiene for Nurses*, still discussed purification of air as a key practice alongside bacteria and disinfection.[78] Indeed Lister's practices were initially based on airborne germs in dust, but John Burdon Sanderson, University College, speculated in 1871, when Lister introduced carbolic spray into his antiseptic tool kit, that germs were easily killed by drying in the air, and he questioned the importance of wounds being contaminated by atmospheric matter in 1875 and 1881.[79] Germs in the air were found to be 'far too few and fragile' and levels of 'aerial sewage' could not be easily determined.[80]

The Sanitary Officers' reports reveal that Andrewes and his successors had a busy and varied role on top of work as the hospital Pathologist, with responsibility for recording hazards, practical microbiological analysis and problem solving, including the introduction of new equipment. Although the admission of highly infectious bacterial diseases declined at Barts in the twentieth century, there was much continuity in the role, and there were still activities relating to cross infection from diphtheria and the smells caused by insanitary conditions well into the twentieth century. Yet, alongside these epidemiological and bacteriological tasks, there were also jobs which have traditionally been associated with matrons and nurses, including instructions regarding the disinfection of wards and bedding. So how did the matrons' tasks compare, considering they have previously been perceived as having the key responsibility for infection prevention and control?

The duties of the Matron

The power of the matrons in major hospitals in the late nineteenth century has been explored by historians. The most striking example is the case of Margaret Burt, whose intervention into hospital and nursing management at Guy's Hospital in 1879–1880 was controversial, as discussed by the historian Keir Waddington. Burt argued for better meals and uniform dress for nurses and the alteration of their work to include the removal of menial roles. The new arrangements which she and the Treasurer introduced were so contentious that they were discussed in the national press, especially as a nurse was subsequently convicted for manslaughter by undertaking diagnosis and treatment of a woman for hysteria with a cold bath, which was said to have killed her by causing tubercular and inflammatory disease of the brain. Doctors opposing the new nursing system used this tragedy to argue that they should control nurses and regain some authority, despite the convicted nurse acting on the advice of an 'old' sister, rather than a nurse trained within the new system.[81]

With particular relevance for this chapter, Susan McGann has included two Barts Matrons within her collective biography of Matrons. Ethel Manson, later Ethel Bedford Fenwick after marriage, was Matron of Barts from 1881 to 1887. A formidable character, she fought for the registration of nurses for decades, establishing many organisations along the way, including the Royal British Nurses' Association and the International Council of Nurses, on which she served as the first President.[82] By the time Manson resigned in 1887, in order to marry, the nursing school was amongst the best in the world. From 1906, students from the Salpêtrière in Paris travelled to Barts to gain experience there.[83] Barts Matrons were powerful within their profession; with her successor at Barts, Isla Stewart, Bedford Fenwick formed the Matrons' Council of Great Britain in 1894, with Stewart as the first Chair. Stewart was Matron at Barts from 1887 to 1910, and amongst other nursing leadership roles, in 1901, she gave the opening address at the first International Council of Nurses meeting. In 1906 she was appointed as a member of the Army Nursing Board.[84]

Barts was pioneering in educating nurses about bacteriology. Stewart recommended that nurses should be taught bacteriology and its bearing on surgery, and particularly asepsis, within the revised curriculum in 1894.[85] She co-authored a textbook in 1899 which included chapters explaining contagion and disinfection, and the 'production of surgical cleanliness', that is asepsis, with a discussion of microorganisms.[86] A further new nursing scheme was introduced at Barts in 1906, which included nine lectures on 'elementary bacteriology' during the third year of training.[87] In comparison, nursing education at St Thomas' Hospital, London, and the Royal Infirmary of Edinburgh (RIE), touched on putrefaction and germ theories from the mid-1870s, but it was not until 1895 that bacteriology was taught explicitly at the Glasgow Royal Infirmary, the first of four hospitals studied by Claire Jones *et al.* (the other hospitals being St Thomas' and King's College Hospitals in London, and the RIE).[88]

The Matron's 'charge' (job description) from Manson's time reveals more of the tasks which were relevant to infection control and prevention at Barts. Beyond training, supervising and recruiting the nurses, and looking after the linens and the tradesmen's accounts, the Matron's charge included visiting every ward four times per week, checking the staff were performing their respective duties, ensuring patient comfort and care, securing 'clean and wholesome' wards and ensuring 'sobriety, good order and decorum'. She was additionally required to inform the Clerk of any suspected insanitary conditions she encountered.[89]

Rather than the Matron appearing at management meetings in person, her historical voice can be detected in communications to the Treasurer and Almoners' Committee or medical committees. As Matron, Manson was expected to write a report for the Treasurer and Almoners every Thursday. For example, in 1882 she argued for more reasonable hours of work for nurses. In 1891, she reported that twenty to twenty-five patients were admitted with diphtheria per year in 1881–1884, but that this had increased since 1887, with sixty-three in that year and 119 in 1890. Nurses were contracting diphtheria and other infectious diseases.[90] In 1892, Stewart recommended that each sister should be present for the operations of patients from her own ward, rather than the Sister of Abernethy Ward attending all male operations, and the Sister of Lucas Ward attending female operations, as was the current practice. Her idea was accepted; Sister Abernethy continued to be responsible for the operating theatre, but she no longer had to attend all of the operations.[91] Geoffrey Bourne, who studied at Barts, revealed in his memoir the activities relating to infection prevention which were part of the role of 'Sister Surgery' (the name for the Sister in Charge of the nursing staff). She had to listen out for surgical patients who had acquired measles, diphtheria or whooping cough. Meanwhile, the theatre sister and her team sterilised equipment and counted swabs.[92] Sister Abernethy's voice can also be heard within the minutes: in 1892, her views were acknowledged as she was given permission to increase the number of articles to be washed; she could send thirty articles for washing rather than twenty-four, and other nurses working in the operating theatre could send twenty-four articles instead of eighteen.[93] Demonstrating teamwork, in 1905, along with the Treasurer and the Sanitary Officer, the Matron asked for sanitary alterations to the South Block including impermeable flooring in the lavatories and plumbing. Along with several ward sisters, they considered and reported upon the redesign of the bathrooms and lavatories for the block.[94]

Despite Matron's responsibility for cleanliness, the cleaning of wards was not wholly within her remit. In 1868, a decision was made to employ scrubbers to relieve the nurses of cleaning the wards and the staircases, with the Treasurer and Almoners' Committee recommending to the House Committee that the expenditure was worth paying because the nurses would be able to provide 'more unremitting attention' to patients than their current duties allowed and the 'efficiency' of hospital nursing would be increased. It was argued that many people who wanted to offer themselves as nurses 'shrink from accepting it' because of the 'laborious work of scrubbing Wards and staircases'.[95] From at least 1870, laundry was contracted out, although some was still done in-house. Yet, Matron had some control over the situation; she complained repeatedly about the condition of the linen returning from the washing contractor, and the hospital changed the contract for the nurses' linen to another contractor. In light of her frequent complaints, Mr Oswald was called to meet with the Treasurer and Almoners' Committee twice so they could impress 'upon him the importance of all the articles sent to him being washed thoroughly clean', and at both meetings Oswald promised to prevent future causes for complaint. But the contract for other washing continued until a new hospital laundry was constructed at Swanley in 1885.[96] In 1884, further movements to contract out cleaning were made. Mrs Ross, the nurse in the outpatient room, was advancing in age, and her duties of scrubbing the outpatient and waiting rooms were to be given to Mrs Logan, 'the Contractor for the Scrubbing'.[97] Barts was much later than Guy's in abolishing nurses' scrubbing. This occurred in 1857 at Guy's to attract a 'better class' of woman for nursing.[98]

In May 1892, it was the Sanitary Officer, not the Matron, who raised the point that more cleaning was necessary. He recommended more frequent cleaning of the floor of the surgery, and it was decided that three times a week would be suitable.[99] In July 1892, the temporary arrangement of Mrs Logan providing the scrubbers for the operating theatre, supervised by the Sister of the Surgery, ended, and Mrs Bartlett was to be paid to organise a 'sufficient number of women for scrubbing the floor of the Surgery', including its entrance, the House Physicians' and House Surgeons' rooms, the dispensary and the basement three times per week; the forms and stools in the surgery twice a week; and further rooms once a week. Bartlett was to provide all the materials, and to personally superintend the work.[100] This was happening at the same time as radical changes were being made to the theatres: glazed white tiling, painting, reflooring, hand basins and a better drainage system.[101] In June 1893, the Sanitary Officer also recommended that if a patient suffered from diphtheria, scarlet fever or septicaemia, the bedstead had to be removed from the ward and repainted. For other infectious diseases it should be cleaned on the ward with disinfectant, being taken apart as far as possible. The disinfector attendant had been appointed by the hospital in 1894 to take charge of disinfection of the bedding and clothing in the hospital.[102] However, this demonstrates continuity with the pre-bacteriological period; Lindsay Granshaw refers to practices in the 1860s of disinfecting wards and beds with chemicals such as carbolic acid.[103]

With the Sanitary Officer's appointment in 1892, the contracting out of cleaning and laundry services, plus the appointment of the disinfector attendant, the Matron's role in prevention of infection was limited at Barts. As knowledge of sepsis and germs developed during the late nineteenth century, her influence was gradually eroded from the late 1860s when cleaning was contracted out, and particularly from the early 1890s, with the coordination of infection prevention and control taken over by a doctor trained in public health. This was in spite of the leadership roles which Manson and Stewart had within their wider profession as Matrons. These women lost control of key tasks in the nineteenth century, long before the period leading up to the Second World War, which has been cited by Wildman and Hewison as the transition to centralisation of infection prevention and control services.[104] At Barts, the Matron's responsibilities in reporting disease and looking after the supplies and linens of the hospital, as delineated in her charge, had already been reduced during a much earlier period.

Conclusion

A huge amount of investigations into ward and post-operative infections were recorded in the Sanitary Officers' reports between 1892 and 1939, and this chapter has provided snapshots of this work. At Barts, pathologists implemented infection prevention and control policy and practices within the hospital, playing a powerful role in investigating cross infection long before phage typing. Although there were changes, such as exclusive measures of searching for carriers who may have transmitted disease from the first decade of the twentieth century, there was also continuity throughout the period in terms of searching for the causes of cross infection from infectious disease, with inclusive measures of suggestions for improvement of hospital structures, and environmental matters such as commenting on foul smells.

This research has revealed that, at least at Barts, the role of a hospital pathologist could be much broader than laboratory diagnosis and research, and that there were important connections between the implementation of this new role and the existing staffing framework, including the Matron. Yet, the Matrons had already begun to lose control from the 1860s to 1880s, with less responsibility for cleanliness and laundry, but even more so after the introduction of the Sanitary Officer and the disinfector attendant in the early 1890s. Therefore, despite the leadership roles of Barts' Matrons Manson and Stewart within their profession, they could not take charge of the control of infection within their own hospital.

Acknowledgements

Thank you very much for the assistance of archivists at St Bartholomew's Hospital and for permission to quote from the records, particularly to Katie Ormerod who alerted me to the Sanitary Officers' reports. The research and writing for this chapter were undertaken whilst working at King's College London, Imperial College London and the University of Hull. I am very grateful for insightful comments from editor Fay Bound Alberti, and for feedback from audiences at three conferences: 'Learning from Lister' at the Royal Society, Royal College of Surgeons and King's College London in 2012; the European Association for the History of Medicine and Health Conference in Lisbon in 2013; and 'From Microbes to Matrons: The Past, Present and Future of Hospital Infection Control and Prevention' at the Royal College of Surgeons in 2016. Many thanks to the conference organisers and funders for support in attending the events in 2012 and 2016, especially the Leverhulme Trust, and to the University of Hull for funding my travel to Lisbon. This chapter furthers research undertaken for my PhD, funded by the Arts and Humanities Research Board/Council (grant number 103736) and within my book, Rosemary Wall, *Bacteria in Britain, 1880–1939* (London: Pickering and Chatto, 2013).

Notes

1 S. Wildman and A. Hewison, 'Rediscovering a history of nursing management: from Nightingale to the modern matron', *International Journal of Nursing Studies*, 46 (2009), 1651.

2 *Ibid.*, 1653 and 1655.

3 Peter Ardern, *When matron ruled* (London: Robert Hale, 2002), 161.

4 T. H. Pennington, 'Listerism, its decline and its persistence: The introduction of aseptic surgical techniques in three British teaching hospitals, 1890–99', *Medical History*, 39 (1995), 35–60, especially 58; Graham A. J. Ayliffe and Mary P. English, *Hospital infection: From miasmas to MRSA* (Cambridge: Cambridge University Press, 2003), 221.

5 Kathryn Hillier, 'Babies and bacteria: Phage typing, bacteriologists, and the birth of infection control', *Bulletin of the History of Medicine*, 80 (2006), 750–751 and 760–761.

6 Ayliffe and English, *Hospital infection*, 187.

7 *Ibid.*, 192–193.

8 Central Health Services Council and Standing Medical Advisory Committee, *Staphylococcal infections in hospitals* (London: Ministry of Health, 1959), 26, in Hillier, 'Babies and bacteria', 755.

9 Rosemary Wall, *Bacteria in Britain, 1880–1939* (London: Pickering and Chatto, 2013), 13–40; Rosemary Wall, 'Using bacteriology in elite hospital practice: London and Cambridge, 1880–1920', *Social History of Medicine*, 24 (2011), 777–788.

10 See Keir Waddington, *Medical education at St. Bartholomew's Hospital 1123–1995* (Woodbridge: The Boydell Press, 2003), 132–135 for the reception at Barts. For the reception of Lister's ideas by surgeons, see Michael Worboys, *Spreading germs: Disease theories and medical practice in Britain, 1865–1900* (Cambridge: Cambridge University Press, 2000), 161–192; and Christopher Lawrence and Richard Dixey, 'Practising on principle: Joseph Lister and the germ theories of disease', in Christopher Lawrence (ed.), *Medical theory, surgical practice* (London: Routledge, 1993), 153–215. See Lindsay Granshaw, '"Upon this principle I have based a practice": The development and reception of antisepsis in Britain, 1867–90', in John V. Pickstone (ed.), *Medical innovations in historical perspective* (Basingstoke and London: Macmillan Academic and Professional, 1992), 17–46, especially 23–24 and 38–42 for important context regarding the variety of methods of cleanliness already practised in London before Lister's publications on antisepsis in the 1860s, and reasons for rejecting or modifying Lister's methods.

11 Pennington, 'Listerism, its decline and its persistence', 50.

12 Waddington, *Medical education*, 132, citing Frederick Andrewes, 'The beginnings of bacteriology at Bart's, being part of an address to the Abernethian Society', *St Bartholomew's Hospital Journal*, 35 (1928), 101.

13 Waddington, *Medical education*, 133; Worboys, *Spreading germs*, 163.

14 Granshaw, '"Upon this principle"', 30–31, citing Holmes Coote, 'On the treatment of wounds', *St Bartholomew's Hospital Reports*, 6 (1870), 113.

15 Granshaw, '"Upon this principle"', 31.

16 *Ibid.*, 20 and 31–32.

17 *Ibid.*, 37–38. See Victor Medvei and John Thornton (eds), *The Royal Hospital of Saint Bartholomew, 1123–1973* (London: St Bartholomew's Hospital, 1974), for dates when people worked at the hospital, including a useful chronology, 385–390.

18 Waddington, *Medical education*, 133.

19 Thomas Smith, 'Clinical lectures on Lister's treatment of wounds and abscesses by the Antiseptic Method', *Lancet* (25 Mar 1876), 453 and 455; (1 Jul 1876), 5, and Thomas Smith, 'Conclusions from a personal experience of Lister's antiseptic treatment during three years of hospital practice', *St Bartholomew's Hospital Reports*, 14 (1878), 137–139, both cited and discussed in Jerry L. Gaw, *'A time to heal': The diffusion of Listerism in Victorian Britain*, Transactions of the American Philosophical Society, 89:1 (Philadelphia: American Philosophical Society, 1999), 106–107 and 116.

20 Keir Waddington, *Charity and the London hospitals, 1850–1898* (Woodbridge: The Boydell Press, 2000), 105.

21 Claire L. Jones, *The medical trade catalogue in Britain, 1870–1914* (London: Pickering and Chatto, 2013), 120–121 and 157.

22 Waddington, *Medical education*, 133–135; Worboys, *Spreading germs*, 187.

23 Waddington, *Medical education*, 135; Charles Barrett Lockwood, *Aseptic surgery* (Edinburgh: Young, J. Pentland, 1896), cited in Thomas Schlich, 'Asepsis and bacteriology: A realignment of surgery and laboratory science', *Medical history*, 56 (2012), 332; Worboys, *Spreading germs*, 187.

24 Lockwood, *Aseptic surgery*, 193, cited in Schlich, 'Asepsis and bacteriology', 333.

25 Laura Newman, 'Making germs real: germs, the germ sciences, and the British workplace, c. 1880–1940' (PhD dissertation, King's College London, 2018), 64–74.

26 St Bartholomew's Hospital Archives (SBHA), SBHB/HA/3/19, Treasurer and Almoners' Minute Book (T and A), Jul 1891–Dec 1892, 11 Feb 1892, 156–159.

27 SBHA, SBHB/HA/3/19, T and A, Jul 1891–Dec 1892, 7 Apr 1892, 194.

28 *Ibid.*, 16 May 1892, 221; 21 Jul 1892, 254.

29 M. H. G. [initials only], 'Obituary: Sir Frederick Andrewes', *British Medical Journal*, 1 (5 Mar 1932), 451.

30 Wall, *Bacteria in Britain*, 17–20; F. L. H. [initials only], 'Obituary: Dr R. G. Canti', *Nature*, 137 (15 Feb 1936), 262–263; R. A. Shooter, 'Lawrence Paul Garrod', in Gordon Wolstenholme (ed.), *Lives of the Fellows of the Royal College of Physicians continued to 1983* (Oxford: IRL Press, 1984), 203.

31 M. H. G., 'Obituary: Sir Frederick Andrewes', 451–452; H. H. Dale, 'Andrewes, Sir Frederick William', in *Oxford Dictionary of National Biography* (Oxford: Oxford University Press, 1949, revised 2004), doi. org/10.1093/ref:odnb/30416.

32 SBHA, SBHB/HA/3/19, T and A, 19 Jul 1891–Dec 1892, 10 Nov 1892, 306. See Graham Mooney, *Intrusive interventions: Public health, domestic space, and infectious disease surveillance in England, 1840–1914* (Rochester, NY: University of Rochester Press, 2015), 139–141, for more information about the Washington Lyon steam disinfector.

33 SBHA, SBHB/HA/3/20, T and A, Jan 1893–Aug 1894, 16 Mar 1893, 52.

34 Quotations from Jones, *The medical trade catalogue*, 61 and 63. Jones notes that aseptic products were marketed more widely in 1893 but that non-aseptic equipment continued to be advertised alongside them at least until 1914, 61–65. Pennington proposed that the disinfector was Lockwood's idea as he could not find evidence to suggest otherwise when a steam steriliser and boiler for instruments were purchased by 1893. See Pennington, 'Listerism, its decline and its persistence', 51.

35 Waddington, *Charity and the London hospitals*, 102–105.

36 Pennington, 'Listerism, its decline and its persistence', 55.

37 SBHA, SBHB/HA/6/8/3/1, Sanitary Officer's Reports (SOR), 3 Jul 1901, 7–9.

38 *Ibid.*, 7 Jun 1905, 87–88.

39 *Ibid.*, Quarterly Report 1 Jul to 30 Sep 1917, 9 Oct 2017, 270–271.

40 *Ibid.*, 5 Apr 1904, 58.

41 For example, *Ibid.*, 7 Jun 1905, 85–87.

42 *Ibid.*, 20 Apr 1907, 122; 10 Oct 1910, 159; Quarterly Report 1 Jul to 30 Sep 1917, 9 Oct 2017, 270–271.

43 *Ibid.*, Quarterly Report Oct to 31 Dec 1901, 18.

44 B. Abel-Smith, *The hospitals 1800–1948: A study in social administration in England and Wales* (London: Heinemann, 1964), 38, 45 and 126–127; SBHA, St Bartholomew's Hospital, *Statistical tables of the patients under treatment in the wards of St Bartholomew's hospital, 1880–1920* (1913 and 1918 are missing).

45 SBHA, SBHB/HA/6/8/3/1, SOR, 13 Jan 1915, 236; Quarterly Summary Jan–Mar 1928, 384.

46 *Ibid.*, 6 Aug 1902, 31–32.

47 *Ibid.*, 17 Jul 1903, 47–48.

48 *Ibid.*, 7–20 Jul 1908, reported on 30 Jul 1908, 139.

49 *Ibid.*, 19 Mar 1910, 155.

50 *Ibid.*, 13 Jan 1913, 198.

51 *Ibid.*, 7 Aug 1907, 126–128.

52 Debbie Palmer, *Who cared for the carers?: A history of the occupational health of nurses, 1880–1948* (Manchester: Manchester University Press, 2014), 19–20.

53 Pennington, 'Listerism, its decline and its persistence', 52.

54 SBHA, SBHB/HA/6/8/3/1. SOR, Quarterly Report 1 Apr–30 Jun 1903, 27 Jul 1903, 47–48.

55 *Ibid.*, 1 May 1907, 123–124.

56 John Andrew Mendelsohn, 'A bacteriological approach to controlling typhoid,' in Deborah Brunton (ed.), *Health, disease and society in Europe, 1880–1930: A sourcebook* (Manchester: Manchester University Press, 2004), 185–188.

57 SBHA, SBHB/HA/6/8/3/1, SOR, 27 Dec 1904, 74.

58 For example, *Ibid.*, 1 Sep 1911, 179.

59 SBHA, SBHB/HA/6/8/3/1, SOR, 4 Jun 1912, 188–189.

60 *Ibid.*, Quarterly Report, 1 Apr to 30 Jun 1918, 278.

61 *Ibid.*, 29 April 1922, 316–317.

62 For example, *Ibid.*, 31 Jul 1922, 329–330.

63 J. Andrew Mendelsohn, '"Typhoid Mary" strikes again: The social and the scientific in the making of modern public health', *Isis*, 86 (1995), 273, for quotation and a further discussion on this turn in combatting typhoid; Lloyd G. Stevenson, 'Exemplary disease: The typhoid pattern', *Journal of the History of Medicine and Allied Sciences*, 37 (1982), 161–162.

64 SBHA, SBHB/HA/6/8/3/4, SOR, Malcolm Donaldson to Maxwell [no initial], 26 May 1939.

65 Worboys, *Spreading germs*, 37–38; see Nancy Tomes, *The gospel of germs: Men, women, and the microbe in American life* (Cambridge, MA, and London: Harvard University Press, 2002 [1998]), 51–52 for a discussion of sanitarian beliefs, particularly with regard to plumbing,

and 78–80 for more on sewer gas and disinfectants. See also Granshaw, '"Upon this principle"', 17–18.

66 Granshaw, '"Upon this principle"', 19.

67 See Wall, *Bacteria in Britain*, 128; for references in the minutes, see Addenbrooke's Hospital Archives, Addenbrooke's Hospital Minutes (AHM) 31, Weekly Meeting, Report on the Drainage of Addenbrooke's Hospital, 24 Jan 1883; Weekly Meeting, 21 Feb 1883; AHM33, Weekly Meeting, 15 Sep 1886; Weekly Meeting, 9 Dec 1887.

68 SBHA, SBHB/HA/6/8/3/1, SOR, 'Report on the condition of the water-closets in the nurses home', 19 Apr 1907, 122–123.

69 Tomes, *Gospel of germs*, 51.

70 Roger S. Tracy, *Handbook of sanitary information for householders* (New York: D. Appleton, 1884), 63–64, cited by Tomes, *Spreading germs*, 59.

71 Tomes, *Gospel of germs*, 163 and 237–238.

72 Plymouth and West Devon Record Office, 606/1/7, SDEC General Committee Minutes, 23 Sep 1909, cited in Palmer, *Who cared for the carers?*, 28.

73 SBHA, SBHB/HA/6/8/3/1, SOR, 'Report on the condition of the water-closets in the nurses home', 19 Apr 1907, 122–123.

74 *Ibid.*, 13 Apr 1911, 171–172.

75 Worboys, *Spreading germs*, 38–39.

76 SBHA, SBHB/HA/6/8/3/4, SOR, Report on Quarter Ending 31 Mar 1939, 1–3.

77 Alison Bashford, *Purity and pollution: Gender, embodiment and Victorian medicine* (Basingstoke: Macmillan, 1998), 128.

78 H. W. G. Macleod, *Hygiene for nurses* (London: Smith Elder, 1911), cited by Bashford, *Purity and pollution*, 139.

79 Tomes, *Gospel of germs*, 67; Worboys, *Spreading germs*, 158; Granshaw, '"Upon this principle"', 35 and 42.

80 Worboys, *Spreading germs*, 158.

81 Keir Waddington, 'The nursing dispute at Guy's Hospital, 1879–80', *Social History of Medicine*, 8 (1995), 211–230.

82 Susan McGann, *Battle of the nurses: A study of eight women who influenced the development of professional nursing* (London: Scutari Press, 1992), 136–142.

83 *Ibid.*, 60 and 74.

84 *Ibid.*, 58 and 65–69.

85 *Ibid.*, 62.

86 Isla Stewart and Herbert E. Cuff, *Practical nursing* (Edinburgh and London: William Blackwood and Sons, 1899), Chapters 15 and 16, and 221, cited in Rosemary Wall and Christine E. Hallett, 'Nursing

Practice and infection control: In the laboratory

and surgery: Professionalisation, education and innovation', in Thomas Schlich (ed.), *The Palgrave handbook of the history of surgery* (Basingstoke: Palgrave Macmillan, 2018), 161.

87 McGann, *Battle of the nurses*, 63.

88 See Claire L. Jones, Marguerite Dupree, Iain Hutchison, Susan Gardiner and Anne Marie Rafferty, 'Personalities, preferences and practicalities: Educating nurses in wound sepsis in the British hospital, 1870–1920', *Social History of Medicine*, 31 (2018), 584–591.

89 Winifred Hector, *The work of Mrs. Bedford Fenwick and the rise of professional nursing* (London: Royal College of Nursing London, 1973), 29 and Appendix A, 67–69.

90 *Ibid.*, 29–32.

91 SBHA, SBHB/HA/3/19, T and A, 19 Jul 1891–Dec 1892, 24 Mar 1892, 181–182; 14 Jul 1892, 249.

92 Geoffrey Bourne, *We met at Bart's: The autobiography of a physician* (London: Friedrich Muller Limited, 1963), 61 and 65.

93 SBHA, SBHB/HA/3/19, T and A, 19 Jul 1891–Dec 1892, 24 Nov 1892, 312.

94 SBHA, SBHB/HA/6/8/3/1, SOR, 7 Jun 1905, 85–87.

95 SBHA, SBHB/HA/1/23, Board of Governors 1866–1872, House Committee, 13 Oct 1868, 207–208. The scrubbers were employed for six months in the first instance to trial the scheme, House Committee, 13 Oct 1868, 208. The agreement was continued with a higher rate paid to Mrs Law in 1871, T and A, 26 Jan 1871, 79.

96 SBHA, SBHB/HA/3/14, T and A Oct 1880 to Oct 1883, 21 Oct 1880, 2; 16 Jun 1881, 76; 28 Jul 1881, 89; 12 Apr 1883, 272; 26 Apr 1883, 276; SBHB/HA/3/15, T and A 1 Nov 1883 to 31 Dec 1885, 16 Apr 1885, 226. SBHB/HA/3/11, T and A, 6 Jan 1870 to 23 Jul 1874; 7 Jul 1870, 37–38, see continuing arrangement 6 Jul 1871, 109; 3 Jul 1873, 243.

97 SBHA, SBHB/HA/3/15, T and A, Nov 1883–Dec 1885, 17 Jan 1884, 27.

98 Waddington, 'Nursing dispute', 214.

99 SBHA, SBHB/HA/3/19, T and A, Jul 1891–Dec 1892, 16 May 1892, 221, and 9 Jun 1892, 231.

100 *Ibid.*, 23 Jun 1893, 236.

101 *Ibid.*, 24 Nov 1892, 1 Dec 1892, 315–316.

102 SBHA, SBHB/HA/3/20, T and A, Jan 1893–Aug 1894, 8 Jun 1893, 96; 16 Mar 1893, 52.

103 Granshaw, '"Upon this principle"', 19.

104 Wildman and Hewison, 'Rediscovering a history of nursing management', 1655.

9

Infection control from the laboratory to the clinic: John H. Bowie and the Royal Infirmary of Edinburgh, *c.* 1945–1970

Susan Gardiner

Since the early 2000s, medical historians have shown a growing interest in the role of the bacteriologist in the twentieth-century hospital. Collectively, scholars suggest that in the 1950s, bacteriologists emerged as authorities on hospital infection and its control. Rising rates of hospital infection, and antibiotic-resistant infections in particular, led bacteriologists to play key roles in guiding the debate and in formulating new strategies for infection control. Kathryn Hillier, for example, suggests that the introduction of 'phage typing' – a diagnostic technique used to identify bacterial strains and trace the source of outbreaks – provided bacteriologists with an effective method by which they could trace and counter the spread of the '80/81' Staphylococcal pandemic of the mid-1950s.[1] Phage typing contributed to changing perceptions of bacteriological work, and as a result, the status of the bacteriologist 'was raised from mere technician to infection-control expert'.[2] Thereafter, bacteriologists advised on best practice and helped to produce infection control manuals.[3] Similarly, Flurin Condrau asserts that, while the bacteriological profession had long concerned itself with the phenomenon of antibacterial resistance, the increasing relevance of antibiotic resistance in the 1950s 'catapulted' bacteriologists to the centre of conversations about infection control.[4,5] Condrau and Robert Kirk suggest a tension between the expert opinions of the bacteriologist and the views of the clinician on how best to deploy antibiotics, emphasising the hospital as an arena in which these two professional groups debated the best use of these powerful but problematic drugs. Such discussions, they note, explain why bacteriologists began to play an important role in patient care.[6] Graham Ayliffe and Mary English briefly highlight the formation of infection control committees in response to the increasing incidence of Staphylococcal infections in the mid-twentieth century. Bacteriologists, they explain, took up new posts as infection control officers and, in conjunction with the new committees, played an important part in developing new infection control procedures.[7]

Focusing on the years between approximately 1945 and 1970, this chapter will provide a more in-depth exploration of the day-to-day work of bacteriologists in the mid-twentieth-century hospital than has hitherto been achieved, further unpacking their role in the control of infection.[8] In doing so, it focuses on one particular hospital – the Royal Infirmary of Edinburgh (RIE) – where hospital staff witnessed many important developments in infection control and where aspects of infection control practice soon became exemplary. Such an exploration is important in gaining a fuller understanding of why bacteriologists came to be viewed as authorities in that area.

Sydney Selwyn emphasises the importance of infection-related work undertaken in Scotland in the eighteenth, nineteenth and early twentieth centuries and the fact that many developments in infection control during that period were driven by Scots – or, as with Joseph Lister, by individuals working in Scotland.[9] Using the RIE as a case study and expanding Selwyn's work further into the twentieth century, this chapter therefore provides a unique insight into hospital infection and control in twentieth-century Scotland.

This chapter is divided into two sections. First, it explores infection control in the mid-twentieth century as manifest in everyday laboratory work at the RIE. This section addresses the ways in which laboratory work changed and grew in significance during the period under analysis, and the reasons behind this trend. It focuses on developments in antibiotic sensitivity testing and, subsequently, on the growing demand for bacteriological specimen examinations for other purposes. Secondly, this chapter discusses the increasing influence of bacteriologists in the clinical sphere, demonstrating that they played an important part in – and were often crucial to – the implementation of a range of new ward-based anti-infection strategies. This was particularly evident in the area of sterile supply. As such, this chapter represents an important counterbalance to the historiography of hospital infection control in the twentieth century, a historiography which is dominated by discussions of antibiotic resistance.

A particular focus is the work of John H. Bowie, Senior Bacteriologist to the RIE between 1949 and 1974.[10] The key argument is that, in the mid-twentieth-century hospital, bacteriological work took on greater significance for infection control and became increasingly multi-faceted. Bacteriologists performed many important functions, and those functions lay at the heart of numerous developments in infection control procedures in both laboratory and clinic. Such a broad remit explains why they became authorities on infection control.

Infection control in the laboratory

The 1950s and 1960s witnessed the increasing significance of laboratory work to infection control at the RIE. This was partly the result of the introduction of new and improved protocols for antibiotic sensitivity testing. Changes in that area ensured that such tests became part and parcel of laboratory work and imperative to infection management in the wards.

The testing of bacterial specimens for resistance to antimicrobials has long since been the duty of the bacteriologist. Antibiotic sensitivity testing arose in the years prior to the Second World War as a method of predicting when penicillin therapy would be most effective in a patient with any given infectious disease. These laboratory tests were crucial because penicillin was, at this stage, costly and in limited supply. As such, it had to be deployed efficiently. An early method of sensitivity testing was developed in 1929 by Alexander Fleming, in the laboratories of St Mary's Hospital, London, when Fleming was still experimenting with the *Penicillium* mould. Using the agar diffusion technique – more commonly known as the 'ditch plate' technique – Fleming cut a long strip in an agar plate, which he filled with a mixture of agar and an extract of *Penicillium*. Once this mixture solidified, he streaked microbic cultures at right angles across the ditch and was able to observe lanes of inhibition. New methods of sensitivity testing arose in the 1940s, involving filter paper impregnated with antibiotics and then discs.[11]

As antibiotic therapy expanded in the 1940s and 1950s, sensitivity testing was a means of finding the right antibiotic to prescribe in treatment. However, the practice was not widespread. Christoph

Gradmann suggests that sensitivity tests sometimes accompanied the deployment of sulphonamide drugs in the mid-1940s, but that antibiotic sensitivity tests were performed only very occasionally in that decade and in the early 1950s. Much of this can be explained by the relative infrequency with which resistance was actually encountered in hospitals during that period.[12]

At the RIE, in the early years of penicillin, the extent to which sensitivity tests were performed and their overall efficacy were both limited. Ena Ross, who began her nurse training at the RIE in 1945, recalled that, at that time, sensitivity tests were performed not before but during treatment; if the bacterium proved insensitive to penicillin, treatment was simply stopped.[13] Some clinicians lagged behind their bacteriological colleagues in recognising both the need to use antibiotics correctly and the importance of sensitivity testing. Surgeon Iain Ferguson Maclaren implied that some bacteriological and clinical staff's views on using antibiotics were somewhat at odds in those early days. As he remarked, 'and perhaps I'm being unfair but in retrospect, it seems to me that there wasn't much attention given to the proper ways of using the antibiotics. I may say our hospital bacteriologists were always saying, you know, "Using the antibiotic in this way is not really [appropriate]".'[14] Obstetrician Philip Roger Myerscough explained that, across the health service but particularly within general practice, 'the academically-oriented doctors' were the first to realise the necessity of such testing.[15]

The post-war era witnessed the arrival of numerous different antibiotics, including broad-spectrum drugs like chloramphenicol and chlortetracycline, and the triple therapy for tuberculosis, consisting of streptomycin, isoniazid and para-aminosalicylic acid.[16] The explosion of antibiotic therapy both complicated the sensitivity test and further underlined its importance. Writing in the *Edinburgh Medical Journal* in 1952, bacteriologist John Bowie and his colleague J. C. Gould explained that, by then, doctors generally agreed 'in principle' on the need to establish the sensitivity of the causative agent before administering an antibiotic, but that 'inadequate laboratory resources, inconveniently situated laboratories or delay in the receipt of laboratory advice' posed major issues and often rendered sensitivity tests impractical.[17] 'Bacteriological data', they wrote, 'not only serve as guides to the drug of choice, and alternatives, but also as an indication of the adequate dose'.[18]

Myerscough recalled that, when met with a severe case of infection, time pressures often forced doctors into making 'a semi-blind choice' as regards the likely causative organism and its potential sensitivity and, in turn, an appropriate antibiotic. Doctors typically waited around two days to receive the results of a sensitivity test and, if necessary, they altered the course of treatment.[19] The amount of time taken to receive these results reflected the relatively arduous nature of bacteriological work during this period and the lengthy process of developing and analysing the infecting organism in the laboratory, and then returning the results. Thus, commitment to sensitivity testing grew slowly during the 1940s and early 1950s, particularly among clinicians. But, practical concerns and the increasingly complex nature of antibiotic therapy explain the relative inefficacy of the methods of sensitivity testing at that time.

Together with Gould in 1952, Bowie introduced a new and improved method of antibiotic sensitivity testing for the laboratory workers, which led to more effective courses of therapy in the wards. Maintaining an emphasis on speed, standardisation, simplicity and replicability, the two bacteriologists introduced a modified version of the 'paper disc method' – a method they regarded as being faster, more accurate and more easily reproducible compared to the ditch plate technique.[20] They standardised numerous aspects of the method, providing specific details as regards, for example the period of bacterial cultivation (eighteen to twenty hours) and the temperature (37 degrees Celsius); the type of filter paper used to prepare the paper discs ('Whatman No. 1'); the size of the discs (just short of 7 mm in diameter); the process of sterilising the discs (organised into lots of 100, each lot being placed into containers and sterilised for one hour, in a hot air oven at a temperature of 150 degrees Celsius); the amount of antibiotic-in-sterile water solution contained in each disc (0.01 ml) and container (1 ml); the strength of the antibiotic per disc (in the case of penicillin, 1 unit); the methods of both storing and sterilising the tweezers used to transfer the paper disc on to the Petri dish (storing in 70 per cent alcohol and flame-sterilised between each use); and the process of incubating each Petri dish (37 degrees Celsius for between eighteen and twenty hours) before measuring the extent of growth/inhibition. Thereafter, they measured the diameter of the zone of inhibition in millimetres, in contrast to the conventional method of measuring the radius.[21]

A particularly important aspect of Bowie and Gould's work was that they produced standard definitions of degrees of sensitivity. For five of the most commonly used antibiotics (penicillin, streptomycin, chloromycetin, aureomycin and terramycin), they performed repeat examinations of the zones of inhibition using antibiotic solutions of varying strengths, using the resulting data to create standard graphs which measured the zone of inhibition in direct correlation to the potency of the antibiotic solution. These graphs could then be utilised, in future tests, to determine the strength of the antibiotic necessary for treatment.[22] Their examinations demonstrated that a paper disc containing 1 unit of penicillin, for example, typically resulted in a zone of inhibition of 30.5 mm. The concentration of the penicillin solution in the Petri dish always decreased as the distance from the paper disc increased, and, 30.5 mm from the paper disc, the strength of the solution in the culture medium was typically recorded at 0.03 units of penicillin per ml. The minimum concentration required to inhibit the *Staphylococcus*, therefore, was 0.03 units. Similarly, a zone of inhibition of 10 mm typically meant that approximately 1.5 units per ml were required to inhibit growth.[23] Depending on the strength of the solution needed to counter the bacterium, Bowie and Gould could categorise each strain as either 'sensitive', 'relatively resistant' or 'resistant' to the antibiotic: those inhibited by penicillin at a strength of up to 0.3 units per ml were classed as sensitive; relatively resistant bacteria were inhibited when penicillin was deployed at a strength of up to 1 unit per ml; and, when more than 1 unit per ml was required to thwart growth, the bacterium was classified as resistant. In keeping with Bowie and Gould's emphasis on simplicity, when feeding the results back to the clinic, the data was expressed using any one of these three terms. They held that precise levels of sensitivity were required only in cases of septicaemia, or for the purposes of research work.[24]

Bowie and Gould's new methods of sensitivity testing had an immediate impact on laboratory procedures, both at the RIE and further afield. By 1954, the 'Edinburgh Standard Disc Diffusion Technique' (ESDDT) was standard procedure for all routine sensitivity tests at the RIE, and results could be achieved within just twenty-four hours.[25] C. J. Smith describes Bowie's work with Gould as 'pioneering'.[26] Indeed, the method soon found application across the Scottish capital.[27] Annual reports suggest an increasing uptake of antibiotic sensitivity tests in the 1950s and into the 1960s. The managers commented in their 1961–1962 report that the workload of the laboratory had trebled in the last decade, owing partly to an acute rise in the number of 'additional' tests performed on bacteriological specimens, such as sensitivity tests and also phage typing.[28] More will be said on the increasing workload of the bacteriologists in due course. Gradmann highlights that the significance of Bowie and Gould's research was that it addressed the need for international standards in resistance diagnostics in the early 1950s.[29] But the bacteriologists went one step further, for they had already begun the process of remedying this lack of standardisation. Their new procedure could be performed in the laboratory with relative ease, speed and accuracy, leading to an increase in the uptake of this type of test and, in turn, more effective treatment plans for patients.

In the years following the introduction of the ESDDT, the position of the laboratory in matters surrounding infection control continued to strengthen, and the nature of laboratory work continued to change. A new and specially designated infection control committee provided Bowie and his bacteriological staff with a platform on which they could create greater demand for bacteriological expertise, widen the scope of laboratory work and demonstrate their infection control know-how. The committee was, initially, an ad hoc group formed around May 1958 'to enquire into the incidence of hospital infection and the methods of combating it'.[30] It was founded in the wake of startling evidence of infection at the hospital which had surfaced just three months previously. In February 1958, a special article on wound infection had appeared in the *Lancet*. Based on a study of 673 clean wounds of patients admitted to four of the RIE's surgical charges in 1956, J. S. Jeffrey and S. A. Sklaroff established an infection rate of 26.1 per cent. This figure was almost twice as high as that recorded at the Bristol Royal Infirmary in 1957 (13.6 per cent).[31] With the report leaning on the 'bacteriology and advice' of Dr Bowie, Maclaren recalled that 'it was a pretty shattering piece of information'.[32] The ad hoc committee initially comprised members of staff from various branches of hospital practice, including general surgery; neurology; ear, nose and throat; obstetrics and gynaecology; and nursing. T. B. M. Durie and R. W. Tonkin, two bacteriologists, also served on the committee.[33] By June 1960, by which point the committee had been re-branded the 'Hospital Infection

Committee' (HIC), Professor Robert Cruickshank (Bacteriologist in Chief and Chair of Bacteriology at Edinburgh University) had joined, accompanied by Bowie.[34] Maclaren and Myerscough also soon joined.[35] With the bacteriologists well represented from the moment of the committee's inception, they were well placed to express their interest in – and increasingly exert their influence on – the sphere of infection control.

Through the HIC, and Bowie in particular, the late 1950s and 1960s was a period when the bacteriological testing of patient specimens continued to form an increasingly important part of bacteriological work, indicative of a growing significance of the laboratory to infection-related concerns in the clinical sphere. Figure 9.1 illustrates that bacteriological testing became increasingly imperative to

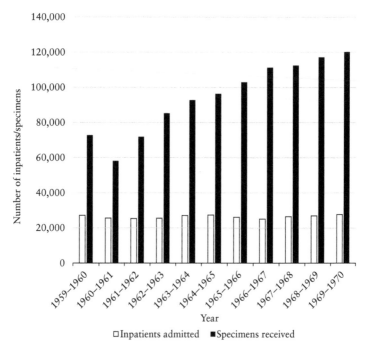

Adapted from: Lothian Health Services Archive, LHB2/3/3-13, Royal Infirmary of Edinburgh and Associated Hospitals annual reports, 1958-70

Figure 9.1   Bacteriological testing at the Royal Infirmary of Edinburgh, 1959–1970.

everyday laboratory work and to infection control at the RIE from the late 1950s onwards. In the ten years between 1959/1960 and 1969/1970, the number of specimens received in the bacteriology laboratory each year rose from 72,741 to 120,100, or by 65.1 per cent. This pattern cannot be explained by any change in annual inpatient admissions. Indeed, in the same period, admissions to the wards remained fairly constant. The number of tests performed on these specimens also rose substantially, from 699,386 in 1959/1960 to 1,108,550 in 1969/1970.[36]

The increasing demand for bacteriological tests, initiated in the 1950s by the ESDDT and by phage typing, continued into the 1960s due to three other important trends: a growing emphasis on infection surveillance; the increasing specialisation of care; and a greater awareness of exactly who constituted an infection risk. Jeffrey and Sklaroff's work marked the beginning of a preoccupation with the rate of surgical infection at the infirmary. In turn, bacteriological testing for the purposes of infection surveillance featured increasingly in laboratory work, and the Bacteriology Department was placed under increasing pressure to meet the demands that it faced as a result. Indeed, as the managers commented in 1958, 'the ever increasing demand for bacteriological investigation placed an almost intolerable strain upon the laboratory staff and will reduce the standard of work maintained by the Department unless urgent action is taken to improve existing laboratory facilities'.[37]

By the time the HIC was in operation, infection surveillance remained high on the agenda. Late in 1958, the Board of Management granted £2,500 to the committee to explore the incidence of surgical infection.[38] At a meeting in January 1961, by which point these funds had been spent, Bowie called for the investigatory work to continue. However, over and above his permanent staff, he required six additional temporary technicians in order to carry out the laboratory work that such studies entailed.[39] Later in that year, the committee endorsed a new system of infection surveillance based on the keeping of 'Infection Cards'. They advised that the registrar should complete one such card for each surgical patient, sending it to the superintendent upon their discharge from hospital. Each card contained details on the operative procedure and the state of the wound. Although clinicians' uptake on the Infection

Card scheme was initially poor, the situation improved gradually. By November 1961, the surgical staff had returned only 315 cards from a possible 2,377. Then, at the HIC meeting in January 1962, the superintendent commented that, between 1 October 1961 and 11 January 1962, he received some 1,203 cards out of a possible 4,570. This figure represented a marked improvement on previous returns.[40]

The rising demand for laboratory expertise can also be explained by the increasingly specialised nature of patient care at the RIE and the setup of new facilities in which infection control and surveillance were paramount. These facilities included a new Kidney Transplant Isolation Suite, a Renal Isolation Unit and an Assisted Respiration Unit, all of which were in operation by 1963.[41] Indeed, the 1961–1962 annual report partly attributed the rise in the number of bacteriological specimens received in the laboratory in that year to the patients receiving care in some of these units and in other areas of the hospital. Because of the high susceptibility of these patients to infection, it was standard procedure to take specimens not only from the patients themselves, but also from members of staff and from the ward environment. Bacteriological specimens were taken even before an infection became clinically manifest. The result was that over 100 specimens could be taken in connection with any one patient in just one day.[42]

The influence of laboratory workers in infection control continued to strengthen with the introduction of new procedures for the bacteriological screening of hospital staff and other personnel. In the early 1950s, the laboratory typically received around thirty specimens for bacteriological examination each day.[43] This is in stark contrast to the position by February 1962, when the Bacteriology Department was examining an average of 226 specimens per day. Of these, twenty-two belonged to members of the RIE staff. Thirteen specimens had been taken from the technical staff; five belonged to the medical staff; three were received from the domestic staff; and the bacteriologists also examined an average of one specimen from animal house attendants each day. The HIC met that month in the wake of an outbreak in the theatre of Wards 17/18. Members of the Bacteriology Department presented the HIC with a series of recommendations to reduce the risk of infection in the theatres. They prompted the committee to consider introducing regular bacteriological examinations for theatre staff who performed – or were present during – lengthy surgical procedures.[44] Bowie later recommended that, in addition to the medical examinations that were routine at the beginning of their post, newly employed theatre orderlies should also attend at the laboratory for examinations of the skin, nose and perineum. Such tests were not limited to those directly employed at the infirmary. Indeed, Bowie also suggested that tradesmen should submit to similar examinations if they were brought into the theatre to carry out work in the vicinity of staff members who were already under the bacteriologists' watchful eye.[45] The introduction of the ESDDT is therefore just one example of how the nature of bacteriological work changed and took on greater significance during the period under analysis. New methods of infection surveillance, the rise of new specialties which prioritised infection control and new procedures for monitoring hospital staff all contributed to the growing demand for laboratory expertise.

In the clinic

The HIC also provided Bowie and his colleagues with a medium through which they could engage with the more overtly clinical aspects of infection control, a situation which they certainly used to their advantage. Much in the way that Hillier suggests, the knowledge and expertise of the bacteriologist increasingly filtered out of the laboratory and into the wards during the 1950s and 1960s.[46] It is worth noting that discussions around the use (and indeed misuse) of antibiotics did surface during meetings of the HIC, but rarely.[47] Rather, the committee adopted a more holistic approach to the subject of hospital infection control in which antibiotics played a relatively minor role. Discussions relating to methods for the disposal of soiled dressings, ward design, new infection control technologies and, above all, sterile supply, all demonstrate that Bowie in particular came to possess a commanding influence on clinical procedures and protocols.

The committee first broached the issue of soiled dressings disposal in November 1959, when Miss Cordiner, the Lady Superintendent of Nurses, highlighted the infection risk posed by the existing system and suggested that new gas incinerators should be installed in the wards.[48] In June 1960, a small sub-committee comprising Bowie, Surgeon Maclaren, Miss Cordiner and the House Steward were tasked with the responsibility of considering ways in which the system could be improved. As such, Bowie suggested that there should be a named individual responsible for supervising and educating the staff involved in disposing of used dressings. The committee soon endorsed Bowie's suggestion, while recommending a seven-day service for the collection and delivery of linen.[49] Following the Wards 17/18 theatre outbreak early in 1962, Bowie provided a report on tests of the theatre's filters. These tests traced the outbreak to materials which were present in the filters before being dispersed into the atmosphere of the theatre. These filters were found to be defective because they could be easily bent, allowing the air to avoid passing through them. The relevant alterations were soon carried out.[50]

The bacteriologists on the HIC were frequently called upon to test and assess various new infection control technologies. For example, in July 1962, the hospital staff trialled a new disposable bedpan machine in the maternity wards. But Bowie found that the new device represented a major infection hazard; it dispersed traces of faecal matter into the atmosphere of the room![51] Maclaren later recalled that Cruickshank, Bowie's senior, was a 'great support' to the HIC.[52] In 1960, Cruickshank, along with two other members of the committee, arranged for a controlled trial of face masks in order to establish whether they had any effect in reducing the frequency of Staphylococcal infections in the surgical wards.[53] Cruickshank later formed part of a small sub-committee whom the HIC prompted to consider appropriate methods for sterilising the skin before operative surgery.[54] In March 1963, another bacteriologist, Dr Durie, worked with Maclaren to explore the efficacy of tincture of iodine as a skin-sterilising agent, finding it to be successful in lowering the rate of wound infection following partial gastrectomy.[55] Two years later, when the hospital pharmacist presented a report on the subject of antiseptics, the committee considered that he, alongside members of the bacteriological and nursing staffs, should explore their relative costs and effectiveness.[56]

A striking example of the growing command of the bacteriologist in infection control in the clinical setting is the profound changes made in the area of sterile supply. An increasing awareness of the deficiencies of sterilisation procedures in the 1950s provided the stimulus for new and improved methods that were implemented early in the following decade. Bowie's pioneering work in this area placed the hospital at the front of an international shift towards the centralisation of sterilisation procedures. According to Smith, it was in matters pertaining to sterilisation procedures in hospitals that Bowie became a 'world authority'.[57] Until then, at the RIE, it was customary for each surgical ward or unit to have its own operating theatre, its own set of instruments and its own autoclave in which to sterilise those instruments. This setup led to variation in the types of instruments that found favour within each ward. It was the duty of the senior theatre nurse to sterilise all of the equipment needed in that theatre. The high degree of autonomy afforded to each ward or unit as regards theatre protocol meant that the chief of each ward was, according to Myerscough, 'a little god in his own kingdom, and the hospital tended to function as [twenty] cottage hospitals rather than one unity'.[58] The existing arrangement therefore encouraged a disparate set of practices in theatres, both in terms of sterilisation methods and the instruments which found favour at each site.

Throughout the 1950s, Bowie became increasingly aware of the deficiencies of the then-present setup and managed to convince the clinical staff of the need for a radical change in sterilisation procedures. Anxieties about the sterility of surgical equipment grew in parallel to rising rates of infection. This was no coincidence. As Maclaren recalled, in the 1950s, the RIE was beginning to encounter problems with antibiotic-resistant Staphylococcal bacteria.[59] Over an eight-month period between 1958 and 1959, Maclaren recorded seven deaths in Wards 7/8 resulting from a Staphylococcal 'super-infection' which was resistant to most antibiotics.[60] Another report from the period shows that by 1959, 56 per cent of RIE personnel were known to be Staphylococcal nasal carriers – 93 per cent of those organisms were penicillin-resistant, 50 per cent were streptomycin-resistant and 45 per cent were tetracycline-resistant.[61]

Bowie knew that issues with sterilisation procedures were not confined to his own hospital but, rather, indicative of a much wider problem. Speaking before the British Pharmaceutical Society, in 1955, Bowie expressed the opinion that the vast majority (approximately 90 per cent) of sterilisers in British hospitals were outdated and unfit for purpose, this figure 'includ[ing] representatives of all developmental stages in design since 1870'.[62] The result was that sterility could not be guaranteed in the preparation of surgical goods. While poor technique on the part of those operating the autoclaves was partly responsible, the issue was generally one of poor autoclave design and maintenance.[63] Three years later, Bowie's sentiments were largely echoed in a report of the Nuffield Provincial Hospitals Trust which emphasised that a combination of poor technique and outdated equipment grossly undermined the sterility of goods used in six separate NHS hospitals.[64] At the RIE, Bowie conducted a review of the performance of the hospital's autoclaves, which were approximately ten to fifteen in number. The autoclaves were becoming increasingly obsolete and ineffective, sometimes leaving theatre staffs no alternative but to use autoclaves belonging to other theatres.[65] According to Maclaren, Bowie's discovery 'created a considerable furore'.[66] Indeed, both oral and documentary evidence suggests that the growing awareness of the deficiencies in sterilisation methods prompted both the seminal Jeffrey and Sklaroff paper and the founding of the HIC.[67]

Through the HIC, Bowie led discussions about improving procedures for sterile supply. In April 1960, in the wake of a recent visit to hospitals in mainland Europe and North America, he produced a report on his findings on sterilisation procedures overseas. He learned that instruments, fluids and utensils were typically distributed to the wards in packs and arranged into 'sets' or 'trays' which had been assembled and sterilised in a Central Sterile Supply Department (CSSD).[68] The CSSD was, in essence, a centralised location dedicated to the preparation and sterilisation of surgical goods, negating the need for goods to be prepared at the ward or departmental level.[69] In 1963, a second report of the Nuffield called for CSSDs to be established across the British hospital system, and they outlined the costs, practicalities, advantages and drawbacks of such a move.[70] They suggested that the CSSD 'should produce for the hospitals it serves all sterile requirements other than theatre surgical instruments, bedpans and urinals, pharmaceuticals and bedding'.[71] According to Monica Baly, the move towards central sterile supply was in keeping with the much wider aim of the National Health Service (NHS) of improving hospital supplies and equipment more generally through standardisation. But sterile supply was given precedence in light of the concerns surrounding cross infection and sterility.[72]

By the time of the Nuffield report of 1963, the RIE had already begun the process of centralisation. Three years previously, Bowie suggested that a centralised system of sterile supply had at least two key advantages. First, since members of the nursing staff were no longer required to sterilise and prepare surgical equipment themselves, they were 'freed to pursue their proper professional duties'.[73] Similarly, the Nuffield report maintained that one of the two main aims of the CSSD was to alleviate the burden of nursing work, allowing for a greater emphasis on patient care. Early estimates suggested that the removal of sterilising duties could save approximately four hours of nurse labour per day; this figure excluded the time saved in actually applying and/or changing dressings. The Nuffield report framed the saving in nurse labour as partly offsetting the huge costs involved in establishing and running a CSSD.[74] For Bowie, another advantage of the CSSD related to the greater efficacy of the methods by which surgical goods were prepared. Lay staff, he noted, prepared surgical goods in a centralised location and adhered to standardised protocols under the guidance of hospital workers with varying areas of expertise: surgeons, nurses, pharmacists and bacteriologists.[75] These comments again reflected the main aims of the CSSD as laid out by the Nuffield report, which held that a centralised, standardised and controlled sterile supply system would result in a lower rate of infection in the hospital.[76]

In June 1960, when Bowie submitted his report on central sterile supply to the HIC, the committee immediately endorsed the setup of a CSSD for the RIE, providing that a suitable location was available. Such facilities, they envisaged, would serve the surgical wards.[77] But they initially struggled to find an appropriate venue which satisfied the Board of Management.[78] This had much to do with pressures on accommodation at the hospital. However, in May 1961, a central sterile 'section' was opened following a reorganisation of the premises.[79] From the moment that these facilities first appeared at the RIE, the issue of sterile supply was firmly in the territory of the bacteriologist. Indeed, in the financial year 1960/1961, the Department of Bacteriology delivered fifteen papers on matters pertaining to central sterile supply, sterilisation and hospital infection to external organisations across the UK.[80] The service proved hugely popular at the RIE. In October 1962, Bowie reported to the committee that the average number of packs of surgical goods sterilised each day increased from thirty-six in July 1960 to 639 in September 1962. In the latter month, the seven-day service sterilised, prepared and issued some 19,186 caskets and packs to all areas of the hospital.[81]

While improvements made in sterile supply is a particularly strong example of the growing influence of the bacteriologist in clinical procedures for infection control, it was in the area of sterile supply to the theatres that this trend was most striking. Despite the growing popularity of the CSSD in the British hospital, the sterilisation of theatre instruments was a separate issue. Indeed, from the laboratories of the Belfast City Hospital in 1960, V. D. Allison commented in the *British Medical Journal* that, while the CSSD's purpose was to provide the wards, theatres and other areas of the hospital with ready-to-use, sterile equipment, theatre instruments continued to be processed in the theatres themselves.[82] According to the 1963 Nuffield report, CSSDs could provide the theatres with items such as gowns, towels, drapes, dressings, bowls and utensils, but they also envisaged that the theatres would continue to prepare and sterilise their own instruments.[83] At the RIE, aside from ongoing concerns about infection, improvements in sterile theatre supply were prompted by a large-scale reconstruction project that was planned for the hospital. E. F. Catford writes that, with the nationalisation of the health services on the horizon, the need for reconstruction work to meet the demands expected of the new service first became apparent in the aftermath of the Second World War. Although plans for the rebuilding work were first drawn up in 1955, another twenty years would pass before such work began.[84] In the midst of the planning for the new RIE, in September 1961, the South-Eastern Regional Hospital Board created a working party to offer guidance on the reconstruction of the operating theatres. Its main concerns for planning were the importance of environmental asepsis; reducing the length of time between operations and the time taken to prepare the theatre for emergency procedures; and the need to economise in the use of theatre staffs.[85]

Working with Anna R. Gordon (Theatre Superintendent and fellow HIC member), F. John Gillingham (Professor of Surgical Neurology) and Ian D. Campbell (Deputy Senior Administrative Medical Officer of the South-Eastern Regional Hospital Board), Bowie developed a new system of sterile theatre supply that met each of the aforementioned requirements.[86] The team described this system in the *British Medical Journal* in 1963. Their suggestion was that all of the sterile articles required in the operating theatres – including all fabrics such as dressings, drapes and towels and, most significantly, all instruments – should be processed in a central facility known as the 'Theatre Service Centre' (TSC). The trays would be standardised according to the nature of the procedure, and their contents would be arranged in the order that the surgeon required them. A thoracotomy, for example, would have its own tray. The auxiliaries who worked in the TSC would be trained to prepare the trays using lists and photographic aids. The trays, mounted on trolleys, would then be distributed to the operating theatres, ready for use. When the operation reached its conclusion, the trays would be returned to the TSC to be processed again.[87]

In developing the trays, Bowie collaborated with Chief Technician, James Dick. Bowie had already worked with Dick in other projects aimed at improving sterilisation procedures. Most notably, this included the Bowie-Dick Autoclave Tape Test, a procedure used across the world to test the efficiency of dressings sterilisers.[88] During preliminary trials of the tray system at the RIE and in the absence of a specially designated area for preparing the trays for theatre (i.e. in the absence of a TSC), they were processed in the central sterilisation department and then set in the operating theatre.[89] Early trials indicated that the new tray system was immensely popular with both the surgeons and nurses working in the participating theatres. Not only was it a considerable time-saver; indeed, it saved up to fifty minutes of trolley-setting time before surgery and, in emergency cases, all sterile articles could be made available to the theatre staffs in a matter of seconds. But the tray system also reduced levels of tension among members of the nursing staff, 'since with experience they gain confidence in the certainty that everything will be ready as soon as the surgeons are ready to begin'.[90] The theatre staff working in the individual suites expressed their desire to continue with the tray service, which they viewed as an improvement on the old system of sterilising the theatre instruments separately from other goods.[91]

The HIC was generally receptive to Bowie's pre-set tray system and his vision for a centralised facility in which the trays could be processed. The July 1962 meeting of the committee adjourned when its members visited the Nurses' Teaching Unit for a demonstration of the new tray system.[92] By November of that year, the committee was receiving indications from the Regional Board that a suitable facility for pre-setting the trays would soon be provided.[93] Thus, in August 1964, an experimental TSC opened under the supervision of Sister S. B. R. Scott. Initially, it provided sterile materials to three of the theatres.[94] Lorna Numbers began her nurse training at the RIE in 1965. She described the TSC as 'a big showpiece' and remembered that films were shown to those who were interested.[95] The trays were colour-coded according to the procedures for which they were intended. It was the duty of the theatre sister to order the trays needed for the following day, and the trays were transported to and from the TSC through 'a system of internal lifts'.[96] Maclaren described Bowie as the 'moving spirit' behind the pre-set tray system; the system was 'the great result' of the HIC and 'a great innovation [which] meant you could have absolute confidence in the sterility of the equipment you were using'.[97] Myerscough remembered that the HIC was responsible for deciding the contents of each tray. It was no easy task getting surgeons on the committee to agree on both the exact instruments that were used and the manner in which they were laid out on the tray. As he recalled, 'one of the great achievements of that committee was that they knocked everybody's head together'.[98] He also explained that the nurses on the HIC were crucial in dealing with the practicalities involved, including the weight of the trays. He suggested that tackling the practical issues was important when gathering support for the trays.[99] Bowie's new system therefore had two significant implications. Not only did it represent an advance from the perspective of infection control, but it also affected the very manner in which surgeons performed operations. In fostering greater standardisation in theatre practice, it symbolised the end of the old system in which, as mentioned previously, 'each chief was a little god in his own kingdom'.[100] From a clinician's perspective, the new system was 'a total revolution'.[101]

As the decade progressed, the TSC continued to expand, and Bowie's ideas about sterile supply rapidly spread southwards and beyond. Its staffing initially comprised a supervisor, a steriliser attendant, two tray assemblers and a seamstress.[102] In the financial year 1966/1967, the service attracted some 239 visitors. The number of tray assemblers had already increased to twelve, and it was supplying all of the general surgical theatres and the thoracic surgery theatre.[103] In March 1967, the TSC processed 935 trays. By March of the following year, this figure had increased to 1,036 trays.[104] Supply rose substantially thereafter. During the financial year 1969/1970, 14,738 trays, 11,589 packs of instruments and over 200,000 pieces of linen were prepared in the TSC, and the Regional Board gave the green light for it to be expanded to serve the entire hospital.[105] According to Ayliffe and English, following its introduction, the Edinburgh pre-set tray system was modified and adopted in all CSSDs.[106] Indeed, in 1969–1970, visitors came to the TSC from across the globe, from Switzerland to Australia. 'Visitors from England', the managers stated, 'are now few because many Theatre Service Centres have already developed there.'[107] The work done with regard to sterilisation procedures at the RIE is again a reflection of the bacteriological profession's increasing command over ward-based procedures for infection control. Not only were Bowie's endeavours in the 1950s important in raising awareness of the need for change in that area, but also his work in the following decade revolutionised sterilisation practices and procedures in hospitals worldwide, at the same time bringing greater standardisation to the methods by which surgeons performed operative procedures.

Conclusion

This work builds on a budding historiography on hospital infection and its control in the twentieth century by offering a fuller understanding of the work of bacteriologists in the mid-twentieth-century hospital, and by providing a unique exploration of the control of infection in Scottish hospitals. In doing so, it both encompasses and moves beyond discussions of antibiotics to demonstrate the holistic approach to infection control adopted by bacteriological staff at the RIE. That such a comprehensive overview of the work of one particular group of laboratory staff can be provided is one of the merits of the case study approach. Between 1945 and 1970, routine laboratory work became increasingly important to infection control at the RIE. The introduction of a relatively speedy, standardised and reliable method of antibiotic sensitivity testing in 1952 – a test which was adopted in hospitals across Edinburgh soon after its introduction at the RIE – led to an increase in demand for that particular type of laboratory test. Largely in connection with the HIC, the demand for laboratory work continued to increase late in that decade and into the 1960s. After the Jeffrey and Sklaroff report, infection surveillance among patients became an increasingly crucial part of routine laboratory work. The founding of new specialist units within the hospital – units which prioritised infection control – also created greater need for laboratory services and bacteriological knowledge. The scope of everyday laboratory work broadened further with the extension of surveillance protocols to new staff groups and to other personnel who were in some way connected to the hospital, further underlining the importance of the laboratory to infection control.

At the regular meetings of the HIC, Bowie and his bacteriologists also exerted a profound influence on methods for infection control in the wards and theatres, with antibiotics taking a backseat in committee discussions. This chapter has explored their role in the development of clinical methods for infection control, discussing new methods for the disposal of soiled dressings, ward design, the testing of infection-related technologies and the implementation of new systems of sterile supply to the wards and theatres. Bowie was crucial to the development of the TSC and pre-set tray system. This was a particularly significant innovation which revolutionised systems of sterile supply to theatres in hospitals across the globe, while fostering greater standardisation of the ways surgeons carried out operations. In sum, in the period 1945 to 1970, bacteriological work grew in significance and expanded into new areas. That the field of infection control increasingly became bacteriological territory was due to the bacteriologists' ability to offer both their guidance and their expertise on infection control concerns as manifest in numerous ways in both the laboratory and clinic. To use Hillier's terminology, Bowie in particular represented the archetypal infection control 'expert'.[108]

Notes

1 K. Hillier, 'Babies and bacteria: phage typing, bacteriologists, and the birth of infection control', *Bulletin of the History of Medicine*, 80 (2006), 733–761.

2 *Ibid.*, 760.

3 *Ibid.*

4 F. Condrau, 'Standardising infection control: antibiotics and hospital governance in Britain 1948–1960', in C. Bonah *et al.* (eds), *Harmonizing drugs: Standards in 20th-century pharmaceutical history* (Paris: Editions Glyphe, 2009), 343–355.

5 It is important here to distinguish between 'antibacterial resistance' and 'antibiotic resistance'. Not all antibacterial agents – for example, antiseptics and sulphonamide drugs – are classed as antibiotics. The phenomenon of antibiotic resistance began with the advent of resistance to penicillin, the first antibiotic drug.

6 F. Condrau and R. G. W. Kirk, 'Negotiating hospital infections: The debate between ecological balance and eradication strategies in British hospitals, 1947–1969', *Dynamis*, 31 (2011), 385–405.

7 G. A. J. Ayliffe and M. P. English, *Hospital infection: From miasmas to MRSA* (Cambridge: Cambridge University Press, 2003), 192–193.

8 This work is based largely on the author's PhD thesis which focuses on infection control in two Scottish hospitals between approximately 1928 and 1970. See S. Gardiner, 'Answering Ackerknecht: Infection control practice in Scottish hospitals in the early "Antibiotic Era", 1928–1970' (PhD dissertation, University of Glasgow, 2017). See Chapter 7 of the thesis in particular.

9 S. Selwyn, 'Hospital infection: The first 2500 years', *Journal of Hospital Infection*, 18, Supplement A (1991), 5–64.

10 C. J. Smith, 'The bacteriology laboratory at the Royal Infirmary', in C. J. Smith and J. G. Collee (eds), *Edinburgh's contribution to medical microbiology* (Glasgow: Wellcome Unit for the History of Medicine, 1994), 129–146.

11 D. Amsterdam, 'Principles of antibiotic testing in the laboratory', in A. Balows, W. J. J. Hausler, M. Ohashi and A. Turano (eds), *Laboratory diagnosis of infectious diseases* (New York: Springer, 1988), 22–38; A. Fleming, 'On the antibacterial action of cultures of a penicillium, with special reference to their use in the isolation of *B. influenzae*', *British Journal of Experimental Pathology*, 10 (1929), 226–236.

12 C. Gradmann, 'Sensitive matters: The World Health Organization and antibiotic resistance testing, 1945–1975', *Social History of Medicine*, 26 (2013), 555–574.

13 Interview with Ena Ross by Susan Gardiner, 29 Apr 2015.

14 Interview with Iain Ferguson Maclaren by Susan Gardiner, 27 Feb 2015.

15 Interview with Philip Roger Myerscough by Susan Gardiner, 6 Mar 2015.

16 S. B. Levy, *The antibiotic paradox: How miracle drugs are destroying the miracle* (New York: Plenum Press, 1992), 45–46; R. Porter, *The greatest benefit to mankind: A medical history of humanity from antiquity to the present* (London: HarperCollins Publishers, 1997), 457–458.

17 J. C. Gould and J. H. Bowie, 'The determination of bacterial sensitivity to antibiotics', *Edinburgh Medical Journal*, 59 (1952), 178–199.

18 *Ibid.*, 195.

19 Interview with Philip Roger Myerscough.

20 Gould and Bowie, 'The determination of bacterial sensitivity', 179–181, 194. Gradmann writes that the paper disc method was first introduced in the 1940s. The procedure involved placing a paper disc containing an antibiotic on a Petri dish in which the microorganism had previously been grown. Thereafter, the bacteriologist observed the bacteria's sensitivity or resistance to the antibiotic by measuring the extent of bacterial growth or inhibition around the antibiotic. Initially, the procedure was largely non-standardised, with great variation in, for example, the size of the paper disc, the quantity of antibiotic and the period of observation. See Gradmann, 'Sensitive matters', 562.

21 Gould and Bowie, 'The determination of bacterial sensitivity', 179–181.

22 *Ibid.*, 180–184.

23 *Ibid.*, 180–182.

24 *Ibid.*, 190–191.

25 *Ibid.*, 178; J. H. Bowie, 'The clinical laboratory aspect of antibiotic therapy', *Edinburgh Medical Journal*, 61 (1954), 1–16.

26 Smith, 'The bacteriology laboratory', p. 141.

27 See, for example: P. N. Edmunds, D. N. Nicholson and D. M. Douglas, 'Two cases of listerial meningitis in infants', *British Medical Journal*, 2:5038 (1957), 188–191; W. P. U. Kennedy, A. T. Wallace and J. McC. Murdoch, 'Ampicillin in treatment of certain gram-negative bacterial infections', *British Medical Journal*, 2 (1963), 962–965.

28 Lothian Health Services Archive (hereafter LHSA), LHB2/3/5, Royal Infirmary of Edinburgh and Associated Hospitals (hereafter RIEAH) annual report, 1961–1962, 64.

29 Gradmann, 'Sensitive matters', 563.

30 LHSA, LHB1/80/61, letter from Medical Superintendent S. G. M. Francis, 15 May 1958.

31 J. S. Jeffrey and S. A. Sklaroff, 'Incidence of wound infection', *Lancet*, 271:7016 (1958), 365–368.

32 *Ibid.*, 368; interview with Iain Ferguson Maclaren.

33 LHSA, LHB1/80/61, Ad Hoc Committee on Hospital Infection minutes, 18 November 1959; LHSA, LHB2/3/2, RIEAH annual report, 1958–1959.

34 LHSA, LHB1/80/61, Hospital Infection Committee (hereafter HIC) minutes, 20 Jun 1960; C. J. Smith, 'Professor Robert Cruickshank', in Smith and Collee, *Edinburgh's contribution*, 84–98; LHSA, LHB2/3/2.

35 Interview with Iain Ferguson Maclaren; interview with Philip Roger Myerscough.

36 LHSA, LHB2/3/3–13, RIEAH annual reports, 1958–1970.

37 LHSA, LHB2/3/1, RIEAH annual report, 1948–1958, 51.

38 LHSA, LHB1/80/61, HIC minutes, 16 Jan 1961.

39 *Ibid.*

40 *Ibid.*, 15 May 1961; 20 Nov 1961; 15 Jan 1962.

41 LHSA, LHB2/3/4, RIEAH annual report, 1960–1961, p. 26; LHSA, LHB2/3/6, RIEAH annual report, 1962–1963, 66.

42 LHSA, LHB2/3/5, 63–64.

43 *Ibid.*, 64.

44 LHSA, LHB1/80/61, HIC minutes, 19 Feb 1962.

45 *Ibid.*, 18 Apr 1962.

46 Hillier, 'Babies and bacteria', 737.

47 LHSA, LHB1/80/61, HIC minutes: 20 Jun 1960.

48 LHSA, LHB1/80/61, Ad Hoc Committee minutes.

49 LHSA, LHB1/80/61, HIC minutes: 20 Jun 1960; 18 Jul 1960; 17 Oct 1960.

50 *Ibid.*, 19 Feb 1962; 18 Apr 1962; 18 Jun 1962.

51 *Ibid.*, 16 Jul 1962.

52 Interview with Iain Ferguson Maclaren.

53 LHSA, LHB1/80/61, HIC minutes, 20 Jun 1960.

54 *Ibid.*, 20 Feb 1961.

55 *Ibid.*, 15 Mar 1963.

56 *Ibid.*, 14 Jun 1965; LHSA, LHB2/3/9, RIEAH annual report, 1965–1966, 19.

57 C. J. Smith, 'Appendix D: Staff and associates of the University Department of Medical Microbiology', in Smith and Collee, *Edinburgh's contribution*, 211–281.

58 Interview with Philip Roger Myerscough.

59 Interview with Iain Ferguson Maclaren.

60 LHSA, LHB1/80/61, I. F. Maclaren, 'Interim report on study of surgical infections in the general surgical charges of the Royal Infirmary' (*c.* June 1959).

61 LHSA, LHB1/80/61, James Murdoch, memorandum on Staphylococcal infection at the RIE (16 Apr 1959).

62 LHSA, LHB1/80/21, J. H. Bowie, 'Modern apparatus for sterilisation', in *An address given to an evening meeting of the Pharmaceutical Society of Great Britain in Edinburgh on February 16, 1955* (London: The Pharmaceutical Press, 1955), 3.

63 *Ibid.*, 22–23.

64 Nuffield Provincial Hospitals Trust, *Present sterilizing practice in six hospitals* (London: Nuffield Provincial Hospitals Trust, 1958).

65 Interview with Philip Roger Myerscough; interview with Iain Ferguson Maclaren.

66 Interview with Iain Ferguson Maclaren.

67 *Ibid.*; interview with Philip Roger Myerscough; Jeffrey and Sklaroff, 'Incidence of wound infection', 365; LHSA, LHB1/80/61, letter from Medical Superintendent S. G. M. Francis, 15 May 1958.

68 LHSA, LHB1/80/21, report on sterile supply, from J. H. Bowie to Medical Superintendent Francis, 20 Apr 1960, 1.

69 Ayliffe and English, *Hospital infection*, 141–143.

70 Nuffield Provincial Hospitals Trust, *Central sterile supply: Principles and practice* (London: Oxford University Press, 1963).

71 *Ibid.*, 2.

72 M. E. Baly, *Nursing and social change* (London: Routledge, 3rd edition 1995), 199.

73 LHSA, LHB1/80/21, report on sterile supply, 1.

74 Nuffield, *Central sterile supply*, 1, 55–64.

75 LHSA, LHB1/80/21, report on sterile supply, 1.

76 Nuffield, *Central sterile supply*, 1.

77 LHSA, LHB1/80/61, HIC minutes: 20 Jun 1960; 18 Jul 1960.

78 *Ibid.*, 18 Jul 1960; 17 Oct 1960.

79 LHSA, LHB2/3/4, 25, 62.

80 *Ibid.*, 62.

81 LHSA, LHB1/80/61, HIC minutes, 15 Oct 1962.

82 V. D. Allison, 'Hospital central sterile supply departments', *British Medical Journal*, 2:5201 (1960), 772–778.

83 Nuffield, *Central sterile supply*, 82–85.

84 E. F. Catford, *The Royal Infirmary of Edinburgh 1929–1979* (Edinburgh: Scottish Academic Press, 1984), 119–130.

85 J. H. Bowie, F. J. Gillingham, I. D. Campbell and A. R. Gordon 'Hospital sterile supplies: Edinburgh pre-set tray system', *British Medical Journal*, 2:5368 (1963), 1322–1327.

86 *Ibid.*; LHSA, LHB1/80/61, HIC minutes, 20 Feb 1961.

87 Bowie *et al.*, 'Hospital sterile supplies', 1322–1327.

88 *Ibid.*, 1324; Catford, *The Royal*, 167–168.

89 Bowie *et al.*, 'Hospital sterile supplies', 1324–1325.

90 *Ibid.*, 1324.
91 *Ibid.*
92 LHSA, LHB1/80/61, HIC minutes, 16 Jul 1962.
93 *Ibid.*, 19 Nov 1962.
94 LHSA, LHB2/3/8, RIEAH annual report, 1964–1965, 82.
95 Interview with Lorna Numbers by Susan Gardiner, 27 Apr 2015.
96 *Ibid.*
97 Interview with Iain Ferguson Maclaren.
98 Interview with Philip Roger Myerscough.
 99 *Ibid.*
100 *Ibid.*
101 *Ibid.*
102 Catford, *The Royal*, p. 168.
103 LHSA, LHB2/3/10, RIEAH annual report, 1966–1967, 80.
104 LHSA, LHB2/3/11, RIEAH annual report, 1967–1968, 84.
105 LHSA, LHB2/3/13, RIEAH annual report, 1969–1970, 108.
106 Ayliffe and English, *Hospital infection*, 143.
107 LHSA, LHB2/3/13, 108.
108 Hillier, 'Babies and bacteria', 733.

Part V

Into the future

10

Infection prevention and control in the twenty-first century: the era of patient safety

Neil Wigglesworth

This chapter focuses on infection prevention and control (IPC) towards the end of the twentieth century. Like Alistair Leanord's contribution to this volume, it offers a senior participant observer account of the shifting nature of infection control policies, though it focuses on England rather than Scotland. It considers how past events might influence current and future policy, especially with regard to the role of IPC in methicillin-resistant *Staphylococcus aureus* (MRSA). Thus, it begins with a consideration of MRSA in the late 1990s into the early 2000s and the ways in which that outbreak produced a sea change in the roles and responsibilities of infection specialists. It goes on to consider how and why IPC strategies have engaged with the wider patient safety agenda. And, finally, it explores what possible futures we might see for IPC in England, in the light of recent historical experience.

The MRSA outbreaks of the 1990s

I have worked in infection control, with a nursing background, for more than twenty years. IPC had its 'fifteen minutes of fame' or infamy in the latter part of the last century, when MRSA and *Clostridium difficile* (*C. diff*) became a huge media and political issue in the 1990s and through the 2000s. This period of intense concern was characterised by a massive increase in MRSA. The data I am using in this chapter comes from England and Wales, but the situation was essentially the same across the United Kingdom from the early 1990s to the turn of the century.[1] At the same time, or shortly after, there was a marked increase in *C. diff*. So, these were two significant problems that emerged roughly over the same time frame.

The media reaction to infection outbreaks was immediate and dramatic, and continues in more recent newspaper accounts of 'superbugs' and hospital infections.[2] From the perspective of a specialist working in the field, these reports were often wildly exaggerated and unhelpful. When the *C. diff* outbreak occurred, there was a similar media response, and the headlines were full of news about superbugs; essentially, 'MRSA ate my granny' would be a consolidated version of these headlines during this period. The effect of this media coverage was to induce fear and anxiety in patients and their families.

The inflamed media response also led to various governmental responses, and some significant and high-profile investigations and inspections that culminated in the work of the Francis Inquiry.[3] I am going to focus here on the response of the English National Health Service (NHS), though there are similar stories that could be told by colleagues working in other parts of the UK. For example, there was a reduction in MRSA bacteraemia (i.e. the presence of MRSA bacteria in the blood) in England between 2001 and 2013. This reduction in reported MRSA cases reflects a whole raft of governmental interventions that were brought in in the wake of the 1990s outbreaks. Multiple forms of legislation, new roles and guidelines were introduced after the media furore surrounding MRSA, and this seems to be characteristic of the process by which government policy is formed. Developments in IPC tend to follow some kind of 'happening' or incident. Other examples include the infamous outbreak of Salmonella food poisoning at the psychiatric hospital, Stanley Royd, in Wakefield, and the Stafford Legionnaire's Disease outbreak in the 1980s.[4]

It is important to note the progress made in the UK due to policy developments around IPC; overall, we have seen a reduction in MRSA bacteraemia that is both dramatic and probably unique in the world. One of the reasons, undoubtedly, for the investment in IPC was that it became a crucial issue for organisations, and chief executive jobs were on the line. For the first time in history, significant resources were found to tackle the problem, and there was a considerable expansion in teams equipped to undertake the work. It also changed the nature of those teams, with antimicrobial pharmacists becoming an integral part of an IPC team. There was a sea change in the roles and responsibilities of infection control specialists within NHS organisations, which enabled such dramatic effects.

This recent historical example begs the question: what might bring the next development in IPC? And how do we sustain that development once a crisis is over? I do not believe, from my personal and professional experience, that we will have any future outbreak as large as the MRSA and C. *diff* episodes discussed here, at least in the UK. Ebola was a big issue internationally – and received a similar tenor of media reaction to MRSA – but it did not have the same impact in the UK as these home-grown events did. Our current challenge, of course, is antimicrobial resistance, which is a global problem. Professor Dame Sally Davies has put antimicrobial resistance on the risk register for the UK because it requires a UK-wide response rather than an English response.[5] To contextualise its significance, this puts antimicrobial resistance on the same footing as terrorism in terms of its threat to the UK population.

It is unclear yet whether raising the status of antimicrobial resistance in this manner will give more power to IPC. Moreover, the new superbug that is being addressed is not MRSA but carbapenem-resistant Enterobacteriaceae (CRE) or carbapenemase-producing Enterobacteriaceae (CPE); multi-resistant bacteria that potentially threaten untreatable infections in the future (carbapenems are antibiotics used for the treatment of infections caused by multidrug-resistant bacteria.) The resistant organism *Candida auris* has also caused severe illness in hospitalised patients across the world. Professor Dame Davies, the Director of the Centers for Disease Control and Prevention (CDC), Prime Minister David Cameron and the forty-fourth President of the US, Barack Obama, all noted how dangerous antibiotic-resistant bacteria are, especially carbapenem-resistant bacteria. Statistical reports from Public Health England highlight the rise of CPE according to UK data.[6] The statistics are crude because they are based on specimens sent to Public Health England as a reference laboratory, but it is clear that the incidence of carbapenem-resistant bacteria has significantly increased in the past few years.

Despite some bias where there have been outbreaks in specific parts of the country such as the experience with *Klebsiella pneumoniae* carbapenemase (KPC) in the northwest of England, the overall increase is clear. Most hospitals are now seeing occasional cases, and some hospitals are experiencing clusters. The pattern looks rather like MRSA did before the last series of outbreaks, and that is troubling because carbapenem-resistant bacteria are much harder to treat. In this context, the nightmare scenario is running out of drugs to combat infections. In Italy, for example, when the laboratories were recently surveyed for last-line antibiotics for these bacteria, almost half of the CPE isolates were resistant.[7] IPC is crucial in preventing antimicrobial resistance, as noted in the UK five-year antimicrobial resistance strategy. What concerns me, however, is that IPC is receiving less attention than more dramatic, headline-hitting themes such as surveillance and public information and new drugs development. The reasons for this are unclear; it might well be, as Sally Sheard suggests in her contribution to this volume, that hygiene has a low status.

This is also an important point to make in relation to nursing. Of the range of activities involved in IPC, those that relate to nursing are receiving a disproportionately low level of attention. One might argue that this is because nursing does not attract the same levels of research funding that new drugs might, or other innovations in IPC. There are certainly traditional hierarchies at work that mitigate against nursing being given the same status as physician- and surgeon-led care. There is a danger, as a result, that the nursing strategies that have made a difference in the past, in combatting outbreaks of MRSA for instance, will be overlooked in the future and when other bacteria are involved.

A final point must be made in relation to finance. After the 2010 general election, and the global economic crisis, spending on the NHS has decreased in real terms and will continue to do so in the foreseeable future. This is important because the 1990s and 2000s saw significant financial investment in addressing the problems discussed in this chapter; this may not be an option in the current financial climate, where we are going to need to do more for less.

Patient safety in the UK

For the last ten years, interest in patient safety in the UK has produced something of a revolution in healthcare; one of the reasons for this shift is a recognition that historically, we have reached the limits of our effectiveness in key areas. Widespread education, policy and initiatives from governments as well as attempts to enforce diligence and increase efficiency have done all they can. We therefore need other approaches to go further in terms of improving quality and safety in healthcare. Another stimulus for the patient safety movement is the realisation that healthcare is potentially dangerous; Rene Amalberti and Lucien Leape have compared the risk of fatality per encounter in healthcare with practice in other industries, such as nuclear and airline industries and the European railways.[8] The writers discovered that healthcare was roughly as safe as mountain climbing and bungee jumping. This is obviously a crude comparison because people coming to hospital are usually sick and some die *because* they are sick, but nevertheless, people also die because they have contact with healthcare practices.

The point of this analogy is not to suggest that healthcare is comparable to a nuclear plant, but to indicate that we can learn from other industries about the reliability of processes and general safety. By way of illustration, let us consider the Keystone Intensive Care Unit (ICU) project, which was a very large, multi-centre intervention around intensive care units in the United States.[9] This patient safety collaborative included 108 ICUs and used the quality improvement approaches of the Institute for Healthcare Improvement (IHI). The main interventions of the Keystone project were care bundles, which means applying the five most important interventions, according to the evidence, for any given problem. In the example I am discussing, the problem was bloodstream infections (BSIs) from intravenous (IV) devices and ventilator-associated pneumonia, which are typical intensive care issues. Healthcare bundles work as follows: the targeted interventions are put into an easy to understand, simple to follow, set of instructions for everyone to follow and check off. All five interventions must be checked off and followed; it is all or nothing in terms of their success.

In addition to healthcare bundles, the Keystone units sought to improve organisational safety culture, especially the intensive care safety culture in the identified units. There are few details about what was implemented, besides training a couple of leaders on each unit, unfortunately. But we know that improving safety culture can reduce infection risks.[10] The results were dramatic; the most famous of these is around catheter-related BSI. The Keystone project reduced the median catheter-related BSI in these 108 ICUs to zero. Catheter-related BSI is arguably a totally preventable infection if managed appropriately. Some infections are less preventable; pneumonias, for instance, can be hard to prevent in some patients.

Nevertheless, the Keystone project did manage to prevent many instances of BSI: there was a dramatic reduction in the mean from 7.0 to 2.0 of BSI, but the median was reduced to zero, because many of the units had no infections at all. The Keystone unit work on safety connects to my own work in Salford a few years ago, based on the IHI initiatives used in infection control in the US. We undertook an IHI patient safety collaborative using their model for improvement in patient safety quality improvement to reduce *C. diff*.[11] We undertook this work – which was effective in getting results – at a time when *C. diff* infections were generally reducing, so it is difficult to assess the contribution of our interventions to the overall reduction. Nevertheless, it is an example of the ways quality improvement approaches are becoming established in healthcare settings and influencing the way we think about reducing infections.

There is, however, an important distinction to be made here between policy in England and in Scotland and Wales. In Scotland and Wales, the IHI Model for Improvement is used as the primary model for quality improvement and patient safety programmes. In England, NHS England has undertaken several patient safety initiatives, such as the Safer Patient Initiatives and the Sign Up for Safety approach, but they are less based on this particular, collaborative model for improvement discussed here. Why does this matter? Professor Elaine Larsson and colleagues at the Columbia School of Nursing have undertaken a systematic review looking at safety culture in organisations, making comparisons with compliance in basic infection prevention precautions. They identified seven studies that compared safety culture measurement with standard precautions compliance; all seven studies showed a statistically significant relationship between patient safety culture in an organisation, and compliance with basic infection control. The study didn't measure actual outcomes or infection levels. They measured the processes of infection control, such as the use of gloves and aprons and hand-washing. And, what the study suggests is that a good patient safety culture produces better compliance with infection controls, which in turn leads to fewer infections.

Human factors and ergonomics and the future of infection control

I want to conclude this essay with some thoughts on the future of infection control, and my own current professional interest, which is human factors and ergonomics (HFE) – the practice of designing products, systems and processes that take proper account of the interaction between them and the people who use them to optimise human performance. In 2013, I co-authored a thought paper for the Health Foundation charity on the possibility of engaging HFE in healthcare to improve IPC.[12] HFE combines psychology and engineering to design tasks, systems and organisations around people, rather than the other way around. It is essentially the opposite of behaviour change approaches, which approaches infection control from a different direction. HFE seeks to adapt systems and organisations to the people within them, while behaviour change approaches try to adapt people to the systems and organisations in which they work. A further benefit of HFE is that it acknowledges the complex sociotechnical aspects of modern healthcare.

Professor Pascale Carayon has published extensively on human factors in healthcare. Her systematic review examined how commonly HFE approaches are used in the design of patient pathways and systems in healthcare to improve quality and safety.[13] It identified twelve projects where HFE was used consistently, which demonstrates HFE is being used in healthcare, but infrequently.[14] Evidence from those twelve projects provide examples of HFE in practice. These include the example of practice in a laminar flow operating theatre. The laminar flow theatre has a clean air curtain that comes straight down over the operating theatre from a box in the ceiling. For the theatre to work properly, all the surgical instruments need to be placed beneath the curtain; outside the curtain they are not in clean air. However, prior to the intervention in this study, instruments were being placed outside the area of the curtain. Lights were also being placed beneath the curtain, where they blocked the airflow.

To understand why this was happening, HFE researchers examined everyday practice in the airline setting, looking at the movement of people and vehicles and aircraft, and how movement was encouraged by clearly defined floor markings. They experimented by clearly marking the floor in the operating theatre: a line was placed where the air curtain was. By implementing that simple change, surgical placements in the theatre were improved from 10 per cent to 60 per cent; a significant improvement but still not perfect. The reason why there wasn't a 100 per cent improvement was found in HFE. The area outlined by the floor markings, and covered by the air curtain, simply was not big enough. The canopies themselves were designed thirty years ago, when there was arguably half as much equipment as there is today.

The laminar flow theatre provides a good example of the ways HFE needs to take account of human factors in developing IPC policies. Another research project was based on the redesign of a patient's surgical pathway through the hospital system. The researchers followed a patient's journey and made recommendations based on HFE principles, from admission to pre-op, operative, post-op, recovery, ICU and discharge. They used their findings to create a workable checklist of elements that the staff need to check off by following the patient's progress. This is called the Surgical Patient Safety System (SURPASS).[15]

There have been some interesting results on implementation of SURPASS at intervention and control hospitals, with the outcome measure being post-operative complications. In the intervention hospitals, the range of post-operative complications was lower, thus increasing patient safety. For infection complications, a category called 'Infection as a Whole' was used, which is unfortunately not very specific; buried in that category is surgical site infection. Overall results showed a statistically significant reduction in infection found in the intervention hospitals, compared to the control hospitals, which improved post-surgical outcomes.

Key HFE work has also been published in *Infection Control & Hospital Epidemiology* that focuses on design. Experts undertook simulations with a range of staff and departments, dealing with how to put on and remove protective clothing: gloves, aprons and masks used in high-risk infections like Ebola, and some viral respiratory infections, including Severe Acute Respiratory Syndrome (SARS).[16] Their analysis included human factors analysis of the personal protective equipment (PPE); looking at the equipment itself, how it works as a system and how it is used. This identified several weaknesses in the design of PPE that could be rectified by HFE experts, including a lack of clarity about whether a garment was the right way out; making this more apparent – by changing the colours of the PPE so that insides were blue and outsides green, for instance – would eliminate any confusion. Additionally, the PPE used wasn't designed well as a system: the gloves didn't fit the gowns; the zips were badly designed so that self-contamination was made possible through wrestling to unfasten the clothing; the excessive stretchiness of plastic aprons could cause splashing; and so on. These flaws could have been avoided if HFE experts were consulted prior to the manufacturing process, so there are clearly significant economic and practical benefits to be had from bringing this expertise into healthcare. We might consider, then, whether in this era of co-production with clients and patients and the consumerist nature of healthcare, IPC policies should be integrated with the wider patient safety agenda. The contrary argument, however, is the risk that IPC could be subsumed into the patient safety agenda and lose its identity, eventually leading to a diminution of the specialty and its related benefits.

Notes

With thanks to John Otter, Julie Storr and Claire Kilpatrick.

1 For further information on the data used in this chapter, see the Reflections on Infection Prevention and Control blog, https://reflectionsipc.com/ (accessed 11 May 2020) and Public Health England, www.gov.uk/government/organisations/public-health-england/about/statistics (accessed 11 May 2020).

2 See, for instance, S. Borland, 'Rise of superbug that is almost untreatable as 2,000 cases of infection are now recorded a year', *Daily Mail*, 22 Apr 2017, www.dailymail.co.uk/news/article-4434346/Rise-superbug-untreatable.html; and L. Rogers, '10 million lives could be lost to superbugs – so how far have we got in the race to beat them?', *Telegraph*, 2 Apr 2018, www.telegraph.co.uk/health-fitness/body/10-million-lives-could-lost-superbugs-far-have-got-race-beat/ (accessed 23 May 2017).

3 www.health.org.uk/about-francis-inquiry (accessed 23 May 2017).

4 www.stokesentinel.co.uk/legionnaires-outbreak-28-patients-died-disease/story-16590072-detail/story.html (accessed 23 May 2017).

5 F. Walsh, 'Antibiotics resistance "as big a risk as terrorism" – medical chief', BBC News, www.bbc.com/news/health-21737844, 11 Mar 2013.

6 For further information, see www.gov.uk/government/organisations/
   public-health-england/about/statistics (accessed 11 May 2020).

7 M. Monaco, T. Giani, M. Raffone *et al.*, 'Colistin resistance super-
   imposed to endemic carbapenem-resistant Klebsiella pneumoniae:
   a rapidly evolving problem in Italy, November 2013 to April 2014',
   Eurosurveillance, 42 (2014), www.eurosurveillance.org/ViewArticle.
   aspx?ArticleId=20939 (accessed 23 May 2017).

8 R. Amalberti, Y. Auroy, D. Berwick and P. Barach, 'Five system barriers
   to achieving ultrasafe health care', *Annals of Internal Medicine*, 142
   (2005), 756–764.

9 www.ncbi.nlm.nih.gov/books/NBK43708 (accessed 23 May 2017).

10 A. J. Hessels, V. Genovese-Schek, M. Agarwal *et al.*, 'Relationship
   between patient safety climate and adherence to standard precautions',
   American Journal of Infection Control, 44 (2016), 1128–1132.

11 M. Power, N. Wigglesworth, E. Donaldson *et al.*, 'Reducing Clostridium
   difficile infection in acute care by using an improvement collaborative',
   British Medical Journal, 341 (2010), c.3359.

12 J. Storr, N. Wigglesworth and C. Kilpatrick, 'Integrating human factors
   with infection prevention and control' (London: Health Foundation,
   2013).

13 A. Xie and P. Carayon, 'A systematic review of human factors and ergonomics (HFE)-based healthcare system redesign for quality of care and
   patient safety', *Ergonomics*, 58 (2015), 33–49.

14 *Ibid.*; D. F. de Korne, J. D. H. van Wijngaarden, J. van Rooij *et al.*, 'Safety
   by design: Effects of operating room floor marking on the position of
   surgical devices to promote clean air flow compliance and minimise
   infection risks', *British Medical Journal Quality & Safety*, 18 Aug 2011.
   doi: 10.1136/bmjqs-2011-000138.

15 E. N. de Vries, M. W. Hollmann, S. M. Smorenburg *et al.*, 'Development
   and validation of the SURgical PAtient Safety System (SURPASS) checklist', *British Medical Journal Quality & Safety*, 18 (2009), 121–126.

16 T. A. Herlihey, S. Gelmi, C. J. Flewwelling *et al.*, 'Personal protective equipment for infectious disease preparedness: A human factors
   evaluation', *Infection Control & Hospital Epidemiology*, 37 (2016),
   1022–1028.

11

Infection control and antimicrobial resistance: the past, the present and the future

Alistair Leanord

This chapter explores, from a senior participant observer perspective, the emergence of recent policy in infection control in Scotland, and the ways in which this differs in England. With specific reference to methicillin-resistant *Staphylococcus aureus* (MRSA) and *Escherichia coli* (*E. coli*), it considers the reasons why policy and implementation can lag behind knowledge about infection control. It begins with an account from Scotland in 2002 which traces the following fifteen years during which infection control became a priority area for government policy. It also considers the ways in which migration and localism have become key concepts in policy development. Finally, this chapter ends with some reflections on the future of infection control, based on experience, evidence and developing technologies.

Background

The emergence of a national system of control is often reactive; a 'call to arms' that provides the first stage of a policy cycle. In this context, the inciting event was a significant salmonella outbreak in a Scottish hospital.[1] In response to this specific outbreak, the Scottish government commissioned a report that produced a series of recommendations.[2] The Scottish government subsequently established a Healthcare associated infection (HAI) taskforce, to develop a range of initiatives within Scottish healthcare to reduce the risk of HAIs. That taskforce developed codes of practice and identified roles and responsibilities to deal with and prevent future infection outbreaks. There were various complex politico-economic questions to work around, including debates around contracting out domestic services. Surveillance systems were developed, as well as targets that still exist today, as part of a long, complex process to deal with hospital-based infections.

It took us five years to enact the recommendations of the task force, evidence from which was used in the development of the Point Prevalence Survey (PPS); point prevalence referring to the proportion of a population that has a condition at a specific point in time. Scotland has used a PPS to look at levels of HAIs and anti-microbial use since 2005/2006. This methodology has been used to assess every hospital for HAIs at five-year intervals. The latest PPS in Scotland in 2016 was reported in 2017. This European-based initiative has been in use since the 2000s and was used in Scottish hospitals to provide a gap analysis of the systems used to control HAIs. One of the most significant recommendations was around standardisation. The Scottish healthcare system started the 'hand hygiene' campaign and participated in the PPS, using the results of the gap analysis to develop a further set of initiatives around infection control.

After a decade of policy work that had taken place from 2002 to 2012, the Scottish healthcare system ended up with a portfolio of around forty projects. My personal reflection of that time is that Scotland entered a period of *stasis*, where there were so many different projects on the go that it was difficult to identify the key elements fundamental to the promotion of infection control. There was certainly a sense, from politicians and civil servants, that the *more* that was being done the better; one could argue that the desire to show more and more activities took away, in some respects, from the core effort of controlling infections. I have observed this trend happen more recently, with the UK Antimicrobial Resistance (AMR) strategy (2013–2018).[3] This is a relatively young strategy development, and within the first two years, no fewer than 117 initiatives were identified. As a result, the central plank of the AMR policy was being diminished; some of the initiatives were highly significant and others less so. The recommendation of the High Level Steering Group, which has the strategic overview of the programme, was to highlight the most important work. In Scotland, this included the 'Cleanliness Champions' programme, which has subsequently been embedded into undergraduate nursing and undergraduate medical courses. There is also a national HAI compendium, which means there is one single infection control manual for Scotland that is freely available on the Internet. This is a remarkable shift from when I worked as an infection control doctor in the 1990s: my colleagues and I used to borrow other people's manuals, replacing one Health Boards name for another. Now there is a single centrally controlled and regularly updated manual for use by all hospitals.

The creation of a single, web-based manual is one of the areas where Scotland differs from England; south of the border, separate manuals still predominate.[4] Another significant development in Scotland has been the strengthening of infection control precautions in a large-scale awareness-raising campaign which has produced significant effects. There has been a consequential reduction in antimicrobials being prescribed in primary care. General practitioners (GPs) have been quick to take the message on board. As an anecdotal aside, I started as a GP in the early 1990s, and I used prescriptions of antimicrobials to reduce anxiety in mothers of toddlers even if there was no objective evidence of infection. I generally prescribed amoxicillin for the children, and the only real discussion was whether they preferred the banana or strawberry flavour. Adults were offered tetracycline, because there was no resistance to it in those days and it was underused. This is not considered best practice nowadays! So clearly there has been a sea change in the use of certain classes of antibiotics, and that can be linked to an adhered-to national prescribing policy. *C. diff* and MRSA rates have been reduced in Scotland in much the same way as they have in England.

Developing proactive infection control policies

Today, the drive-in policy is to be proactive rather than reactive in dealing with infection control. As noted already, by 2012 my colleagues and I found ourselves with forty or so projects that were not all being delivered on. Having learned from that process, we have become more strategic about policy development and identifying the factors that make a difference. The current five-year strategy, that will take Scotland to 2021, benefits from the latest PPS published in 2017, and it will implement the gap analysis that has previously been shown to be successful in highlighting areas of the healthcare system on which to focus. We have started some long-term pieces of research that will evaluate how effective the measures and interventions taken as part of the overall national strategy have been. I can share some data from the Scottish PPS, 2005/2006–2017, and wish to bring out some key points. First, gastrointestinal infection (GI) reduced between 2005 and 2017, and that is almost certainly a result of the effort put into controlling *C. diff* infection and, to a lesser extent, norovirus infections.

However, urinary tract infections (UTIs) increased over the same period. That increase is echoed in the increasing prevalence of *E. coli*, another organism which has become more commonplace. There have been significant differences in the predominant organisms that cause HAIs over the period studied. It will also be important to consider emergent threats from the next PPS. In this volume, Neil Wigglesworth indicates what some of these might be: *S. aureus*, for instance, which is a very common organism. And while we have seen reductions in MRSA, the same cannot be said about *S. aureus* that are not MRSA. At present, we are unsure why we have seen reductions in MRSA while the numbers of MSSA (methicillin-sensitive *S. aureus*) have stayed static over a ten-year period.

Although I am focusing on Scotland in this chapter, the data here refers to all four countries in the UK, and therefore the shifts that I am discussing are relevant across the board. To refer to Table 11.1, there has been a reduction in GI and *C. diff* across the UK. This reflects the fact that there has been a systematic and joined-up approach to infectious disease control across the nation. This development was effected by several interconnecting policies, agendas and guidelines that were enforced through political will, substantial investment, target setting, surveillance, guidelines, campaigns and legislation. This evidence shows that governments must *enact* change. It is not sufficient to advise or to provide guidelines; they need to implement obligatory standards and public health legislation. They also need to provide sufficient financial support, which can be challenging during a global economic crisis. In an ideal world, governments would provide financial support for countries to build teams and implements structures, irrespective of how challenging this may be financially.

Table 11.1   Distribution of HAI types in acute adult inpatients (including independent hospital inpatients) in 2005, 2011 and 2016

Distribution of HAI types 2005–2016 (percentage)

	2005	*2011*	*2016*
Urinary tract infection	19.7	23.1	24.5
Pneumonia	8.8	17.6	22.4
Surgical site infection	15.9	19.2	16.5
Laboratory confirmed BSI	4.4	9.7	8.7
Skin and soft tissue infection	11	4.1	7.2
Eye, ear, nose or throat and mouth infection	12.5	9.0	5.5
Gastrointestinal tract infection	15.4	6.8	5.1
Systemic infection	0.2	3.4	3.2
Central/peripheral venous catheter	N/A	2.5	3
Bone/joint infection	0.5	0.5	0.8
Cardiovascular system	0.9	0.2	0.8
Central nervous system infection	0.2	0.7	0.4
Reproductive tract infection	1.4	0.5	0.4

Sources: Health Protection Scotland, *Scottish national point prevalence survey of healthcare associated infection and antimicrobial prescribing 2016* (Health Protection Scotland, 2017 [Report]); Health Protection Scotland *Scottish national point prevalence survey of healthcare associated infection and antimicrobial prescribing 2011* (Health Protection Scotland, 2012 [Report]); J. Reilly *et al.*, 'Results from the Scottish National HAI Prevalence Survey', *Journal of Hospital Infection*, 69 (2008), 62–69

In the early twenty-first century, all areas of the health service, including government departments, are operating in a very tight financial environment which in many cases means doing more with less. Crucially, there are significant differences in the levers that can be used to effect change between Scotland and England. The government in England used fiscal means to encourage attainment of targets. In Scotland, by contrast, we did not have a monetary response to attaining targets, using instead monitoring undertaken by professional groups, and the emphasis was on the carrot, rather than the stick. Although both countries used different approaches, each saw significant reductions in the incidence of *C. diff*. The attainment of the desired outcome was still central to how each country tackled the issue of *C. diff* reductions; each, however, put in place a mechanism for achievement that both knew worked.

The implementation of targets

Targets have been immensely helpful in combating infection. NHS Scotland and the Scottish government's Health Directorates have issued four groups of targets, collectively known as HEAT targets: Health Improvement; Efficiency; Access to Treatment; and Treatment. These guidelines were developed by groups of experts who determined through discussion what is doable. An 'achievable target' ideal is then passed on to civil servants. The current target is to achieve a reduction of the rate of *C. diff* infection (CDI) cases in patients aged fifteen and over to 0.32 cases or less per 1,000 total occupied bed days.

What is difficult and uncertain about the process of target setting is that there is no certainty what definitively works in infection control. There is a thin evidence base on much of what is carried out, and across the UK we are not achieving the target in *S. aureus* control. That does not mean there is no reduction in infection; in fact, there has been a significant reduction. However, the reduction in overall *S. aureus* bacteraemais has been due almost exclusively to a reduction of MRSA and not MSSA, and hence we will not meet the overall target. What is important to note, moreover, in relation to Scotland, is that these targets will change. The Scottish government is moving towards new measures that involve standards, as opposed to targets. This is an important political distinction: a target is something you hit; a standard is something you maintain.

By contrast to the relative lack of progress in reducing all *S. aureus* infections, we have seen a significant shift in the occurrence of MRSA. Indeed, there has been an almost 90 per cent reduction in MRSA since 2005, when its magnitude was first realised. This is a clear result of a multi-modal intervention, bringing together codes of practice, Cleanliness Champions, performance management, hand hygiene and MRSA guidelines. Crucially, it is not possible to identify one single act by which that 90 per cent reduction was made possible; that is not how infection control works. This is partly because not every single intervention is evidence-based, and partly because there is never 100 per cent compliance.

There is always slippage in the system, not least because of human error. And when reflecting on the success of infection control over a ten-year period, it is just not possible to identify those *specific* interventions that created change. A similar argument can be made about infection control within wards that have an outbreak, only that experience is condensed into a few days or weeks rather than years: once there is an outbreak, every possible response is mobilised, from screening to surveillance, from cleaning to changing prescriptions. When the outbreak passes, there might be great relief, but no certainty about what worked.

To elaborate on this point, I want to turn to some evidence from 2003. Figure 11.1 shows a local strain of MRSA in Glasgow, when I was a trainee. At the early stages of the MRSA outbreak, cases were rare enough to be reported in the medical literature as case series, something that myself and many trainees did at the time. After a few years, MRSAs were everywhere and no longer worthy of individual reports in the medical literature! What I want to show from this graph, however, is the context of what happened. If we look at the decline of MRSA, we can see that this is part of an epidemic curve of twenty-five years. Within that time, we have worked hard to eradicate MRSA for at least a decade. There is also the question of policy lag – the amount of time it takes for policy to be developed and implemented once a problem has been recognised.

The reality is that for a long period of time, probably from 1991 to 2003, nothing effective was in place in Scottish hospitals. It was only from 2003, as I have said earlier, that we started measuring

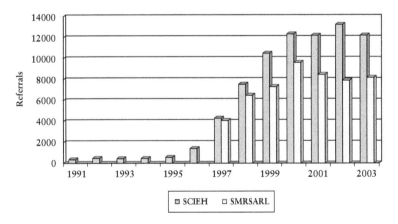

Figure 11.1   MRSA in Scotland. SMRSARL=Scottish MRSA Reference Laboratory; SCIEH=Scottish Centre for Infection and Environmental Health. Since 2005 SCIEH has been Health Protection Scotland (HPS).

rates of MRSA, and only two years later that we began to do anything effective to combat it. Once MRSA became a political priority,
then effective investment and resources went into tackling it as a
national priority area.

Inspections and standards

I would like to turn now to the current landscape of standards,
and the state of reactive policy around inspections. Inspections are
a means of assessing and enforcing good behaviour, but I do not
believe that they are effective.[5] The value of inspections is prin-
cipally to show that governments are taking infections seriously.
In Scotland, the Healthcare Environment Inspectorate (HEI) is an
independent body that reports publicly. It was established by the
government in 2009 as a response to the Vale of Leven *C. diff* outbreak that took place a year earlier. It was important politically for
the government to be seen to act, and the HEI implemented wide-
ranging inspection measures that included leadership, education,
communication, surveillance, antimicrobial prescribing, infection
control policies, maintenance of invasive devices, decontamination and equipment acquisition. Inspections are not announced in
advance, and the inspectors undertake around twenty-four inspections around the country in any one year.

What we find when we consider the feedback on these inspections, including the most recently reviewed outbreaks in Stoke
Mandeville, Maidstone, Tunbridge Wells, Northern Ireland and the
Vale of Leven, is a similar cluster of causal circumstances. These
include a lack of organisational governance, lack of awareness in
terms of what individuals should be doing about infection control, poor uptake and lack of compliance around infection control
procedures, and inadequate facilities that include poor building
stock. Sometimes surveillance systems are inadequate or not timely
enough, or communication is lacking between organisations. I
have had an experience, in one of the Scottish hospitals in 2014,
when inspectors turned up unannounced and went directly to the
Accident and Emergency unit. There they found basic standards of
hygiene lacking, such as blood spots not cleaned on the underside of
trolleys. These human errors in the system of infection control are

difficult to prevent, and create a significant and disproportionate amount of paperwork.

The future of infection control: localisation and migration

What does the future look like, for infection control in the current landscape? In my view, it can be encapsulated in two themes: localisation and migration. Firstly, localisation: there has been a move away from central government and downward control, towards local delivery planning and local quality improvement programmes. England is ahead of Scotland with the Public Health Profiles (PHP) Fingertips system of presenting local data, which is an open and transparent system. This local emphasis is extremely important in being able to address the pertinent issues on the ground within a particular region or hospital.

There has been a significant reduction in hospital *C. diff*, and a slight reduction in community *C. diff*, changing the proportion of community cases as part of the whole (see Figure 11.2).

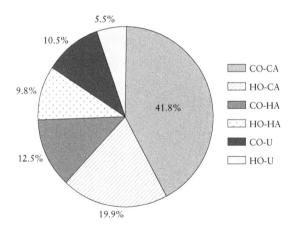

Figure 11.2   Relative frequency (%) of patients within each of the epidemiological categories (n=256). CO-CA=community-onset, community-associated; HO-CA=hospital-onset, community-associated; CO-HA=community-onset, hospital-associated; HO-HA=hospital-onset, hospital-associated; CO-U=community-onset, unknown; HO-U=hospital-onset, unknown.

Approximately 30 per cent of C. *diff* cases in the UK and Scotland are now coming out of the community. Moreover, there is usually no association with healthcare in these cases, and no association with recent antibiotic use, which we know to be one of the triggers. It has generally been assumed that these community C. *diff* infections are mild, but we now know that the risk of mortality associated with community C. *diff* infections is higher than cases associated with healthcare, even if the absolute numbers are lower. Moreover, outbreaks that used to be seasonal, for instance norovirus, also known as winter vomiting disease, happen all the time now, closing wards and putting pressure on hospital beds all year round.

In the Scottish system, we are still encountering a significant number of HAI outbreaks – around a hundred per year – most of which are gastrointestinal, though a significant proportion are respiratory (see Figure 11.3). Of these cases, the gastrointestinal incidents will almost certainly be norovirus outbreaks, and the respiratory cases are likely to be viral. Respiratory Syncytial Virus (RSV) is a significant problem, especially in children, and there are still influenza cases routinely causing outbreaks. Biologically, we won't see an end to these kinds of outbreaks – largely because hospitals collect people in a close environment, and some degree of contagion is inevitable.

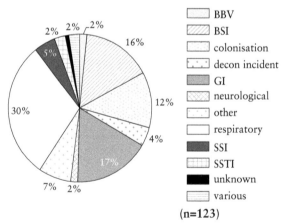

(n=123)

Legend BBV = blood borne virus; BSI = blood stream infection;
decon incident = decontamination incident; GI = gastrointestinal outbreak.

Figure 11.3 Types of HAI outbreak and incident 2016–2017.

However efficient we are about keeping infection numbers down, we will always have outbreaks. All we can do in these terms is to stay on top of the epidemic curve and to act quickly.

However, new and emerging HAIs are more challenging. *E. coli* is a significant problem, as discussed already. It is in this organism that we see a relatively high proportion of resistance, especially in carbapenemase-producing bacteria. There is, moreover, a difference between Scotland and England in the number of these very resistant carbapenemase-producing bacteria, with thousands of cases in England and only just over 100 cases reported in Scotland. In my view, this reflects the early curve of the MRSA graph, where there were a smattering of cases and then an exponential rise over a twenty-five-year-period. Given that it took UK healthcare a generation to get on top of MRSA once we had a clear strategic focus, we need to make sure we are as proactive in the early stages of controlling resistant *E. coli*. We are now using guidelines that were produced in 2013, and we are on top of implementing policy in Scotland and in the UK as a whole.

Policy and implementation must go hand in hand; the unpredictability and speed of infection means that it is as important to implement a policy quickly as it is to develop the policy itself. An implementation lag can happen because policy is difficult to implement, or because it's not being supported financially, or even because there is patient resistance. MRSA screening was simple: it involved a discreet nose swab. *E. coli* screening, by contrast, requires a rectal swab, and the insertion of that swab into the rectum. Swabs must have visible faecal material present. Understandably, some patients are reluctant to undergo this screening test. If we find a resistant *E. coli* in a patient, there is presently no effective means to de-colonise the patient. So, even something as simple as screening highlights multiple ethical, social and behavioural issues that need to be considered, sometimes in a short time frame.

Historically, moreover, patients stayed in hospital wards for longer than they do today; I remember at the start of my career (thirty years ago) seeing the same patients in a ward for a week or more. Today, patients are kept in for no more than two and a half days. What we are seeing is the second part of my prediction for future infection control: migration – the migration of healthcare, and the migration of our problems into the community. The situation will be different across the UK. In Scotland, we are undergoing a redesign of healthcare where there is an integration of healthcare and social care into the same healthcare body, a unified health board. With the council and the health board being united, the goal is for a seamless patient pathway from acute hospital into residential care and then into social care. There may be delivery problems in the future, but that is the model in principle.

I would like to conclude by considering the future of infection prevention. If we look at the Study on the Efficacy of Nosocomial Infection Control (SENIC) project, it suggests that 30 per cent of HAIs were preventable with an infection control team.[6] So, how much infection is preventable now? We undertook a piece of work into this question in Scotland, looking at a range of bloodstream infections (BSIs), catheter-related BSIs, skin and soft tissue infections, UTI and pneumonias, and ventilatory-associated pneumonias. We concluded that up to 50 per cent of HAIs *are* preventable if all the standards and provisions discussed in this chapter are put in place. It is important to know that this is an achievable target.

The past teaches us that assumptions we have regarding the causation of infection control incidents will change as new evidence of transmission events, treatments and emerging pathogens comes to light. The broad body of already embedded infection control practice, although in many cases not heavily evidence-based, has stood the test of time and is still fit for purpose in the practice of modern healthcare. What will change will be the evolution of practice, still based on the basic principles of infection control, but with a firmer scientific foundation that will allow us to finesse our interventions.

There is still a long way to go in developing policy and implementation around HAIs, and new technologies have a role to play. These include whole genome sequencing, on which a Scottish research team are collaborating with the Sanger Institute in Cambridge. My colleagues and I used to manually create dendograms to show the clustering of associations between infectious organisms; today, there exists whole genome sequencing that can be linked to clinical outcomes to make inferences and produce hypotheses. We are now able to look at the genetic structure of organisms such as *E. coli*, see how they are related to each other and which genetic groups they fall into, as well as detecting whether one strain might be linked to a certain disease or medical interventions such as catheterisation.

This will be the start of personalised medicine for infections. To date we have seen personalised medicine being developed in genetics and cardiac medicine as well as in mental health, and I believe that it has a role to play in infection control. Because of (near) real-time sequencing and data linkages, we can undertake targeted infection control and management. We can identify which *E. coli* are particularly aggressive and those which might be easier to control. This development will allow us to use different management algorithms when necessary. So, there are exciting times ahead in the field of infection control, though we can't take any gains for granted. As the Danish expression says, 'it's tough to make predictions, especially about the future'.

Notes

1 Watt Group Report, *A review of the outbreak of salmonella at the Victoria Infirmary* (2002), www.webarchive.org.uk/wayback/archive/20180517133344/http://www.gov.scot/Publications/2002/10/15658/12294 (accessed 18 January 2021).

2 From the Preface of the Watt Group Report: 'the outbreak of Salmonella infection in the Victoria Infirmary was a tragic episode for the patients who died and their relatives. It also had an impact on the Hospital and its staff. It is, therefore, particularly important to ensure that appropriate lessons are learned for the future both in the Hospital itself and in the wider NHS.'

3 www.gov.uk/government/uploads/system/uploads/attachment_data/file/244058/20130902_UK_5_year_AMR_strategy.pdf (accessed 18 January 2021).

4 *National Infection Prevention and Control Manual*, www.nipcm.hps.scot.nhs.uk (accessed 18 January 2021).

5 *Healthcare Improvement Scotland: inspecting and regulating care, NHS Hospitals and Services*, www.healthcareimprovementscotland.org/our_work/inspecting_and_regulating_care/nhs_hospitals_and_services/find_nhs_hospitals.aspx (accessed 18 January 2021).

6 R. W. Haley, D. Quade, H. E. Freeman and J. V. Bennett, 'Study on the efficacy of nosocomial infection control (SENIC) project: Summary of study design', *American Journal of Epidemiology*, 111 (1980), 472–448.

Conclusion: using the past

Marguerite Dupree, Anne Marie Rafferty
and Fay Bound Alberti

Like Virginia Berridge in her influential writings on history and health policy, which bring together historians and policymakers,[1] the contributors to this volume demonstrate how history can enrich our understanding of current issues of hospital infection control, including antimicrobial resistance (AMR), and inform perspectives on the future. As Berridge points out, 'history is a discipline which … can add dimensions which others cannot. It can give an overview of the complexity of policy issues and their change over time; other social science disciplines tend to label and categorise, to neaten things up, or to deal with small sections of an issue.'[2] History can show us the importance of understanding particular sets of circumstances; the interest groups, which help form policy and practical responses; the need to look behind stereotypes; and, why particular groups take particular stances. It can remind us that responses are time-dependent and can change; changing constellations of interests can achieve change in policy; and different national histories and contexts still mean much.[3] Thus, this volume concludes with both an overview of how the contributors utilise history, and discussions of key themes arising from the chapters: change and continuity, or the mixture of the old and new in practice and policy; the roles of bacteriologists; nurses and nursing; blame and responsibility; economics; and the hospital and community.

Uses of history

Contributors emphasise the use of history to provide a framework for coping with complexity. Flurin Condrau, for example, using the neonatal and Asian Flu Pandemic examples from the 1950s and 1960s, shows how a historical approach can successfully intertwine political, institutional, professional histories, and 'draw together seemingly unrelated fields of inquiry to shed light on complex interactions between the communities and hospitals involved in problems of Staphylococcal infection'.[4]

Another feature of history, as Pamela Wood argues, is the long view, which teaches an understanding of the context in which healthcare practices take shape and 'creates an awareness that knowledge continues to change', though alongside continuities. Historical analysis allows us to 'distinguish between issues that are enduring and those that are transient', offering new perspectives regarding preventing and managing wound infection. She points, for example, to warnings in 1904 about over-reliance on antiseptics and concerns in 1921 that the wearing of rubber gloves could make nurses careless about handwashing. Similarly, Jennie Wilson demonstrates the unintended consequences of the more recent widespread use of non-sterile gloves among healthcare workers to protect themselves as much as the patients.[5] As Wood suggests, the long view of a historical approach reveals that 'over-reliance on any method obscures other measures to prevent or control infection' and can lead to unintended consequences.[6]

Similarly, the importance of investigating alternative approaches and their rationales in the past emerges clearly from the volume. Thomas Schlich, for example, points to the 'misuse of history' in the history of surgery, which has been 'shaped by underlying teleological principles which take the present state of things as the quasi-natural outcome of history', and makes the 'fluidity and contingency of technical change invisible', sanitising and streamlining 'the diversity of new and old surgical technologies and the technical creativity that went into these technologies'. He challenges the histories produced by the victors. He stresses the importance of questioning the belief in the superiority of the new, of avoiding anachronistic explanations such as resistance, inertia and blindness, and of recognising complexities. Schlich argues it is essential to try to understand the rationales that were motivating contemporaries, such as Halstead. Such a broader historical 'perspective makes it possible to appreciate ... the diversity of technologies today ... to take notice of alternative forms of understanding and solving problems and ... to beware ... of "overblown claims of a one best way" of dealing with technical, surgical and medical challenges'.[7]

Change and continuity

With a historical perspective highlighting changing and enduring issues, it is not surprising to find current concerns emerging in earlier contexts in the chapters. A striking example is Susan Gardiner's account of J. H. Bowie's development of sensitivity testing. Initially, in the mid-1940s, testing of the sensitivity or susceptibility of bacteria to penicillin and determination of dosage took place during the administration of penicillin: if the infection was not sensitive, penicillin treatment ceased. With the introduction of other antibiotics in the later 1940s, Bowie developed the Edinburgh paper disk method and standardised measures, producing results within twenty-four hours to inform antibiotic choice and dosage *before* administration. Sounding remarkably similar is one of the ambitions in the UK's new twenty-year vision for antimicrobial resistance, that is 'ensuring all decisions to use antimicrobials are informed by a diagnostic test, clinical decision support tool or relevant data and where antimicrobial treatment is indicated, prescribe and administer the right agent promptly to reduce harm from sepsis'.[8]

The difficulties of implementing and maintaining changes in practice is a recurrent theme, particularly in the chapters focusing on the last fifty years. As Susan Macqueen remarks, 'looking back on my experiences, and the changes that have occurred in infection prevention and control, one thing is clear: it takes a long time to change practice' and maintain standards, thus the need for audits and monitoring.[9] Alistair Leanord echoed the sentiment, when he pointed to the 'question of policy lag', that is the amount of time it takes for policy to be developed and implemented once a problem has been recognised. He sees the dramatic decline of methicillin-resistant *Staphylococcus aureus* (MRSA) by 90 per cent in the ten years from 2005 as part of an epidemic curve of twenty-five years from *c.* 1990: 'from 1991 to 2003 nothing effective was in place in Scottish hospitals; only from 2003 when the rates of MRSA started to be measured and from 2005 did we start to do anything effective'.[10]

Macqueen, Leanord and Neil Wigglesworth all emphasise the immense importance of 'political will' and effective financial investment and resources in bringing about the changes in infection prevention and control (IPC) that has led to the dramatic decline in MRSA and *C. diff* since 2003. According to Macqueen, 'where there is a political will there is a way'; Alistair Leanord observed that 'once MRSA became a political priority then effective investment and resources went into tackling it as a national priority area'; and, Wigglesworth argued that 'reduction in reported MRSA cases reflects a whole raft of governmental interventions that were brought in in the wake of the 1990s outbreaks'.[11]

A pattern of policy formation and change in practice emerges in England and Scotland in the recent past, featuring local outbreaks, media attention, high-profile investigations and inspections, multiple forms of new guidelines and legislation, which 'produced a sea change in the roles and responsibilities of IPC specialists' and new prominence for IPC in hospital governance.[11] Local outbreaks begin the process, for example an outbreak of Salmonella at Great Ormond Street Hospital (GOSH) in 1980 led directly to Susan Macqueen's appointment as the hospital's first infection control nurse (ICN). The local outbreaks often attracted immediate and dramatic media attention highlighting individual cases, which led to government enquiries, recommendations and new guidelines for surveillance, for example the Stanley Royd Hospital food poisoning outbreak (where metal-topped kitchen tables were found to be wiped off with same mop head used to clean floors) and the Stafford District Hospital outbreak of Legionnaires' Disease in the 1980s, or MRSA and *C. diff* outbreaks in the 1990s.[12]

Reports, guidelines and legislation in England were crucial, as was sufficient funding.[13] Highlighting again the importance of government intervention, Macqueen pointed to the 2003 Department of Health report and initiative, *Winning Ways*, which ensured IPC was in the clinical governance structure by introducing a Director of Infection Prevention and Control (DIPC) designated in each organisation, who had corporate responsibility for the IPC strategy and team, reporting directly to the chief executive and board with authority to challenge clinical hygiene practice and antibiotic prescribing decisions and to ensure that additional resources, both personnel and financial, were provided in outbreaks.[14]

Macqueen also shows that guidelines incorporated the results of research, particularly the SENIC studies from the 1980s, which demonstrated the clinical and cost effectiveness of IPC and the Keystone study findings of the effectiveness of evidence-based 'bundles of care'. She points especially to the 2005 Department of Health initiative 'Saving Lives: reducing infection, delivering clean and safe care', which facilitated the 'bundles of care' or high-impact intervention (HII) approach, helping trusts achieve IPC targets by focusing on evidence-based elements of the care process and a method for measuring the implementation of policies and procedures. While she suggests that staff tended to welcome guidelines for cutting through complexities, one of the first bundles was central venous catheter care, and she reveals it took two to three years to educate and remind medical staff to chart whether a catheter line infection was hospital-acquired or not, in order to measure the effectiveness of the care bundles, before recording the information was embedded.[15]

Policies required legislation for enforcement and funding. As Alistair Leanord argues forcefully, 'governments must *enact* change .... It is not sufficient to advise or to provide guidelines; they need to implement obligatory standards and public health legislation.' In England, the Health Act of 2006 introduced the Code of Practice for the prevention and control of infections, and the Health and Social Care Act of 2008 gave power to IPC, using financial penalties to force managers and clinicians to comply and thus maintain a high profile for IPC. Wigglesworth emphasises the importance of this legislation for the dramatic reduction in MRSA, arguing that because chief executive jobs were on the line, IPC became an important issue for organisations. 'For the first time in history', he writes, 'significant resources were found to tackle the problem and there was an expansion of the teams equipped to undertake the work'.[16]

In Scotland, like the rest of the UK, Leanord argues that the reduction in MRSA and *C. diff* reflected a 'systematic and joined-up approach to infectious disease control across the nation', effected by 'several interconnecting policies, agendas and guidelines that were enforced through political will, substantial investment, target setting, surveillance, guidelines, campaigns and legislation'. At the same time, he highlights the differences in the levers used to effect change, between England and the less populous Scotland. Whereas in England, because of the size of population, government used fiscal means to encourage the attainment of hospital-acquired infection (HAI) targets, in Scotland the Scottish government used monitoring undertaken by professional groups. Groups of experts developed four sets of achievable targets, passed the targets on to civil servants, and the government and the National Health Service (NHS) in Scotland issued them as Health Directives with funding, provided 'the emphasis was on the carrot, rather than the stick'.[17] Although both countries used different approaches, each saw significant 90 per cent reductions in the incidence of MRSA and *C. diff* since 2005.

In both countries, the reduction was the result of a 'multi-modal' intervention, bringing together, for example, codes of practice, Cleanliness Champions, performance management, hand hygiene and MRSA guidelines. Both Wigglesworth and Leanord point out that it is not possible to identify one single measure which made the reduction possible, because 'not every single intervention is evidence-based and because there is never 100 per cent compliance. There is always slippage in the system because of human error. It is 'just not possible to identify those specific interventions that created change'.[18] Like IPC in the country as a whole, Leanord suggests IPC within wards that have an outbreak follows a similar pattern – with 'experience condensed into a few days or weeks rather than years: once there is an outbreak, every possible response is mobilised, from screening to surveillance, from cleaning to changing prescriptions. When the outbreak passes there is relief, but no certainty about what worked.'[19]

Unlike the mid-twentieth century when Condrau reminded us of those who believed infection could be eradicated, there now appears to be a consensus that sepsis and other outbreaks will happen and recur. 'Biologically we won't see an end to these kinds of outbreaks – largely because hospitals collect people in a close environment and some degree of contagion is inevitable. However efficient we are about keeping infection numbers down, we will always have outbreaks.'[20] It is now a matter of identifying the outbreak of sepsis in the individual or department or institution as quickly as possible, being as proactive as possible and implementing policies quickly. As Leanord writes, 'we know what to do'. And, as he reminds us, it is not only implementing changes to meet targets, but maintaining practices to change targets into standards.[21] To accomplish such a change, Wigglesworth and Wilson point in the future away from a focus on individual behaviour, to structuring the environment to shape behaviour, using human factors and ergonomics, while Alistair Leanord points toward a future of utilising the techniques of molecular biology to specify the genetics of the organisms infecting individuals to better target treatment and create personalised medicine.

Despite the emphasis on change with government interventions and the transformation in the roles and responsibilities of IPC specialists in accounts of the rapid reduction of MRSA and C. *diff* in the UK, there is a consensus that no single measure stands out, instead a range of measures are required, many of which, for example screening, surveillance, guidelines, strict hygiene practices, inspection, would be familiar in hospitals since the late nineteenth century. It is continuity, as well as change, and the mix of the old and new that create impact.

Bacteriologists

The role of hospital pathologists and bacteriologists in the emerging field of IPC is one of the pre-existing issues within the historiography to which several chapters in this volume contribute new perspectives. There has been a consensus that, before resistance rose to prominence in the 1950s, bacteriologists, although they played a role in diagnosis and prognosis without leaving the laboratory, had little influence on patient care and were confined to the laboratory.[22] Bacteriologists then assumed expert roles in the new field in the 1950s and thereafter, aided by the new techniques of phage typing, when the bacteriologist moved 'to the forefront of hospital management and hospital-based medical care'.[23] Both Cresswell and Gardiner, through detailed examination of the practice of the hospital pathologist and bacteriologist, offer evidence which questions whether it is correct to portray the status of the bacteriologist as shifting 'from mere technician to infection control expert' in the 1950s.[24]

Cresswell and Gardiner do not dispute the fact that bacteriologists emerged as infection control experts in the 1950s, but argue that bacteriologists were always important to infection control regimes, at least since the early 1890s at St Bartholomew's (Barts) and 1920s at the Royal Infirmary of Edinburgh (RIE) and suggest a more gradual change in their status as they rose to prominence. They offer detailed evidence that supports assigning greater importance to pre-1950s bacteriological work. Cresswell illuminates the surveillance and hygiene responsibilities that Andrewes, the Pathologist/Sanitary Officer at Barts, carried out and their differentiation from those of the matron. Gardiner also builds on Condrau's chapter by discussing facets of hospital infection prevention and control strategy other than antibiotic use, showing that bacteriologists engaged effectively in the clinical sphere and influenced both treatment methods and sterilisation procedures. She shows that there was a high degree of collaboration between bacteriologists and clinicians at the RIE in connection with penicillin when it first arrived during the Second World War, with bacteriologists playing an important role in dictating the form that the new treatment took. Bacteriologists were far from confined to the laboratory. Their important work on infection-related concerns should be emphasised, not underestimated.

Hospital bacteriological work became increasingly central to infection control in the hospital and increasingly multi-faceted. This broad remit explains why bacteriologists became authorities on infection control, not just phage typing and not just the increase in AMR in the 1950s. In the period from 1948 to 1970 (and particularly after 1958), less in connection with antibiotics and more with his work on the infection control committees (ICCs) and on sterile supply, Gardiner shows that J. H. Bowie at Edinburgh played a leading role in developing new anti-infection strategies and recommendations, much in the way that Hillier and other historians suggest. For a brief period in Edinburgh before the late 1950s, bacteriologists did think about antibiotics in ways that were different from some clinicians. Also, some clinicians did not immediately welcome Bowie's new pre-set tray system in the early 1960s; nurses were key in harnessing support for it and in winning these clinicians over. Nevertheless, in the late 1950s and increasingly thereafter, the emerging picture is of the senior bacteriologists as the infection control experts and of the acceptance of their advice by other staff groups. Other historians' interpretation of the hospital 'as an arena where professional battles between research, medical practice and public health interests were being contested' did not generally apply to the RIE.[25] In Edinburgh, routine bacteriological work also became increasingly important after 1958, particularly with the rise of new specialities which depended heavily on it. Laboratory work also expanded into new areas, such as the screening of personnel, further cementing the field of infection control as the preserve of bacteriologists.

Nurses and nursing

The central importance of nurses and nursing for hospital infection control in the operating theatres and wards emerges clearly from the contributions in this volume. As Pamela Wood points out, surgical success in the late nineteenth and early twentieth centuries depended on both the surgeon's operative skill during surgery, and on the prevention of sepsis afterwards. 'Pre- and post-operative care was mainly directed at preventing or managing infection and was the relatively new professional sphere of the nurse', requiring arduous work to ensure the clean environment necessary to prevent sepsis: 'rigorous scrubbing of wards, furniture and operating theatres and the sterilisation of equipment and materials through heat', as well as antiseptics and strict standards of personal cleanliness; 'a scouring of all crevices where microbes could lurk'. As Claire Jones highlights, regimes of hygiene, personal cleanliness, antisepsis and asepsis were introduced into wards, into operating theatres and into nursing and medical curricula for the benefit of both patients and staff.[26] It is important to stress that by the early twentieth century surgeons and trained surgical nurses could treat wounds so they healed 'without infection'.[27]

Wood elucidates the hierarchy within the hospital among nurses, organised according to a gradient in the size and type of the particles of 'dirt' targeted, with the higher status, trained nurses in operating theatres coping with the smaller size, invisible microbial causes of 'pus' inside wounds, while probationer nurses, in early career stages, coped with the larger particles of dirt visible in the wards and on the patient's body. Within the operating theatre, the authority shifted gradually from a hierarchy of surgeon and surgical nurses to a 'surgical team' within the operating room by the 1930s. Nevertheless, the association of infection control with nursing remained reflected in the higher rates of compliance with IPC practices, such as handwashing for nurses, than for surgeons/medical practitioners, at GOSH in 2009: 99 per cent compliance for nurses, compared with 76 per cent for surgeons/medical practitioners.

Claire Jones and Susan Macqueen remind us forcefully that, contrary to some historians who have argued that the introduction of antibiotic therapy undermined and redefined the role of the British nurse from the 1940s, there was a continued emphasis on hygiene and preventive measures alongside the use of new drug therapeutics.[28] Increasingly intensive surgical procedures supported by antibiotics, for example transplantation, anti-cancer therapy cardiac surgery, the increasing use of in-dwelling devices and new specialist departments, exposed nurses to new types of cases often with heightened sets of care needs. The removal of sterilising duties to Central Sterile Supply Departments (CSSD) reduced risk of human error and thus patient and staff infection rates, and led to a greater emphasis on patient care and associated stringent aseptic techniques. At the same time, from the 1950s nurses with and without specific infection control titles made profound contributions to the new ICCs and to the development and everyday running of new systems for sterile supply which Susan Gardiner describes and Susan Macqueen recounts. Finally, Susan Macqueen's experience illuminates the development and practice of the new speciality of ICN and the integration into to governance at local and national levels of infection prevention and control.

Responsibility, reputation and blame

Issues of responsibility and blame for infection prevention and control in the wards and operating theatres emerged from the fatalism of the mid-nineteenth century and are a theme that concerns several chapters and resonates in the present.

In the mid-nineteenth century, although surgeons strove for improvements, a fatalistic attitude dominated discourse around surgery.[29] The surgeon did what he could, but the outcome was hard to predict, in large part due to the difficulties of infection control and prevention of surgical sepsis. From the 1860s and 1870s, with the development of antiseptic and aseptic ideas and methods of infection control, the surgeons came to take responsibility for the outcome. Joseph Lister, for example, blamed himself for poor outcomes and constantly experimented with techniques to improve the outcomes of his 'antiseptic system'; he argued that surgeons who could not reproduce his results were not following his antiseptic principles properly and blame rested with them. Also, instead of nurses, he used resident surgeons and medical students for assistance in the operating theatre; nurses cared for patients in the wards. During the 1880s, surgery started to be seen as the work of a team, including trained nurses, rather than the individual surgeon, and with this change, responsibility and blame came to be passed on to the nurses. Pamela Wood's chapter explores the various ways in which surgeons ascribed responsibility for sepsis to the nurse, while Claire Jones examines blame in the wards and nursing education, from the perspective of the health of the nurses and doctors, as well as patients. Jones demonstrated the great lengths nursing education went to instil attitudes of care and attention to hygiene, including self-care and regulation of behaviour.

Wood concluded from her analysis that 'the history of infection control shows us that a culture of blame is not productive. Septic wounds caused septic relations.'[30] For the present and future, she advocates a 'culture of curiosity' in which it is important to 'discover the reason for any infection so that practice can be improved', and 'with commitment from every health professional to take responsibility for preventing infection, we can develop a culture of exquisite care'.[31]

Similarly, both Wigglesworth and Leanord point to 'no blame' policies arising from the patient safety movement (embodied in the title of the report, *To Err is Human: Building a Safer Health System*[32]) and the importance of such policies in promoting teamwork among staff in the package of measures improving and maintaining standards of hospital infection prevention and control in the past fifteen years.[33]

Reminding us of the wider context of the accountability of the hospital as a whole, Rosemary Cresswell suggested that Frederick Andrewes' prominent role in infection control at Barts arose in part from the concern of the governors that mortality due to HAI not damage the reputation of the hospital among subscribers. Also, as noted previously, Neil Wigglesworth emphasised the importance of the legislation in England, particularly the 2008 Health and

Social Care Act, which made hospital trusts fiscally responsible for meeting HAI targets and threatened the jobs of their heads. Susan Macqueen, too, focused on the accountability of the hospital as a whole, when she argued that 'finding the definitive proof that hospitals were responsible for giving individual patients infections was notoriously difficult'.[34] As the director of IPC for GOSH during the 2000s, she was 'concerned that GOSH did not become [legally] liable'. She asked what evidence would a lawyer look for when a patient made a claim of HAI. Finding that lawyers were focusing on compliance with health and safety guidelines and good practices gave her leverage in persuading staff to follow the many guidelines issued in the 2000s, guidelines which she praises for clarifying a path for staff through the masses of evidence and which continue to perform this role in the UK through the guidelines offered by IPS and National Institute for Health and Care Excellence (NICE).

Economics

Contributors remind us that issues of economy cannot be separated from hospital infection control practices and policies over the period. Supply issues, whether of nurses or penicillin in its early years, or concerns about hospital expenditure, exerted a great influence on methods for infection control and *vice versa*. Susan Gardiner, for example, pointed out that the huge costs of the introduction of CSSDs in the 1960s were considered to be partly offset by savings in the labour of nurses.

Claire Jones also demonstrates that infection control practices cannot be separated from issues of economy. Throughout the hundred years from *c.* 1870 to 1970, hospitals carried the economic burden of looking after their ill staff, often because it was in their financial interest to do so. Hospital governors understood that they not only had a duty of care to their staff, but that it financially benefited them to do so. After all, it was extremely costly to train up a nurse to the required standard over the course of two or three years, particularly when lodging and board were included. To lose their expertise due to illness for any length of time was costly, and getting them back to health was in a hospital's interest. The RIE in 1890 justified building a new nurses' home and convalescent homes for nurses. Costs of caring for nurses with some form of sepsis could be particularly high, as nurses were taken off duty as soon as it was reported and did not return until their hospital could be sure they had fully recovered.

The many guidelines issued in England and Wales in the 2000s required a rethink of the management of infection prevention and control, which Susan Macqueen points out reinforced the economic and clinical message. Also, like the Centers for Disease Control's influential SENIC project in the mid-1980s, which demonstrated the extent of 'preventable' infections and associated cost savings, Macqueen reports the cost of controlling an outbreak at GOSH amounting to £434,623 offered a major incentive for her efforts and those of her colleagues to implement infection prevention measures.[35] Finally, Wigglesworth emphasises the importance of the relatively buoyant national economic context and the government's willingness to fund IPC in response to MRSA and *C. diff* in the 1990s and 2000s, but is pessimistic that funding on a similar scale will be forthcoming in the future in a national context of financial austerity. In particular, he argues that nursing strategies in the past made a difference regarding the dramatic reduction of MRSA, but there is a danger they might be overlooked in future when other bacteria are involved and finance less likely to be available than in the 1990s and 2000s.[36]

Economic considerations and hospital infection receive sustained analysis in Sally Sheard's pioneering chapter. Her method of focusing on the emergence of the recognition among policymakers in both post-war Britain and the United States of a relationship between length of stay in hospital, infection and costs demonstrates the power of a historical approach in combination with current policy considerations, as well as, like Wigglesworth and Leanord on England and Scotland, the utility of international comparisons to illuminate distinctive national features. The recognition of the relationship between length of stay in hospital, infection and costs came earlier in the United States with the introduction in the 1980s of a system of insurance payments by diagnosis related group (DRG). Each DRG had an associated expected length of stay, and a hospital would not be reimbursed if a patient exceeded that length due to an HAI. In the UK, Sheard shows that it was not until the 1990s that researchers were observing that 93 per cent of the total additional cost incurred by surgical patients with an HAI could be attributed to an extended length of stay.[37] In the UK, the shorter lengths of hospital stay for all types of patients, but especially surgical and obstetric, came to be associated with a combination of advances in clinical performance, concerns about increasing NHS costs, the introduction of general management, transition from larger 'Nightingale' wards to small bed units, with implications for nursing and clinical management, linked the concept of 'value for money' in the NHS and the introduction of analyses of cost-effectiveness. However, changes to patient management in hospitals had risks, such as the rise of HAIs. At the same time, the shorter lengths of stay raised questions about the hospital as a site of infection prevention and control.

Hospital and community

This volume focuses on infections caused by bacteria thought to be *acquired* in hospitals, and their prevention and control, yet it is important to note that it begins and ends with chapters stressing the links between hospitals and the community, and the problematic nature of a focus on the hospital alone. Flurin Condrau pointed to the global spread in the 1950s of *S. aureus* 80/81, resistant to all forms of penicillin, and traceable by phage typing, as a turning point and foretaste of the spread of resistant bacteria and 'the ways the idea of hospital infection has blurred rather than helped our understanding of resistance travelling between hospitals and communities'. Nurses, he argued, played a crucial role in the spread of hospital infection as they tended to patients, moving in and out of their wards, and like babies discharged from neonatal wards, carried acquired bacteria out into the community. He highlighted the Asian Flu Pandemic of 1956–1957 as evidence that the community had to be taken into account as a major source of infection to understand HAI. Patients coming into hospitals with compromised immune systems due to viral infection had increased chances of resistant *Staph* infections. Gardiner described how the influence of laboratory workers in infection control increased after the Second World War with the rise of specialities which prioritised infection control and new procedures for the bacteriological screening of hospital staff of all kinds and others, including tradesmen coming into the hospital.[38]

Looking at the current landscape and future challenges for infection control and healthcare delivery, Alistair Leanord highlights the very short lengths of stay in acute hospitals and the migration of healthcare and associated problems of infection control into the community, where surveillance and prevention of individual infection is more difficult. In Scotland, for example, there was a big reduction in hospital cases of *C. diff*, and only a slight reduction in community *C. diff*. Moreover, 30 per cent to 40 per cent of *C. diff* cases in Scotland come from the community with no association with healthcare or previous antibiotics as triggers. Who is going to look after these cases? How are we going to treat them? What are the trigger factors?

Contributors feature another aspect of looking outside the hospital in pursuit of infection prevention and control within hospitals – working with manufacturers. Susan Macqueen recounts the identification of the source of infection in GOSH in 1995–1996 in the wooden tongue depressors from a new NHS supplier using wood from unmanaged forests in China not treated in a hot kiln before production, which led to pressure on manufacturers to produce a cost-effective splint small enough for children. Also, to prevent cross infection from re-used red rubber suction catheters, she worked with manufacturers to ensure that small, soft-ended disposable suction tubes appropriate for newborn babies were manufactured, and to decontaminate ventilator tubes and equipment, she visited a German hospital similar to GOSH to see automated disinfection equipment in use and worked with the German manufacturer to supply the specific needs of GOSH for installation of the new equipment away from the wards and separation of clean and dirty items at ward level and instruction of staff.[39]

Brief overall conclusions

The contributions to this book offer a variety of perspectives focusing on the past, present and future of hospital IPC from scholars at all career stages and current and former healthcare practitioners and policymakers. Contributors investigate practice in hospital settings, as well as the origins and implementation of policies. They integrate historical and contemporary evidence, and illuminate both changing views of the roles of *germs* or microbes in creating infection from the mid-nineteenth century; and the management of the microbes in which the *governance* arrangements of the hospital and staff of all kinds play a prominent role in mediating policy and practice. A number of overall conclusions emerge.

First, although challenges faced at different times were historically contingent, over the 150-year period the establishment and maintenance of standards of hygiene in the hospital environment, in both wards and operating theatres, depended on the education and work of nurses, bacteriologists, cleaners, pharmacists and other hospital staff, as well as surgeons and physicians. Nursing education, practice and strategies in particular, made a difference, including most recently with regard to the dramatic decline of MRSA and C. *diff*, but there is a danger they could be overlooked in future when other microbes are involved.

Second, alongside the risks of sepsis to patients, most hospital occupations carried fundamental health risks. IPC for both staff and patients since the 1990s has benefited from measures adapted from human factors and ergonomics and the patient safety movement, particularly a 'no blame' culture. It is important to remember the century-old reminder in Pamela Wood's conclusion that everyone fails at times, yet when someone makes mistakes, the 'crucial outcome is to learn from the error in order to avoid it in the future'.[40] Yet healthcare today is so fast-paced and overstretched that the capacity to learn is severely compromised. We have been adept at putting many data feedback and learning systems in place, but it takes time to digest the lessons, and that is often where the gap lies.[41]

Third, too much emphasis on one method or technique or policy, such as surgical or non-sterile gloves, drug therapies or shorter hospital stays can lead to overlooking alternative methods and rationales, or to unintended, detrimental consequences. The importance of multiple interventions and, within this, teamwork, stand out. It is not possible to point to just one as crucial for success in reducing infections, since some interventions cannot be evidence-based and because it is so difficult to eliminate human error and not possible to eradicate the 'moving targets' which 'germs' or microbes have come to be seen to pose.

Fourth, political will, government interventions and financial resources since the 1990s, although differing in different parts of the UK, have been crucial in the decline of rates of some HAIs in all parts of the UK. Human factors are important: time, repetition and communications matter. Emotional reactions change; for example, what is found to be disgusting in relation to touching patients, or the fact that babies are often the most common carriers of infection, though gloves are not readily used in the same way they might be with elderly people. Without political will, government interventions and financial resources, it will not be possible to introduce individualised, genome-based treatments, nor maintain the institutional change and development of new arrangements of the hospital environment suggested by the human factors and ergonomics approach, which should not be overlooked in the transformation of practice.

Finally, as many of the authors suggest and Claire Jones clearly articulates, the long view that history provides points to 'a great deal more continuity than change in hospital practice' across the past 150 years. First established in the late nineteenth century, preventative aseptic techniques and the concern with the hospital environment did not disappear, even after the introduction of drug therapies. With the growing threat of methicillin-resistant *Staphylococcus aureus* (MRSA) and antibiotic resistance in the present, the hospital environment and maintaining standards of hygiene have become even more important.[42]

Thus, the current, high profile, international and national calls for increased funding for the development of new classes of antimicrobial drugs, which dominate discussion at present, should not overshadow and neglect the financial, personnel and governance methods necessary to maintain standard infection control precautions in the hospital environment, associated most recently with the dramatic reduction of two very different clinical presentations and problems – MRSA and *C. diff* – in the UK since 2002.

Notes

1   See, for example V. Berridge, 'Why policy needs history (and historians)', *Health Economics, Policy and Law*, 13:3/4 (2018), 1–13, https://doi. org/10.1017/S1744133117000433 (accessed 4 May 2019); V. Berridge,

'History and the future: Looking back to look forward?', *International Journal of Drug Policy*, 37 (2016), 117–121; V. Berridge (ed.), *Making health policy: Networks in research and policy after 1945* (Amsterdam and New York: Rodopi, 2005); V. Berridge (ed.), *Aids in the UK: The making of policy, 1981–1994* (Oxford: Oxford University Press, 1996).

2 Berridge, 'Why policy needs history (and historians)', 11.

3 Berridge, 'History and the future', 120.

4 See Condrau, p. 44, this volume.

5 See Wilson, p. 179, this volume.

6 See Wood, p. 97, this volume.

7 See Schlich, pp. 165, 166, 167, this volume.

8 HM Government, 'Contained and controlled: the UK's 20-year vision for antimicrobial resistance (AMR)' (24 Jan 2019), 10, www.gov.uk/government/publications/uk-20-year-vision-for-antimicrobial-resistance (accessed 31 Jan 2019); a slightly more specific target is included in the UK's new five-year national action plan, see 'Tackling antimicrobial resistance 2019–2024: The UK's five-year national action plan' (24 Jan 2019), 80, https://assets.publishing.service.gov.uk/government/uploads/system/uploads/attachment_data/file/773130/uk-amr-5-year-national-action-plan.pdf (accessed 31 Jan 2019). For a failed attempt to standardise the process of sensitivity or susceptibility testing during the 1960s through the World Health Organization and continuing focus on the paper disk element, see C. Gradmann, 'Sensitive matters: The World Health Organisation and antibiotic resistance testing, 1945–1975', *Social History of Medicine*, 26:3 (2011), 555–574.

9 See Macqueen, p. 143, this volume.

10 See Leanord, p. 263, this volume.

11 See Macqueen, p. 144, Leanord, p. 264, Wigglesworth, p. 248, this volume.

12 See Wigglesworth, p. 247, Macqueen, p. 132, this volume.

13 For a timeline summarising interventions to reduce healthcare associated infections and improve infection prevention and control, 2001 to 2014, see www.health.org.uk/sites/default/files/IPC-TimelineSelectedInterventions.pdf.

14 Department of Health, *Winning Ways – working together to reduce healthcare associated infection in England – a report from the Chief Medical Officer* (2003), https://webarchive.nationalarchives.gov.uk/20040329042309/http://www.publications.doh.gov.uk/cmo/hai/winningways.pdf (accessed 4 May 2019); see Macqueen, p. 142, this volume.

15 See Macqueen, p. 143, this volume; for the Keystone study, see also Wigglesworth, pp. 251–2, this volume.

16 See Leanord, p. 260, Macqueen, p. 142, Wigglesworth, p. 248, this volume.
17 See Leanord, pp. 260–1, this volume.
18 See Wigglesworth, p. 248, Leanord, pp. 262–3, this volume.
19 See Leanord, pp. 262–3, this volume.
20 See Leanord, pp. 266–7, this volume.
21 See Leanord, pp. 260, 261, this volume.
22 K. Hillier, 'Babies and bacteria: phage typing, bacteriologists, and the birth of infection control', *Bulletin of the History of Medicine*, 80 (2006), 733–761; F. Condrau, 'Standardising infection control: Antibiotics and hospital governance in Britain 1948–1960', in C. Bonah *et al.* (eds), *Harmonizing drugs: Standards in 20th-century pharmaceutical history* (Paris: Editions Glyphe, 2009), 352–353. See also Ayliffe and English, *Hospital infection: From miasmas to MRSA* (Cambridge: Cambridge University Press, 2003), 192–196.
23 F. Condrau and R. G. W. Kirk, 'Negotiating hospital infections: The debate between ecological balance and eradication strategies in British hospitals, 1947–1969', *Dynamis*, 31 (2011), 385–405, quotation 401.
24 Hillier, 'Babies and bacteria', 760.
25 Condrau and Kirk, 'Negotiating hospital infections', 403.
26 See Wood, pp. 81, 83, Jones, p. 107, this volume.
27 See Wood, p. 83, this volume.
28 For the argument that antibiotics undermined the role of nurses, see: M. E. Baly, *Nursing and social change* (London: Routledge, 1995) 178–192; P. Starns, *Nurses at war: Women on the frontline 1939–45* (Gloucestershire: Sutton Publishing, 2000), 73.
29 Thomas Schlich, 'Farmer to industrialist: Lister's antisepsis and the making of modern surgery in Germany', *Notes and records of the Royal Society*, 67 (2013), 245–260; http://doi.org/10.1098/rsnr.2013.0032.
30 See Wood, pp. 97–8, this volume.
31 See Wood, p. 98, this volume.
32 US Institute of Medicine, *To err is human: Building a safer health system* (Washington: Institute of Medicine and National Academy Press, 1999); Department of Health, *An Organisation with a memory: Report of an expert group on learning from adverse events in the NHS, chaired by the Chief Medical Officer* (London: Department of Health, 2000).
33 See Wigglesworth, pp. 251–2, Leanord, pp. 262–3, this volume.
34 See Macqueen, p. 140, this volume.
35 *Ibid.*, p. 141, this volume.
36 See Wigglesworth, pp. 248–50, this volume.
37 See, for example, R. Coello, H. Glenister, J. Fereres *et al.*, 'The cost of infection in surgical patients: A case-control study', *Journal of Hospital Infection*, 25 (1993), 239–250.

38 See Condrau, p. 44, Gardiner, p. 229, this volume.
39 See Macqueen, pp. 135, 139, this volume.
40 See Wood, p. 98, this volume.
41 Charles Vincent, Susan Burnett and Jane Carthey, 'Safety measurement and monitoring in healthcare: A framework to guide clinical teams and healthcare organisations in maintaining safety', *British Medical Journal Quality and Safety*, 23 (2014), 670–677; C. Vincent, S. Burnett and J. Carthey, *The measurement and monitoring of safety: Drawing together academic evidence and practical experience to produce a framework for safety measurement and monitoring* (London: The Health Foundation, 2013).
42 See Jones, p. 122, this volume.

Index

Note: Page numbers in **bold** reference tables.
Note: Page numbers in *italics* reference figures.
Note: 'n.' after a page reference indicates the number of a note on that page.

1957 influenza pandemic, hospital-community interaction (1930–1960) 9, 40–41
1990s, MRSA (methicillin-resistant *S. aureus*) outbreaks 247–250

Abel-Smith, Brian 55, 201
Ackerknecht, Erwin H. 28
agar diffusion technique 221
AHA (American Hospital Association) 58–60
Ajemian, Elizabeth 60, 62
Allison, V. D. 234
alternatives to gloves 164–167
Amalberti, René 251
American Hospital Association *see* AHA
AMR (antimicrobial resistance) 1–3, 249
    history 5–6
AMR Historical Foresight project 5
Andrewes, Frederick 16, 193–194, 196, 198–201, 204–206
    Sanitary Officer (St Bartholomew's Hospital) 195–207
antibiotic resistance 131
antibiotic sensitivity testing 221–224
antibiotic therapy 222–223
antibiotics 131, 222
antimicrobial resistance *see* AMR

Antimicrobial Resistance (AMR) strategy (2013–2018), UK 258
antisepsis 83, 87, 153, 164–165
APIC (Association for Practitioners in Infection Control; in 1993, renamed Association for Professionals in Infection Control and Epidemiology) 59, 60,73n.36
Ardern, Peter 194
artificial hyperleucocytosis 160
asepsis 83, 87, 91, 156
Aseptic Firm 197
Asian Flu Pandemic 40–41, 271
Association for Practitioners in Infection Control *see* APIC
Australia, surgical nurse training (1900–1935) 88
autoclaves 231–232
Ayliffe, G. A. J. 5, 62, 64, 75n.58, 195, 219

Bacilli coli 161–162
bacteriological testing at RIE (1959–1970) 226
bacteriological tests 226–227
bacteriologists 194–195, 219–220, 276–278
Bailey, David 119
Bailey, H. 87
Baker, William Morrant 196

Baly, Monica 232
Barber, Mary 37
Bartlett, Mrs 210
Bashford, A. 91, 206
Bennett, John 60
Berridge, Virginia 270,
    286–287n.1–3
Bevan, Aneurin 53
Billroth, Theodor 35
Bishop, E. Stanmore 92–93
blame 279–281
Bloodgood, Joseph 153
bloodstream infections *see* BSIs
Blowers, Robert 58
Body Substance Isolation *see* BSI
Bourne, Geoffrey 209
Bowie, John H. 17, 221, 222–224,
    226, 227, 229, 230, 272
    sterilisation 231–235
    tray system 235–236
Bowie-Dick Autoclave Tape Test
    235
Brachman, Philip 60
Branson, William 112
Brexit 2
BSI (Body Substance Isolation) 174
BSIs (bloodstream infections)
    251–252, **261**, 266, 268
builder's rubbish 206
Burdett, Henry 54
Burt, Margaret 207
Butlin, Henry 196–197

C. *diff* (*Clostridium difficile*)
    infections 4, 247–250, 252, 261
    gastrointestinal infections 260
    infection rates relative to
        national standard *263*
    outbreaks and incidents (2016–
        2017) *266*
    Scotland 265–266
    targets *262*
Callender, George 196
Cameron, David 249
Campbell, Ian D. 234
Candida auris 249
Canti, Ronald 199
Carayon, Pascale 253

carbapenemase-producing
    Enterobacteriaceae *see* CPE
carbapenem-resistant
    Enterobacteriaceae *see* CRE
carbolic acid 153
Castle, Mary 60, 62
Catford, E. F. 234
CDC (Centers for Disease Control
    and Prevention) 10, 58, 59,
    60, 249
Centers for Medicare and Medicaid
    Services *see* CMS
Central Sterile Supply Department
    see CSSD
Central Venous Catheter Care 143
centralisation, RIE (Royal
    Infirmary of Edinburgh) 233
Chambers, M. 88, 95
change 272–276
Chavigny, Katherine 61
Chester, Teddy 55
Childe, C. 88, 94
Church, William 198–199
Clarke, Suzanne 57–58
clean dressings 92
Clean Your Hands campaign 130
cleanliness 89–91
Cleanliness Champions programme,
    Scotland 258–259
clinics, infection control (1945–
    1970) 229–237
CMS (Centers for Medicare and
    Medicaid Services), US 66–67
Coello, R. 65
co-infection 29
Colebrook, Leonard 35
community 8, 9, 11, 27, 28, 33,
    38, 39, 41, 43, 134, 265–267,
    283–284
    hospitals and 27, 29, 30, 36, 43,
        44, 270
Control of Infection Officer 195
convalescence 53–56
Cooke Report (1988) 138
Coote, Holmes 196
Cordiner, Miss 229–230
cost of drug-resistant infections
    2–3

costs
enquiry into 54–55
of HAIs 58–61, 68–70
see also economics
Cottrell, E. M. 131
CPE (carbapenemase-producing Enterobacteriaceae) 2, 18, 249, 250
Craven, D. E. 61
CRE (carbapenem-resistant Enterobacteriaceae) 249
Creed, Edward 120
Cripps, Harrison 196–197
cross contamination, non-sterile gloves 176–177
cross infection 34–35, 117, 134
diphtheria 201–202, 204
typhoid 203–204
Cruickshank, Robert 226, 230
CSSD (Central Sterile Supply Department) 118, 132, 279, 232–233
Cunliffe, A. C. 118
curriculum, surgical nurse training (1900–1935) 85–90, 232–234, 237, 279, 281
Currie, E. 65
Cyllin 201

D&V (diarrhoea and vomiting) 141
Daschner, Franz 63
Davies, Professor Dame Sally xvii, 249
deaths
due to healthcare interventions 4
from superbugs 2
delayed recovery, HAI (hospital-acquired infection) 56–61
delivery of curriculum, surgical nurse training (1900–1935) 85–90
diagnosis-related groups *see* DRGs
diarrhoea and vomiting *see* D&V
Dick, James 235
DIPC (Director of Infection Prevention and Control) 142, 147n.30, 273
diphtheria 201–204
Director of Infection Prevention and Control *see* DIPC

dirt 180–181
pus 84–85
dirty dressings 92
disposal of 17, 229–230, 238
disabilities, due to healthcare interventions 4
disposal of soiled dressings 17, 229–230, 238
distribution of HAI types 2005–2016 (percentage) **261**
ditch plate technique 221, 223
Divens, E. 92
doctors, hygiene practices 120–121
Donaldson, Liam 4
Douglas, Mary 84
DRGs (diagnosis-related groups) 12, 62, 69, 282
drivers of glove use behaviour 179–185
Dubos, René 35
Duncan, Catherine 111, 115
Durie, T. B. M. 225, 230

E. coli 260, 267
early ambulation 53
Easson, Hannah 116
Ebola 249
economics 281–283
HAI (hospital-acquired infection) 67–68
see also costs
Edgerton, David 166
Edinburgh Standard Disc Diffusion Technique *see* ESDDT
efficiency 56
emotion
disgust 185
driver of glove use behaviour 179–180
ENB (English National Board) 137
English, Mary 5, 195, 219
English National Board *see* ENB
Entwisle, I. 113
Escherichia coli 2
ESDDT (Edinburgh Standard Disc Diffusion Technique) 224–225, 229
EU (European Union), AMR (antimicrobial resistance) 2

Feldstein, Martin 55
Fenwick, B. 93
fever hospitals 31–33
Fischer, Janet 61
Fleming, Alexander 57, 221
Flügge, Carl 160
food poisoning outbreak, Stanley
    Royd Hospital 138
Foothills Hospital Wound Study 58
Foucault, M. 28
foul smells 205–206
Frampton, Sally 166
Fraser, Isabella 82
Freeman, Jonathan 60
fumigation 135–136
Fürbringer, Paul 155

Garrod, Lawrence 58, 199, 206
gastrointestinal infections 260
Geddes, Alasdair 62, 75n.58
Giddens, Anthony 186
Gillingham, F. John 234
Girou, E. 175
Givens, C. D. 60
Glasgow Royal Infirmary *see* GRI
Glenister, H. 64
gloves 8, 11, 15–16, 92, 96–97,
    106, 151–157, 159, 172–173,
    186–187, 197, 252, 254–255,
    271, 284, 286
  alternatives to 164–167
  attitudes toward the use of non-
    sterile clinical gloves **182–183**
  drivers of glove use behaviour
    179–185
  misuse of 185–186
  non-sterile gloves 174–178
  risk of cross-contamination and
    appropriateness of glove use
    177
  situations where gloves should
    or should not be worn *177*
  touch sequences during observed
    episodes of care **178**
Gordon, Anna R. 234
Gordon, Louisa 113
GOSH (Great Ormond Street
    Hospital) 129–139, 273, 279,
    281, 284

Central Venous Catheter Care 143
D&V (diarrhoea and vomiting)
    141
decontamination of respiratory
    equipment *136*
decontamination of ventilator
    tubing *137*
DIPC (Director of Infection
    Prevention and Control)
    142, 273
liabilities for HAIs 140
MRSA (methicillin-resistant
    S. aureus) 140–141
S. aureus 140
Salmonella outbreak 273
Gould, J. D. 222–224
Gradmann, Christoph 29–30,
    221–222, 225
Granshaw, Lindsay 196, 211
Great Ormond Street Hospital *see*
    GOSH
GRI (Glasgow Royal Infirmary) 88,
    105–106, 109, 111, 116, 117,
    120, 208
Grimwalde, Mary McLaren 116
Gullan, M. A. 89
Guthrie, Irene 111
Guy's Hospital 18, 85, 89, 210, 207

H2N2 40
Hadley, W. 87
Haegler, Carl 157
Haemophilus influenza 41
HAI (Healthcare-Associated Infection)
    taskforce, Scotland 257–258
HAI (hospital-acquired infection)
    3–6, 10, 12, 14, 19, 51–53,
    172, 175, 187, 257–260, *261*,
    266–268, 275, 280–283, 286
  costs 58–61, 68–70
  delayed recovery 56–61
  impact of healthcare financing
    policies 61–67
  preventing 268
  types of outbreaks and incidents
    (2016–2017) *266*
Haley, Robert 59, 60, 63
Halsted, William 151–154, *154*
hand disinfection 155, 197

hand hygiene 175–178, 185–187, 258
hand washing 130
Handfield-Jones, R. 104
hands, role in transmission
    of healthcare-associated
    infection 172–174
HCAI (healthcare-associated
    infection) 15, 142
Health Act (2006) 142, 274
Health and Social Care Act (2008)
    142, 274
Healthcare Environment
    Inspectorate *see* HEI
healthcare financing policies,
    impact on HAIs 61–67
healthcare interventions, disability
    or death 4
Healthcare-Associated Infection
    (HAI) taskforce, Scotland
    257–258
healthcare-associated infection
    (HCAI) 15, 142
HEAT targets 262
HEI (Healthcare Environment
    Inspectorate) 264–265
Hewison, Alistair 194
HFE (human factors and
    ergonomics) 177, 187,
    253–255, 276
HIC (Hospital Infection
    Committee) 225–228, 232
use/misuse of antibiotics 229
hierarchies of practices, surgical
    nurse training (1900–1935)
    90–92
high impact intervention (HII) 143,
    274
Hillier, Kathryn 29, 36–37,
    194–195, 219, 229
HIPE (Hospital In-Patient Enquiry)
    54, 56
HIS (Hospital Infection Society) 9,
    23n.32
history
    hospital infection control 5–6
    uses of 270–272
HIV (human immunodeficiency
    virus) 174

Hospital Infection Committee *see*
    HIC
use/misuse of antibiotics 229
hospital infection control 51–52
    history and 5–6
    patient safety agenda 3–4
Hospital Infection Society *see* HIS
hospital infections 28–29
Hospital In-Patient Enquiry *see*
    HIPE
hospital management, efficiency
    and effectiveness 53–56
hospital nurseries, hospital-
    community interaction
    (1930–1960) 36–40
hospital stays 53
hospital-acquired infection *see* HAI
hospital-community interaction
    (1930–1960) 28–30
    1957 influenza pandemic 40–41
    background of 30–35
    newborns 36–40
Howard, R. 86, 93
Hubble, Douglas 118
human factors and ergonomics *see*
    HFE
human immunodeficiency virus *see*
    HIV
Humphrey, L. 87
Hunter, Beatrice 55
hygiene practices, doctors 120–121
hypercytosis 160
hyperleucocytosis 160–162

I'Anson, Edward B. 199
iatrogenesis 22n.19
iatrogenic diseases 29
ICLN (infection control link nurse)
    programme 138
ICN (infection control nurse) 9, 57,
    131–132
ICNA (Infection Control Nurses
    Association) 9, 132, 137
ICS (infection control sister) 57
ICUs (intensive care units) 10, 251
IHI Model for Improvement 252
Illich, Ivan 4, 29
immunisation 162–163

inappropriate glove use 184
incidence rate 64
'Infection as a Whole' 254
Infection Cards 227–228
infection control
 future of, Scotland 265–269
 HFE (human factors and
  ergonomics) 253–255
infection control (1945–1970)
 in clinics 229–237
 laboratories 221–229
infection control link nurse
 programme *see* ICLN
  programme
infection control nurse *see* ICN
Infection Control Nurses
 Association *see* ICNA
infection control sister *see* ICS
infection prevention and control,
 hospital infection control *see*
 hospital infection control
Infection Prevention Society *see* IPS
infectious disease 8
infectious disease hospitals 8
influenza 40–41
inspections, Scotland 264–265
intensive care units *see* ICUs
IPS (Infection Prevention Society)
 9, 18, 137, 281
isolation 32–33

Jameson, W. 62, 119
Jeffrey, J. S. 225, 227, 238
Jenner, Edward 129, 159
Jewson, Nicholas 28
John Hopkins Hospital
 Department of Surgery 152
junior nurses 90–91

Kanthack, Alfredo 198–199
KCH (King's College Hospital)
 105–106, 109, *116*, 120,
 200, 208
 staff illness 111, 113–114
 sterilising techniques 118
 wound books 119
Keetley, C. B. 95
Keystone ICU project 10

Keystone Intensive Care Unit (ICU)
 251–252
King's College Hospital *see* KCH
Kirk, Robert 219
Klebsiella pneumoniae
 carbapenemase *see* KPC
knife and fork method of operating
 157
Koch, Robert 129–130, 153, 203
Kocher, Theodor 155
KPC (*Klebsiella pneumoniae*
 carbapenemase) 249–250
Kristeva, J. 84, 90

laboratories, infection control
 (1945–1970) 221–229
laminar flow theatre 253–254
Lane, William Arbuthnot 157
Larsson, Elaine 252
laudable pus 84, 87
Lawrence, William 196
Leape, Lucien 251
Legionnaires' disease 138
length of hospital stays 53–56
link nurse programmes 138
Lister, Joseph 8, 83, 110, 129, 153,
 164–165, 280
localisation, future of infection
 control (Scotland) 265–269
Lockwood, Charles B. 105, 156, 197
Lockwood system 197
London Hospital, diphtheria 203
Lowbury, E. 62, 75n.58
Löwy, Ilana 166
Lucas-Championnière, Just 53
Lückes, E. 82, 113, 203

Maclaren, Iain Ferguson 222, 225,
 226, 230, 231, 232, 236
Macleod, Herbert 206
Maitland, H. L. 95
Manson, Ethel 207–209
Matrons 193–194, 207–211
Maynard, A. 65
McGann, Susan 207
McGowan, John 60
McGregor, A. N. 88, 94
McNeill Love, R. J. 87

Meachen, G. Norman 88
Meade, Agnes 111
medical anthropology 138
medical asepsis 90–91
medical mortality 14, 107–108
Medicare 56
    healthcare financing policies
        61–62
methicillin-resistant *S. aureus see*
    MRSA
methicillin-sensitive *S. aureus see*
    MSSA
Metropolitan Asylums Board 31
miasma 206
miasmatic 205
microbiologists 195
migration, future of infection
    control (Scotland) 265–269
Mikulicz, Johannes 159–164
Miles, A. 94
misuse of: gloves 185–186; history
    271
Miyake, Hiyaki 160
Monk, Katherine 113–114
Moore, Brendan 131–132
mortality, medical mortality 14,
    107–108
Mortimer, E. A. 173
MRSA (methicillin-resistant *S.
    aureus*) 4–5, 18–19, 43, 64,
    122, 140, 142–143, 257,
    259–260, 267, 272, 273
    1990s outbreaks 247–250
    targets 262–264
MRSA screening 267
MSSA (methicillin-sensitive
    S. aureus) 260
multidrug-resistant years 2
multi-modal intervention 275
Murchison, Charles 205
Myerscough, Philip Roger 222–
    223, 226, 231, 236

Nairn, Flora 111
NAO (National Audit Office), UK 66
nappies 133–134
nasal carriers of Staphylococcus
    120

National Audit Office *see* NAO
National Health Service *see* NHS
national system of control 257–258
Neuber, Gustav Adolf 156
New Zealand
    nurses 82
    surgical nurse training (1900–
        1935) 88
newborns, hospital-community
    interaction (1930–1960)
        36–40
newness 166
Newsholme, Arthur 34
Newsom Kerr, Matthew 8, 31
NHS (National Health Service) 4,
    9, 12, 35–36, 28, 42, 54–56,
    63, 65–66, 107, 117–118, 139,
    142, 195, 232, 248–250, 252
NHS England 252
NHS Scotland 262, 275
Nightingale, Florence 8, 30–31, 81,
    108, *109*, 110, 129
Nightingale Home 114
Nightingale Training School, septic
    finger 113
non-sterile clinical gloves *see* NSCG
non-sterile gloves
    problems with 175–178
    in routine clinical practice
        174–175
Norovirus 141
nosocomial infection *see* HAI
    (hospital-acquired infection)
Nosocomial Infection National
    Surveillance Scheme 66
Nottingham patent steam
    disinfectors 200
NSCG (non-sterile clinical gloves)
    175–178
Numbers, Lorna 236
nurses 8, 9, 11–14, 16–18, 43, 51,
    66, 81–88, 143, 151–152,
    173–174, 180–181, 183–184,
    186, 193, 201, 203 205,
    207–211, 229, 233, 235–236,
    270–271, 278–283, 285
    cleanliness 89–90
    health of (1880–1929) 108–115

infection control nurses 9,
131–132
maintaining standards, sharing
responsibility (1930–1965)
115–121
observations on patients *180*
probationer nurses 108
sterilising badges *116*
surgical nurse training (1900–
1935) *see* surgical nurse
training (1900–1935)
Nurses, Midwives and Health
Visitors Act (1979), Britain
137
nursing 278–279
as a profession 82
nursing responsibilities (1880–
1929) 108–115
see also nurses

Obama, Barack 249
Ochsner, Albert 155
Ogle, William 108
O'Neill, Lord 2
Opie, Evie 117
Oxford, M. N. 85, 89

Paget, James 196
Palmer, Debbie 107, 113, 203
paper disc method 223, 240n.20
paraffin 157
Pasteur, Louis 35, 129
pathologists 193–194
St Bartholomew's Hospital
198–199
patient safety, United Kingdom
250–252
patient safety agenda, hospital
infection control 3–4
Payr, Erwin 159
pedagogy, pus 85
penicillin 9, 42, 58, 131, 184, 194,
221–224, 230–231, 272, 277,
281, 283
Pennington, Hugh 195, 200
peppermint tests 205
personal protective equipment *see*
PPE

phage typing 36, 219
Pickstone, John 165
Pinker, Robert 54
Platt, R. 61
Plowman, Rosalind 65–66, 68
Podolsky, Scott 30, 42
Point Prevalence Survey *see* PPS
poison finger 104
policy formation 273
political will 273
Poor Law 8, 31
post-surgical regimes 53–54
PPE (personal protective
equipment) 15, 254–255, 260
PPS (Point Prevalence Survey) 258,
260, **261**
prevalence rate 64
preventing surgical infection
159–164
preventing wound infection
through touch 155–159
proactive infection control policies
259–261
probationer nurses 108
professional drivers of glove use
184–185
Pseudomonas 134
Public Health England 249
pus 81–85, 87

Randers-Pehrson, Justine 152
recovery, delayed recovery, HAI
56–61
Reid, William Henry 120
reputation 279–281
Respiratory Syncytial Virus *see* RSV
responsibility 279–281
Rhizopus microsporus 139
RIE (Royal Infirmary of Edinburgh)
17, 105–106, 109, *112*, 118,
120, 208, 219, 220, 226, 232,
234–238, 277–278, 281
absences of sick nurses 115–116
bacteriological testing *226*
centralisation 233
group portrait (1904) *112*
infection control in laboratories
(1945–1970) 221–229

staff illness 111–112, 115
Staphylococcal super-infections
    231
  wound infections 225
ringworm 203
risk 107
Ristori, B. 86
Robb, Hunter 152
Roberts, J. 65–69
Roemer, Milton 55
role of Sanitary Officer (St
    Bartholomew's Hospital)
    195–207
Rosenberg, Charles 40
Ross, Ena 222
Rotavirus 141
Rountree, Phyllis 36, 37, 38
Royal Infirmary of Edinburgh *see*
    RIE
RSV (Respiratory Syncytial Virus)
    266
Ruddock, Rosaline 111
Rutherford Darling, H. C. 86

S. aureus 3–4, 9, 11, 27, 39–41,
    43, 57–58, 64, 122,131, 140,
    173, 181, 183, 247, 258, 260,
    272, 283
  spread among babies 173–174
  targets 262
Salmonella outbreak
    GOSH (Great Ormond Street
      Hospital) 273
    Victoria Infirmary 269n.2
sanatoriums 34
Sanderson, John Burdon 206
sanitarian practices, 1860s 205
Sanitary Officer (St Bartholomew's
    Hospital) 193
  creating role of 195–207
SARS (Severe Acute Respiratory
    Syndrome) 254
Saving Lives: reducing infection,
    delivering clean and safe
    care 143
Savory, William 196
scarlet fever 33–34, 202
Schimmelbusch, Kurt 105, 155–156

Schleich, Carl Ludwig 158
Schleich paste 158
Scitovsky, Anne 55
Scotland 274–275
  Cleanliness Champions
      programme 258–259
  future of infection control
      265–269
  HAI (Healthcare-Associated
      Infection) taskforce 257–258
  implementing targets 262–264
  inspections 264–265
  proactive infection control
      policies 259–261
Scott, S. B. R. 236
Scottish PPS (2005/2006–2017) 260
Selwyn, Sydney 219
Semmelweis, Ignaz 129, 172
SENIC (Study on the Efficacy
    of Nosocomial Infection
    Control) project 10, 12,
    59–61, 63, 138, 268, 274, 282
sensitivity testing 221–224, 272
sepsis 81, 83, 92, 110–113
  maintaining standards, sharing
      responsibility (1930–1965)
      115–121
  surgical nurse training (1900–
      1935) 86–88
septic finger 104, 110–113,
    116–117
septic wounds 280
Severe Acute Respiratory Syndrome
    see SARS
sewer gas 205
sewer traps 205
Shooter, Reginald 58
Sisters, division of labour 209
Sklaroff, S. A. 225, 227, 238
smallpox hospitals 31
Smith, Brian A. 28
Smith, C. J. 224
Smith, Thomas 196
smoke tests 205
socialisation, drivers of glove use
      behaviour 181–185
soiled dressings disposal 229–230
South Africa, nurses 82

SP (Standard Precautions) 174–175
Spanish Influenza (1918–1920)
    40–41
Spencer, Jane 111
St Bartholomew's Hospital 16–17,
    112, 119, 193–212, 277, 280
    Matrons 207–211
    Sanitary Officer 193–207
St Thomas' Hospital 18, 36, 81,
    90, 105–106, 108–110, 118,
    120, 208
    staff illness 111–115
staff illness 111–115
    maintaining standards, sharing
        responsibility (1930–1965)
        115–121
Stafford District General Hospital,
    legionnaires' disease 138,
    248, 273
Standard Precautions *see* SP
standards
    maintaining standards, sharing
        responsibility (1930–1965)
        115–121
    sensitivity testing 225
Stanley Royd Hospital, food
    poisoning outbreak 138,
    248, 273
Staph 80/81 38–39, 41–43
Staphylococcal infection 28, 29
    maternity units 37–38
    nurses 119
    RIE (Royal Infirmary of
        Edinburgh) 231
Staphylococcus
    hospital nurseries 39
    nasal carriers 120
Staphylococcus aureus 57–58, 131
    evidence of role of hands in
        transmission in newborn
        nursery **173**
sterile supply 231–235
sterilisation 132, 230–235
sterilising techniques *116*, 132–133,
    145n.8, *200*, 223, 230, 235
    imperfections 118
Stewart, Isla 82, 208–209
Stone, P. 67

strategies for preventing wound
    infection through touch
    155–159
Streptococcal infection 28, 29
Streptococci 27, 30, 35, 41, 117
Streptococcus pyogenes 35
Strong, R. 81
Study on the Efficacy of
    Nosocomial Infection Control
    project *see* SENIC project
superadded infection 32
superbugs 2
suppuration 96
surgical asepsis 91
surgical gloves 151–154; *see also*
    gloves
surgical infection, attempts at
    preventing 159–164
surgical mortality rates 196
surgical nurse training (1900–
    1935) 81–84
    curriculum 85–90
    hierarchies of practices 90–92
    surgical relations 93–96
Surgical Nursing and After-
    Treatment 89
surgical patients, HAI (hospital-
    acquired infection) 60
surgical relations 93–96
SURPASS (Surgical Patient Safety
    System) 254
surveillance
    HAI (hospital-acquired
        infection) 57
    Infection Cards 227–228
    Point prevalence survey (PPS)
        258, 260, **261**

Tait, L. 83
targets, implementing 262–264
Tatham, G. 85, 89, 96
Taylor, Bella Dawson 115
Taylor, K. 66
Theatre Service Centre *see* TSC
theatres 6, 8, 12, 15, 65, 83, 91,
    105, 109, 119–120, 197, 199–
    200, 202, 209–210, 228–238,
    253–254, 278, 280, 285

Therapeutic Revolution 35
Thompson, R. E. M. 121
Thursfield, Hugh 203
Titmuss, Richard 55
Tomes, Nancy 205
tongue depressors 139
Tonkin, R. W. 225
touch sequences during episodes of
    care **178**
Tracy, Roger S. 205
tray system, sterilising techniques
    235–236
Trohler, Ulrich 106
TSC (Theatre Service Centre)
    235–237
tuberculosis 34
typhoid 203

UK *see* United Kingdom
UN *see* United Nations
United Kingdom
    AMR (antimicrobial resistance) 2
    AMR (Antimicrobial Resistance)
        strategy (2013–2018) 258
    failures in infection control and
        prevention 3–4
    healthcare financing policies
        63–66
    IPC (Infection prevention and
        control) 248
    MRSA outbreaks 248–249
    National Audit Office (NAO) 66
    patient safety 250–252
United Nations, AMR
    (antimicrobial resistance) 2
United States
    HAI (hospital-acquired
        infection) 58–59
    healthcare financing polices
        impact on HAIs 61–62
    healthcare financing policics
        66–67
    Keystone Intensive Care Unit
        (ICU) 251–252
    Medicare 56

UP (Universal Precautions) 174
urinary tract infections (UTIs)
    260
US *see* United States
UTIs (urinary tract infections) 260

vaccination 159
Verney, Sir Henry *109*
von Bergmann, Ernst 156

Waddington, Keir 195, 196, 207
washing contractors 210
Washington Lyon patent steam
    disinfector 199–**200**
wax 158
Wells, Thomas Spencer 165
West Midlands, tongue depressors
    139
Whitby, M. 181
WHO (World Health
    Organization)
    AMR (antimicrobial resistance) 2
    hand hygiene 175–176
Wildman, Stuart 194
Willett, Alfred 196
Williams, J. D. 62, 75n.58
Williams, Robert 58, 73n.29
Woodall, S. J. 86
Woods, Robert 107
Worboys, Michael 164–165, 196,
    206
World Bank, cost of drug-resistant
    infections 2–3
World Health Organization *see*
    WHO
wound dressings 92
wound infections
    antisepsis 164–165
    RIE (Royal Infirmary of
        Edinburgh) 225
    strategies for preventing
        155–159
wound sepsis 92, 117

zone of inhibition 224